Difficult Decisions in Surgery: An Evidence-Based Approach

Series Editor

Mark K. Ferguson
Department of Surgery
University of Chicago
Chicago, IL, USA

The complexity of decision making in any kind of surgery is growing exponentially. As new technology is introduced, physicians from nonsurgical specialties offer alternative and competing therapies for what was once the exclusive province of the surgeon. In addition, there is increasing knowledge regarding the efficacy of traditional surgical therapies. How to select among these varied and complex approaches is becoming increasingly difficult. These multi-authored books will contain brief chapters, each of which will be devoted to one or two specific questions or decisions that are difficult or controversial. They are intended as current and timely reference sources for practicing surgeons, surgeons in training, and educators that describe the recommended ideal approach, rather than customary care, in selected clinical situations.

More information about this series at http://www.springer.com/series/13361

John Alverdy • Yalini Vigneswaran

Editors

Difficult Decisions
in Bariatric Surgery

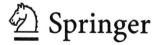 Springer

Editors
John Alverdy
Department of Surgery
University of Chicago
Chicago, IL
USA

Yalini Vigneswaran
Department of Surgery
University of Chicago
Chicago, IL
USA

ISSN 2198-7750   ISSN 2198-7769   (electronic)
Difficult Decisions in Surgery: An Evidence-Based Approach
ISBN 978-3-030-55328-9   ISBN 978-3-030-55329-6   (eBook)
https://doi.org/10.1007/978-3-030-55329-6

This Springer imprint is published by the registered company Springer Nature Switzerland AG
The registered company address is: Gewerbestrasse 11, 6330 Cham, Switzerland

Contents

Part IX The Future

Part I

Introductory Materials

"A Patient, a Surgeon, and an Insurance Agent Walk into a Bar..."

John Alverdy

For a *patient* to make the difficult decision to undergo bariatric surgery, they need to be fully convinced of the following: (1) that they will not, and cannot lose the weight needed to become healthy unless they undergo bariatric surgery (2) that their health is in jeopardy specifically due to their present weight and the co-morbidities that exist because of it and (3) that they trust that the surgery is safe because their surgeon is experienced and works in a high performance environment. For a *surgeon* to embark on the practice of bariatric surgery, he or she needs to be committed to the following: (1) to be willing, above all, to properly evaluate and offer the right operation to a given candidate patient (2) to be himself/herself convinced that the patient's health is in jeopardy and that the surgery proposed is indicated and safe (3) to be confident that their skills, judgment and team are of the highest standard and that their environment is properly equipped to offer state-of-the art bariatric care for the patient both in the short and long term process of care. Finally, for an *insurance company* to offer and support the finances of bariatric surgery, they need to: (1) ensure their customers do not fall prey to unscrupulous practices (2) make sure that the patients are not making rushed decisions to undergo bariatric surgery (3) that resources within their insurance pool are sufficient to support the entire process of bariatric surgery.

Yet if a patient, a surgeon and an insurance agent were to walk into a bar and tell their individual stories over drinks, the discussion could become heated and confrontational. Much angst develops when each participant has to constantly reconcile the wishes of the patient with the judgement of the surgeon and the prerequisites and approval criteria of the insurance company. For many bariatric practices, this reconciliation dance is riddled with unreasonable demands by the insurance company, capitulation of the surgeon's recommendations for one operation versus the

J. Alverdy (✉)
Department of Surgery, University of Chicago, Chicago, IL, USA
e-mail: jalverdy@surgery.bsd.uchicago.edu

© Springer Nature Switzerland AG 2021
J. Alverdy, Y. Vigneswaran (eds.), *Difficult Decisions in Bariatric Surgery*,
Difficult Decisions in Surgery: An Evidence-Based Approach,
https://doi.org/10.1007/978-3-030-55329-6_1

other and purposive obstructionism by family members, reluctant patients and insurance adjusters.

For example, when a patient with a BMI of 50, insulin dependent diabetes mellitus, hypertriglyceridemia and heptatosteatosis is only willing to undergo a sleeve gastrectomy despite being recommended a roux-en Y gastric bypass or a duodenal switch, a difficult decision ensues. Should the patient's wishes be honored as we now practice in the era of shared responsibility and patient participation in their care? Will the decision to operate be dependent on which operation the surgeon is most skilled and comfortable with? Will the decision to operate be a function of which procedure is covered or recommended by the insurance company? The "freedom to operate" in the field of bariatric surgery is often limited by various restrictions placed on the surgeon's experience and judgment that includes those from the patient, the surgeon's training and the patient's insurance status and coverage. As a result there are many "difficult decisions in bariatric surgery" that deserve attention and discussion. We hope the chapters in this book provide information that can not only uncover some of the causes of these problems and dilemmas, but also their potential solution.

Evidence-Based Medicine and Decision Making

2

Grace F. Chao and Justin B. Dimick

2.1 Why Evidence-Based Medicine Matters

Surgeons daily make difficult decisions. These decisions can range from how to counsel an individual patient to how to weigh in on national policy changes. Additionally, these decisions involve multiple stakeholders—patients, families, members of the medical team, policymakers, payors, and communities. Our role as surgeons in these deliberations often requires us to synthesize information that can be complex and incomplete. Bariatric surgery in particular has the added challenge of technology that is constantly evolving. The questions we have to answer have serious implications for patients. *Does laparoscopic sleeve gastrectomy or Roux-en-Y gastric bypass offer better safety, healthcare utilization, or clinical outcomes? Do buttressed staple loads prevent bleeding more that staple loads without reinforcement? When is pregnancy safe for mothers and babies after bariatric surgery? When is too young or too old for bariatric surgery?*

For us to answer these questions rigorously requires an understanding of evidence-based medicine approaches. This chapter will examine evidence-based medicine in the context of bariatric surgery. The rest of this book will explore a number of important and emerging questions in our field. The authors have put together the best supporting evidence available and made recommendations using principles of evidence-based medicine.

G. F. Chao (✉)
National Clinician Scholars Program, Veterans Affairs, Ann Arbor, MI, USA

Department of Surgery, Yale School of Medicine, New Haven, CT, USA
e-mail: grace.f.chao@yale.edu

J. B. Dimick
Center for Healthcare Outcomes and Policy, University of Michigan, Ann Arbor, MI, USA

Department of Surgery, University of Michigan Medical School, Ann Arbor, MI, USA

© Springer Nature Switzerland AG 2021
J. Alverdy, Y. Vigneswaran (eds.), *Difficult Decisions in Bariatric Surgery*,
Difficult Decisions in Surgery: An Evidence-Based Approach,
https://doi.org/10.1007/978-3-030-55329-6_2

2.1.1 A Cautionary Tale

Rigorously evaluating evidence can mean the difference between helping patients and harming them, as the cautionary tale of laparoscopic gastric banding has taught us. The medical field has seen medical reversals throughout history because of studies with design weaknesses recognized after practice patterns had changed—hormone replacement therapy in post-menopausal women, tight glycemic control in the ICU, and routine PSA screening. In bariatric surgery, we have recently seen this in laparoscopic gastric banding.

Banding held great theoretical promise to help patients improve their health. As the most minimally invasive, restrictive procedure at the time, it was thought to be a safe option for bariatric surgery. However, studies published varied widely in their outcomes. Studies reported rates of reoperation ranging anywhere from 4% up to 60% [1–8]. These studies lacked adequate sample size, long-term follow-up, or geographic representation to be able to give a true population estimate.

In order to address this uncertainty over outcomes, researchers used Medicare administrative data with a sample size of 25,042, an average follow-up time of 4.5 years, and national scope [9]. This study revealed high reoperation rates due to failure of weight loss and complications. On average, patients had 3.8 procedures in addition to their index operation. Hospital referral regions had reoperation rates ranging from 5.1% to 95.5%. Additionally, from 2006 to 2013, the proportion of annual spending on the gastric band device due to reoperations rose from 16.4% to 77.3%. Five years prior to this study, the FDA had concluded the existing evidence supported safety and effectiveness of gastric banding [1]. Of note, at that time, the FDA relied heavily on a single-group trial of 149 patients to reach its conclusion. A chapter of this text will delve more into the story of the Lap-Band. However, what we can see for now is that a lack of robust evidence led to many more devices being placed that not only were ineffective, but also exposed patients to the risks of multiple operations and complications, took away valuable time spent on more effective therapy, and increased financial burden on the system. And it was evidence-based medicine that was crucial in eventually identifying these issues.

The goal of research is to produce evidence that accurately describes causal relationships or true phenomena. Evidence-based medicine is the approach to determine how well a study accomplishes this goal. We will next delve into the components that strengthen and weaken the ability of studies to do this. In order to appropriately appraise the evidence available, we must clearly define our question, look for appropriate evidence available, and then critically evaluate this evidence. We will first discuss three key threats to validity that we must always consider in evaluation. We will also introduce Levels of Evidence and the GRADE system. Authors will use the GRADE system throughout this textbook as a strategy for evaluating evidence and subsequent recommendations.

2.2 Defining the Question

The PICO format defines our search question (Table 2.1). For "<u>P</u>atients," we identify the disease and characteristics of interest. The "<u>I</u>ntervention" can be in the form of a procedure or medication. We compare the intervention's outcomes to those of specific "<u>C</u>omparators." Comparators can be no intervention, usual care, or another treatment. Lastly, examples of "<u>O</u>utcomes" of interest are mortality, complication rate, time to event, and costs.

2.3 Threats to Validity

Threats to validity of data are why using an evidence-based medicine approach is important. There are two major types of validity—external and internal validity.

2.3.1 External Validity, Generalizability

External validity, also referred to as generalizability, is our ability to apply the study's conclusions to individuals other than the ones in the sample. This is a deliberation of what kinds of patients and environments (clinical, physical, social, geographic, and financial) we can apply the conclusions of the study. For example, we cannot apply the long-term outcomes of a study of adolescent weight loss after laparoscopic sleeve gastrectomy from centers across the United States to adult patients.

2.3.2 Internal Validity

Looking within the bounds of the study, internal validity is how well the results of a study represent the truth in the study sample. For the remainder of this chapter, we will refer to internal validity as "validity." The three major threats to validity are chance, bias, and confounding. Robust study designs should account for each of these threats.

2.3.3 Chance

This first threat to validity is when findings are due to random error. Chance can distort results in either direction; it can increase the estimated effect or decrease the

Table 2.1 Sample PICO format

P (Patients)	I (Intervention)	C (Comparator)	O (Outcomes)
Patients with Barrett esophagus	Esophagectomy	Endoscopic ablation	Mortality

estimated effect. In order to minimize chance, statistical comparisons must be adequately powered. Power of a study depends on sample size, standard deviation, and magnitude of the treatment effect. This may be a challenge for studies in bariatric surgery with smaller sample size evaluating rare complications (small magnitude of treatment effect). For example, when evaluating whether sleeve gastrectomy or gastric bypass carries a higher risk of reoperation, we may want to examine a randomized control trial. However, the two randomized control trials that study sleeve and bypass outcomes, SM-BOSS (217 patients) [10] and SLEEVEPASS (240 patients) [11], are not adequately powered to look at differences in reoperation rates. These events occur too infrequently for analysis to detect a difference in rates between the two groups; the magnitude of effect of choosing sleeve over bypass or vice versa is too small. To answer this question about reinterventions, we need to increase our sample size; we need a large administrative dataset.

2.3.4   Bias

Bias occurs due to systematic error. Two major sources of error are sample selection bias and systematic measurement error. The major source of sample selection bias in bariatric surgery is in the operation chosen. A patient who undergoes laparoscopic sleeve gastrectomy and a patient who gets a gastric bypass may differ. Patients who undergo gastric bypass may have a higher burden of diabetes than those who elect to have or who are counseled towards sleeve gastrectomy. Another important source of sample selection bias is loss to follow-up. This may happen when examining outcomes in claims data due to patients changing insurance plans. Systematic errors are sources of incorrect measurement that distort study findings in one direction. Systematic measurement error may occur if a study asks diabetic patients after surgery how many days per week they had well-controlled glucose levels. Patients with good post-operative glycemic control may systematically report more days than patients with poor control because they of higher compliance of checking glucose levels. This specific form of systematic bias is recall bias.

2.3.5   Confounding

Finally, confounding is when other variables are associated with both the exposure and outcome. These confounding variables, rather than the one studied, are what truly drive the results. For example, a comparative effectiveness study may show there is a higher risk of myocardial infarction after sleeve gastrectomy compared to gastric bypass. However, this would be an erroneous finding if there was no adjustment in the analysis for significant cardiac history. Surgeons may have counseled patients with a higher risk for myocardial infarction to undergo sleeve gastrectomy rather than gastric bypass. Thus, the findings are confounded by a history of severe cardiac disease.

Table 2.2 Levels of evidence

Level 1	Systematic review of randomized trials
Level 2	Randomized control trial, observational study with dramatic effect
Level 3	Non-randomized controlled cohort
Level 4	Case-control studies, case-series
Level 5	Mechanism-based reasoning

Adapted from the Oxford Centre for Evidence Based Medicine [13]

2.4   Levels of Evidence

In addition to these threats to validity, Levels of Evidence can help us to understand the strength of data for recommendations based on study design. Level 1 provides the strongest evidence for a recommendation. Level 5 designates the weakest evidence. These are reviewed in Table 2.2.

However, there are ways to challenge the premise that the randomized trial is the most rigorous form of evidence. Certain characteristics of observational studies can change the strength of the evidence. As mentioned earlier, randomized control trials in bariatric surgery are often underpowered to study important safety outcomes such as rate of reoperation, a rare event. Thus, it is important to leverage observational studies with innovative approaches. Observational studies using administrative claims data have a large number of patients and accurately track reoperation rates through billing data. When these features are paired with advanced econometrics methods such as instrumental variable or difference-in-differences analysis, observational studies can be robust.

2.5   Grading the Evidence

Building upon the major threats to validity and Levels of Evidence, the GRADE system provides further principles for evaluation of evidence and in many ways is a more extensive list of threats to validity. The GRADE system is a commonly used framework to evaluate data within systematic reviews and meta-analyses. Beyond systematic reviews, it provides principles valuable in broadly evaluating studies and the conclusions drawn from them.

Systematic reviews first pose a specific clinical question with the PICO guidelines. Researchers next identify studies that answer this question. They then pool data from these studies to generate a best estimate of the effect on the outcome of interest. A scoring system lastly classifies recommendations from systematic reviews into four categories as detailed in Table 2.3—High Quality, Moderate Quality, Low Quality, or Very Low Quality.

Initially, randomized control trials begin with a "High Quality" rating and observational studies with a "Low Quality" rating. As noted earlier, the authors believe that observational studies can be even more rigorous than randomized trials depending on features of study design. However, for purposes of the GRADE system, we

Table 2.3 Significance of GRADE levels of evidence

High quality	We are very confident the true effect lies close to that of the effect estimate
Moderate quality	The true effect is likely to be close to the estimate of the effect, but there is a possibility that it is substantially different
Low quality	The true effect may be substantially different from the effect estimate
Very low quality	The true effect is likely to be substantially different from the effect estimate

Adapted from Balshem et al. [14]

Table 2.4 A summary of GRADE's approach to rating quality of evidence

Study design	Initial quality of a body of evidence	Lower if	Higher if	Quality of a body of evidence
Randomized trials	High ⟹	Risk of Bias −1 Serious −2 Very serious	Large effect +1 Large +2 Very large	High (four plus: ⊕⊕⊕⊕)
		Inconsistency −1 Serious −2 Very serious	Dose response +1 Evidence of a gradient	Moderate (three plus: ⊕⊕⊕○)
Observational studies	Low ⟹	Indirectness −1 Serious −2 Very serious	All plausible residual confounding +1 Would reduce a	Low (two plus: ⊕⊕○○)
		Imprecision −1 Serious −2 Very serious	demonstrated effect +1 Would suggest a	Very low (one plus: ⊕○○○)
		Publication bias −1 Likely −2 Very likely	spurious effect if no effect was observed	

From Balshem et al. [14]

Table 2.5 PICO for our GRADE evaluation

P (Patients)	I (Intervention)	C (Comparator)	O (Outcomes)
Adults who underwent laparoscopic sleeve gastrectomy	Bioabsorbable buttressing of staple line	No buttressing of staple line Nonabsorbable buttressing of staple line	Leak rate

begin with the traditional quality levels. The five categories that move studies down in quality level are risk of bias, imprecision, inconsistency, indirectness, and publication bias. Table 2.4 shows these factors as well as categories that increase quality.

To discuss aspects of the GRADE system, we use the clinical question of whether staple line buttressing method affects leak rate from Parikh et al.'s systematic review [12]. The specific clinical question is whether patients who underwent laparoscopic sleeve gastrectomy with bioabsorbable buttressing had different leak rates compared to patients who had no buttressing or nonabsorbable buttressing (Table 2.5). The researchers estimated the effect of buttressing on leak rates using a multivariable regression formulated from a general estimating equation adjusting for bougie size, distance from pylorus, age, and BMI. The researchers conclude that buttressing technique had no significant effect on leak rates. We will next use the GRADE system to analyze the evidence which is also summarized in Table 2.6.

Table 2.6 Summary of threats to validity and GRADE based on Parikh *et al* systematic review

Outcome	Summary of findings Effect estimate adjusted OR (95% CI)	Assessment principles Risk of bias	Inconsistency	Indirectness	Imprecision	Publication bias	Other effects and confounding
Leak rate of bioabsorbable buttressing compared with no buttressing	1.06 [0.49–2.30]	Observational studies—sample selection bias	No significant inconsistency	Direct	No important imprecision	Unlikely	Confounding would not clearly have led to a demonstrated spurious effect
Leak rate of bioabsorbable buttressing compared with nonabsorbable buttressing	2.01 [0.87–4.68]	Observational studies—sample selection bias	No significant inconsistency	Direct	No important imprecision	Unlikely	Confounding would not clearly have led to a demonstrated spurious effect

2.5.1   Risk of Bias

Overall, there were 55 articles with 6578 laparoscopic sleeve gastrectomy patients included that specify buttressing technique. The vast majority are observational studies, and thus we are at risk for sample selection bias. Techniques like instrumental variable analysis to control for unmeasured confounding were not used. Importantly, randomized control trials are not without risk of bias. They include loss to follow-up causing sample selection bias and lack of blinding which can cause measurement error.

2.5.2   Inconsistency

Heterogeneity of conclusions between studies can occur if there are differences in the baseline patient population and how the outcome was measured. In our example, there are differences in how studies identified leak. The reviewers include "leak," "abscess," "staple-line failure or disruption," "infected perigastric hematoma," and "gastro-gastric fistula" as outcomes. These terms are reasonably consistent in describing the same outcome of leak. It is also important to always consider whether search items will miss studies that define an outcome in other terms.

2.5.3   Indirectness

This is when the body of evidence does not directly answer the PICO. The studies in this review are all considered are direct. All studies include adult patients with the same operation, intervention of buttressing technique, and outcome of leak.

2.5.4   Imprecision

Wide confidence intervals signal imprecision since the values at either end suggest very different effect estimates. Our confidence intervals for the odds ratios in the multivariate regression analysis cross 1, meaning there is no difference between bioabsorbable buttressing versus no buttressing or versus non-absorbable buttressing. The lower and upper ends of the confidence intervals for these effects are both near 1. Thus, there is reasonable precision of these findings. Very wide confidence intervals can be due to sample sizes that are too small or events that are too rare.

2.5.5   Publication Bias

Publication bias considers what types of studies are more likely or less likely to be published. In general, studies that do not show an effect are not published and thus are a largely missing portion of our evidence body. Other factors to consider are who sponsored the studies (e.g. industry, academia) and the sample size. Given that the reported outcome is no effect, publication bias is unlikely.

2.5.6   Factors That Can Increase the Quality Assessment

Both magnitude of effect and dose response gradient are not applicable for this clinical question as buttressing technique was found to have no effect and is a non-ordinal categorical variable. For continuous variables, a larger magnitude of effect and greater dose-response gradient strengthens the conclusion that the variable truly has an effect on the outcome. An example of a dose-response gradient would be if a study found that each unit of blood glucose increase above the normal range corresponded to an increasing risk of post-operative infection.

2.5.7   Confounding

In this review, there was significant intraoperative variation in technique that could not be accounted for, such as amount of lateral stretch applied to the stomach and distance the stapler was to the bougie when fired. These are all sources of confounding which could alter the effect on leak rate had they been measured. For our clinical question in which there was no effect, it is unclear whether these confounders would have led to a spurious demonstrated effect. In scenarios in which the evidence does demonstrate an effect, ask if confounding would reduce this effect.

2.6   Putting It All Together

Thus, using the GRADE framework, the evidence would be considered Very Low Quality and does not support recommendations for or against the buttressing options. Table 2.6 summarizes all the GRADE system considerations for this review. The quality of evidence would begin at Low (+ +) per Table 2.4 because it mostly consists of observational studies. The risk of bias is serious because the design did not account for unmeasured confounding such as surgeon preference, comfort, or experience with using different types of staplers (−). The review was consistent, direct, and without serious concern for imprecision or publication bias (no loss of points). Confounders would not clearly have led to a spurious demonstrated effect (no gain of points). Again, while the GRADE system is formally used in evaluating systematic reviews, its principles should be considered when evaluating any type of study.

How much each of these factors discussed influences the strength of the evidence is dependent on the severity of the violation of the study's validity. Chance, bias, confounding, Levels of Evidence, and the GRADE system provide general principles in structuring the surgeon's analysis. We as surgeons can make the best evidence-based recommendations, but any medical decision includes the values of the individuals involved and the healthcare system in which they exist. For example, the above discussion does not consider cost effectiveness, out of pocket costs for the patient, how much risk patients and surgeons are willing to take, etc.

We want to emphasize that observational studies can be rigorous if they employ techniques that account for unmeasured confounding. Examples of robust observational studies are ones that use large administrative claims databases to detect rare occurrences accurately and use instrumental variable analysis to address. Additionally, other quasi-experimental designs such as difference-in-differences analysis can also generate fairly accurate causal estimates.

We hope that this discussion of evidence-based medicine provides you with a foundation for shaping rigorous evaluations of the data available.

References

1. US Food and Drug Administration. Lap-band summary of safety and effectiveness (SSED). https://www.accessdata.fda.gov/cdrh_docs/pdf/P000008S017b.pdf. Published 2011. Accessed December 15, 2019.
2. Anwar M, Collins J, Kow L, Toouli J. Long-term efficacy of a low-pressure adjustable gastric band in the treatment of morbid obesity. Ann Surg. 2008;247(5):771–8.
3. Himpens J, Cadiere GB, Bazi M, Vouche M, Cadiere B, Dapri G. Long-term outcomes of laparoscopic adjustable gastric banding. Arch Surg. 2011;146(7):802–7.
4. Kasza J, Brody F, Vaziri K, et al. Analysis of poor outcomes after laparoscopic adjustable gastric banding. Surg Endosc. 2011;25(1):41–7.
5. Lanthaler M, Aigner F, Kinzl J, Sieb M, Cakar-Beck F, Nehoda H. Long-term results and complications following adjustable gastric banding. Obes Surg. 2010;20(8):1078–85.
6. Stroh C, Hohmann U, Schramm H, Meyer F, Manger T. Fourteen-year long-term results after gastric banding. J Obes. 2011;2011:128451.
7. Victorzon M, Tolonen P. Mean fourteen-year, 100% follow-up of laparoscopic adjustable gastric banding for morbid obesity. Surg Obes Relat Dis. 2013;9(5):753–7.
8. Altieri MS, Yang J, Telem DA, et al. Lap band outcomes from 19,221 patients across centers and over a decade within the state of New York. Surg Endosc. 2016;30(5):1725–32.
9. Ibrahim AM, Thumma JR, Dimick JB. Reoperation and Medicare expenditures after laparoscopic gastric band surgery. JAMA Surg. 2017;152(9):835–42.
10. Peterli R, Wolnerhanssen BK, Peters T, et al. Effect of laparoscopic sleeve gastrectomy vs laparoscopic Roux-en-Y gastric bypass on weight loss in patients with morbid obesity: the SM-BOSS randomized clinical trial. JAMA. 2018;319(3):255–65.
11. Salminen P, Helmio M, Ovaska J, et al. Effect of laparoscopic sleeve gastrectomy vs laparoscopic Roux-en-Y gastric bypass on weight loss at 5 years among patients with morbid obesity: the SLEEVEPASS randomized clinical trial. JAMA. 2018;319(3):241–54.
12. Parikh M, Issa R, McCrillis A, Saunders JK, Ude-Welcome A, Gagner M. Surgical strategies that may decrease leak after laparoscopic sleeve gastrectomy: a systematic review and meta-analysis of 9991 cases. Ann Surg. 2013;257(2):231–7.
13. OCEBM Levels of Evidence Working Group. The Oxford 2011 Levels of Evidence Oxford Centre for Evidence-Based Medicine 2011.
14. Balshem H, Helfand M, Schunemann HJ, et al. GRADE guidelines: 3. Rating the quality of evidence. J Clin Epidemiol. 2011;64(4):401–6.

Part II

Patient Selection

Bariatric Surgery for Uncontrolled Hypertension

3

Kathleen Lak and Jon Gould

3.1 Introduction

Hypertension affects 42.5% of American adults with obesity compared to 15.3% of individuals without obesity [1]. The pathophysiology of hypertension and its close association to obesity is incompletely understood. Genetic and environmental influences lay the groundwork for the complex interplay between the sympathetic nervous system, renal and adrenal function, and their resultant interactions with the endothelium, release of adipokines and overall insulin resistance [2–5]. Uncontrolled hypertension has clinical significance, as it is a risk factor for cardiovascular morbidity and mortality. Although the pathophysiology is multifactorial and interdependent, hypertension as a component to the metabolic syndrome is well established in its negative effects on morbidity and mortality [6]. Hypertension and obesity, as a result, are associated with end organ damage.

The historic treatment for obesity related hypertension has been weight control, in addition to lifestyle changes and medications. Many studies have investigated non-operative management strategies of obesity and hypertension with lifestyle and diet modifications with or without the addition of antihypertensive medications. In this chapter we will discuss hypertension as an indication for bariatric surgery. The implications of bariatric surgery for the management of hypertension itself will be discussed as well as its effects on related comorbid conditions and overall morbidity and mortality.

K. Lak (✉) · J. Gould
Medical College of Wisconsin, Milwaukee, WI, USA
e-mail: klak@mcw.edu; jgould@mcw.edu

© Springer Nature Switzerland AG 2021
J. Alverdy, Y. Vigneswaran (eds.), *Difficult Decisions in Bariatric Surgery*,
Difficult Decisions in Surgery: An Evidence-Based Approach,
https://doi.org/10.1007/978-3-030-55329-6_3

3.2   Search Strategy

PICO table

P (Patients)	I (Intervention)	C (Comparator)	O (Outcomes)
Adult aged (18+) comorbidity hypertension obesity	Bariatric surgery	Medical management	Resolution or improvement in hypertension; improvement in mortality; improvement in cardiovascular disease risk factors

A search strategy based on English language publications from 2000 to 2020 was used to identify relevant articles on bariatric surgery for hypertension. Databases searched include Pubmed, Scopus and Cochrane Evidence Based Medicine. Only full text articles were included. Search terms included "hypertension". "hypertension treatment", "hypertension management", "refractory hypertension", "uncontrolled hypertension", "obesity related hypertension" AND ("bariatric surgery" or "weight loss" or "metabolic surgery" or "antihypertensive") AND ("resolution" or "improvement" or "treatment" or "morbidity" or "mortality" or "cardiovascular outcomes"). Publication types were limited to, meta-analysis, randomized controlled trial, or systematic reviews.

3.3   The Relationship Between Hypertension and Obesity

Hypertension and weight have been shown to be directly correlated with several studies demonstrating a nearly linear relationship. Patients achieving incremental weight loss were found to have concordant improvement in blood pressure. Likewise, studies following patients with weight gain saw predictable elevation of blood pressure measurements [5, 7]. Although the exact relationship is incompletely understood, the relationship between hypertension and obesity is complex and intertwined. The exact method of weight loss is less important in achieving improvement or control of hypertension. In the medical literature, improvement in hypertension has been demonstrated in patients undergoing medical weight loss by intense life-style interventions [7, 8]. Likewise, improvement and resolution of hypertension has been shown after bariatric surgery [9, 10] (Table 3.1).

3.4   Medical Management Versus Surgical Treatment

The basis of treatment for uncontrolled hypertension has been life-style modification and medical treatment to achieve weight loss. However in looking at sustainable and durable treatments, several groups have investigated the role of bariatric surgery in patients that also suffer from obesity. Ikramuddin and colleagues in a randomized control study of 120 participants, directly compared patients with a

Table 3.1 Evaluation of resolution or improvement in hypertension after bariatric surgery

Author, year	N		Weight loss achieved (%EWL)		Resolution of hypertension (%)		Resolution or Improvement of HTN (Resolution only) (%)						Follow-up (months)	Study design (quality of evidence)
			MT	SGY	MT	SGY	MT	SGY	AGB	RYGB	VBG	DS/BPD		
Buchwald et al. JAMA 2004	22,094	All bariatric procedures	–	61.2	–	61.7	–	78.5	70.8 (43.2)	87.2 (67.5)	85.4 (69)	75.1 (83.4)	–	Systematic review and meta-analysis (moderate)
Ikramuddin et al. JAMA 2013.	120	RYGB vs. medical management	7.9	26.1	79.5	84	–	–	–	–	–	–	12	RCT (high)
Vest et al. Heart. 2012	19,543	All bariatric procedures	–	54	–	–	–	62.5	–	–	–	–	57.8	Systematic review (low)
Sarkhosh et el. Obesity Surgery 2012	3997	Sleeve gastrectomy	–	63	–	58	–	75%	–	–	–	–	12	Systematic review (low)
Sjöström et al. NEWJM 2004	4047	Surgical group (variable banding, VBG, RYGB); matched control group non-surgical	0.1	25	21	34							24	
Sjöström et al. NEWJM 2004	1703		1.6	16.1	11	19	–	–	–	–	–	–	120	Prospective controlled trial-not randomized (high)

(continued)

Table 3.1 (continued)

Author, year	N		Weight loss achieved (%EWL)		Resolution of hypertension (%)		Resolution or Improvement of HTN (Resolution only) (%)						Follow-up (months)	Study design (quality of evidence)
			MT	SGY	MT	SGY	MT	SGY	AGB	RYGB	VBG	DS/BPD		
Heneghan et al. ACJ. 2011	16,867	All bariatric procedures	–	52	–	68	–	–	58	60	–	79	34	Systematic review (moderate)
Schiavon et al. Circulation. 2018	100	RYGB + MT versus MT alone	–	–	0	51	–	83.7	–	83 (51)	–	–	12	RCT (high)
Mingrone et al. NEJM. 2012	72	RYGB versus BPD versus MT	–	–	–	–	70	–	–	80	–	85	–	RCT (high)

HTN hypertension, *DS* duodenal switch, *EWL* excess weight loss, *VBG* vertical banded gastroplasty, *RYGB* Roux-en-Y gastric bypass, *RCT* randomized controlled trial, *SG* sleeve gastrectomy, *BPD* biliopancreatic diversion, *MT* medical therapy

BMI of 30–40, treated with laparoscopic Roux-en-Y gastric bypass (RYGB) versus intensive medical therapy. The primary outcomes they investigated were disease control of diabetes, hypertension and hyperlipidemia [8]. They found that those patients in the surgery treatment group reached the primary outcome significant more often than those in the lifestyle intervention group (49% vs. 19%; OR 4.8; 95% CI, 1.9–11.7). Furthermore when regression analysis was performed, weight loss was found to be the factor differentiating the difference in end points between groups.

A systematic review including over 19,000 patients who underwent bariatric surgery from 73 studies performed by Vest and colleagues, demonstrated at 6-month postoperative follow-up, a 63% resolution or improvement in hypertension [11]. Similarly, Sarkhosh et al. reviewed the impact of sleeve gastrectomy on hypertension and found a similar effect with 75% of patients achieving improvement or resolution of hypertension [12]. On univariate analysis the authors describe that age was a negative predictor—suggesting that patient age may impact the effect of bariatric surgery on hypertension resolution. Excess weight loss in this study was a positive predictor. In summary all of these studies support early and high rates of improvement in hypertension and overall cardiovascular events with surgery.

Interestingly, we see similar outcomes when we look at patients on multimodal therapies. The GATEWAY trial investigated the effects of bariatric surgery specifically on patients with hypertension on two or more medications at maximum doses or more than two medications on moderate dosing with a BMI between 30 and 39.9 kg/m^2 [13]. In this non-blinded randomized controlled trial (RCT) patients were randomized to either RYGB with medical therapy or medical therapy alone. At 12-month follow-up, patients in the surgical group had an 83.7% rate of hypertension improvement demonstrated by a $\geq$30% reduction in the number of anti-hypertensive medications required to sustain a normal in office blood pressure compared to 12.8% in the medical therapy alone group. Additionally, 51% of patients in the surgical group had complete resolution of hypertension post-operatively while no patient in the medical therapy group achieved hypertension resolution. Interestingly, in this study hypertension improvement, or resolution for that matter, was achieved at 1 month post-operatively and this effect was sustained over the 12-month period despite ongoing weight loss in the surgical group throughout 12 months. A follow-up analysis on this cohort of patients found that the rate of resistant hypertension, defined as blood pressure that remains above goal despite use of three anti-hypertensive medications of different classes prescribed at optimal doses, was significantly improved in the surgical group compared to the medical group (0% vs. 14.9% in the control group; $p < 0.001$) [14].

With weight loss so closely linked to control of hypertension, sustaining weight loss becomes of utmost importance. Bariatric surgery has been demonstrated to be the best tool for significant, sustained weight loss in severely obese patients [9, 15]. Furthermore, bariatric surgery was found to be superior to intensive medical therapy alone in achieving long-term weight loss and glycemic control [16]. The clinical implications for improvement in blood pressure are not to be discounted. In diabetic patients, hypertension is associated with the development and progression of diabetic complications. The pathophysiology of uncontrolled hypertension and its detrimental effects on end organ function has been well described with systemic macrovascular and microvascular harm [3]. It is incomplete to assess the patient outcomes regarding hypertension without evaluating cardiovascular outcomes in their entirety. And although several systematic reviews and meta-analyses assess the cardiovascular risk factors individually to understand the subsequent impact of bariatric surgery, there are no multicenter clinical trials which prospectively evaluate the cardiovascular outcomes of patients after bariatric surgery.

3.5   Treatment in the Presence of Obesity and Diabetes

The treatment of hypertension can become more complex in the setting of not only obesity but also diabetes. The Look AHEAD trial evaluated patients with type II diabetes and assessed cardiovascular outcomes based on the amount of weight loss achieved by lifestyle interventions [17]. Patients who achieved a 10% total body weight loss were found to have a 20% lower risk of composite death from cardiovascular causes. Likewise, Sjöström et al. demonstrated an overall mortality benefit in the Swedish Obese Subjects study of obese patients who underwent bariatric surgery compared to those receiving conventional medical treatment at an average of 10 years follow-up [18]. In this study, the most common causes of death were myocardial infarction and cancer. The mortality benefit described in this study was achieved in patients matched for diabetes. At 10-year follow-up patients in the surgical group achieved a significantly greater weight loss than those in the conventional medical treatment group.

The STAMPEDE trial, a RCT which aimed to describe the effects of bariatric surgery on the glycemic control and cardiovascular risk factors in diabetic patients also demonstrated a decrease in medications needed to control hypertension [16]. At 5-year follow-up in the surgical group there was a 40.8% decrease in the number of patients who needed ≥3 medications for hypertension control compared to a 13.1% decrease in the intensive medical therapy group. Mingrone et al. also aimed to determine the effects of bariatric surgery on glycemic control in diabetic patients [19]. In their study the rates of hypertension improvement or resolution were significantly increased in the RYGB or BPD groups compared to the intensive medical management group.

The long-term impact on cardiovascular morbidity and mortality after bariatric surgery has yet to be studied in a multi-center controlled trial; however, several systematic reviews have collected data which describes the impact on cardiovascular risk factors such as hypertension, diabetes mellitus, hyperlipidemia, and novel markers such as CRP, albuminuria or proinflammatory markers. In the systematic review by Heneghan et al. a 40% relative risk reduction of 10-year coronary artery heart disease risk based on the Framingham risk score was demonstrated [20]. Across 52 studies, an average 68% resolution rate of hypertension was found. This was in addition to 75% reduction or resolution of diabetes mellitus and 71% rate of resolution or reduction in dyslipidemia. The Framingham heart study found that long-standing hypertension is the underlying factor in the development of heart failure over time. This study found that 91% of patients with heart failure after 20 years of follow-up had hypertension proceeding their diagnosis [21].

3.6 Recommendations Based on the Data

For patients that suffer from hypertension and morbid obesity, bariatric surgery is recommended over medical treatment alone. Bariatric surgery is the best modality treatment for durable long-term treatment of hypertension and lowering the risk of associated cardiovascular events (evidence quality strong, strong recommendation).

3.7 A Personal View of the Data

Hypertension as a single comorbid condition in a bariatric patient is a marker for cardiovascular disease with implications on long-term morbidity and mortality. Evidence to date supports bariatric surgery as the most durable and effective treatment for morbid obesity and long-term weight loss. We know that weight loss is associated with resolution or improvement in hypertension, and that conversely weight regain is associated with an amelioration of this effect. Given the above, we recommend bariatric surgery as one of the most effective options for treating hypertension in morbidly obese patients.

References

1. Wang Y, Wang QJ. The prevalence of prehypertension and hypertension among US Adults According to the New Joint National Committee Guidelines: new challenges of the old problem. Arch Intern Med. 2004;164:2126–34.
2. Narkiewicz K. Obesity and hypertension—the issue is more complex than we thought. Nephrol Dial Transplant [Internet]. 2006 [cited 2020 Jan 6];21(2):264–7. Available from: http://academic.oup.com/ndt/article/21/2/264/1850864/Obesity-and-hypertensionthe-issue-is-more-complex
3. Seravalle G, Grassi G. Obesity and hypertension. Pharmacol Res. 2017;122:1–7.
4. Landsberg L, Aronne LJ, Beilin LJ, Burke V, Igel LI, Lloyd-Jones D, et al. Obesity-related hypertension: pathogenesis, cardiovascular risk, and treatment-a position paper of the the obesity society and the American society of hypertension. Obesity. 2013;21:8–24.
5. Julius S, Valentini M, Palatini P. Overweight and hypertension a 2-way street? Hypertension as a Predictor of Overweight [Internet]. 2000 [cited 2020 Jan 6]. Available from: http://www.hypertensionaha.org
6. Mottillo S, Filion KB, Genest J, Joseph L, Pilote L, Poirier P, et al. The metabolic syndrome and cardiovascular risk: a systematic review and meta-analysis. J Am Coll Cardiol. 2010;56(14):1113–32.
7. Neter JE, Stam BE, Kok FJ, Grobbee DE, Geleijnse JM. Influence of weight reduction on blood pressure: a meta-analysis of randomized controlled trials. Hypertens (Dallas, Tex 1979) [Internet]. 2003 [cited 2020 Jan 6];42(5):878–84. Available from: http://www.ncbi.nlm.nih.gov/pubmed/12975389

8. Ikramuddin S, Korner J, Lee WJ, Connett JE, Inabnet WB, Billington CJ, et al. Roux-en-Y gastric bypass vs intensive medical management for the control of type 2 diabetes, hypertension, and hyperlipidemia: the diabetes surgery study randomized clinical trial. JAMA. 2013;309(21):2240–9.
9. Sjöström L, Lindroos A-K, Peltonen M, Torgerson J, Bouchard C, Carlsson B, et al. Lifestyle, diabetes, and cardiovascular risk factors 10 years after bariatric surgery. N Engl J Med [Internet]. 2004 23 [cited 2020 Jan 6];351(26):2683–93. Available from: http://www.nejm.org/doi/abs/10.1056/NEJMoa035622
10. Buchwald H, Avidor Y, Braunwald E, Jensen MD, Pories W, Fahrbach K, et al. Bariatric surgery: a systematic review and meta-analysis. JAMA. 2004;292:1724–37.
11. Vest AR, Heneghan HM, Agarwal S, Schauer PR, Young JB. Bariatric surgery and cardiovascular outcomes: a systematic review. Heart. 2012;98:1763–77.
12. Sarkhosh K, Birch DW, Shi X, Gill RS, Karmali S. The impact of sleeve gastrectomy on hypertension: a systematic review. Obes Surg. 2012;22:832–7.
13. Schiavon CA, Bersch-Ferreira AC, Santucci EV, Oliveira JD, Torreglosa CR, Bueno PT, et al. Effects of bariatric surgery in obese patients with hypertension the GATEWAY randomized trial (gastric bypass to treat obese patients with steady hypertension). Circulation. 2018;137(11):1132–42.
14. Schiavon CA, Ikeoka D, Santucci EV, Santos RN, Damiani LP, Bueno PT, et al. Effects of bariatric surgery versus medical therapy on the 24-hour ambulatory blood pressure and the prevalence of resistant hypertension: the GATEWAY randomized clinical trial. Hypertension. 2019;73(3):571–7.
15. Health NI of clinical guidelines on the identification, evaluation and treatment of overweight and obesity in adults—the evidence report. Obes Res. 1998;6(2):51S–209S.
16. Schauer PR, Bhatt DL, Kirwan JP, Wolski K, Aminian A, Brethauer SA, et al. Bariatric surgery versus intensive medical therapy for diabetes—5-year outcomes. N Engl J Med [Internet]. 2017 [cited 2020 Jan 6];376(7):641–51. Available from: http://www.nejm.org/doi/10.1056/NEJMoa1600869
17. Look AHEAD Research Group T. Association of the magnitude of weight loss and changes in physical fitness with long-term cardiovascular disease outcomes in overweight or obese people with type 2 diabetes: a post-hoc analysis of the Look AHEAD randomised clinical trial. LANCET Diabetes Endocrinol [Internet]. 2016 [cited 2020 Jan 7];4:913–21. Available from: www.thelancet.com/
18. Sjöström L, Narbro K, Sjöström CD, Karason K, Larsson B, Wedel H, et al. Effects of bariatric surgery on mortality in Swedish obese subjects. N Engl J Med [Internet]. 2007 [cited 2020 Jan 7];357(8):741–52. Available from: http://www.nejm.org/doi/abs/10.1056/NEJMoa066254
19. Mingrone G, Panunzi S, De Gaetano A, Guidone C, Iaconelli A, Leccesi L, et al. Bariatric surgery versus conventional medical therapy for type 2 diabetes. N Engl J Med [Internet]. 2012 [cited 2020 Jan 15];366(17):1577–85. Available from: http://www.nejm.org/doi/10.1056/NEJMoa1200111
20. Heneghan HM, Meron-Eldar S, Brethauer SA, Schauer PR, Young JB. Effect of bariatric surgery on cardiovascular risk profile. Am J Cardiol. 2011;108(10):1499–507.
21. Levy D. The progression from hypertension to congestive heart failure. JAMA. 1996;275(20):1557.

Diabetes as an Indication for Bariatric Surgery

4

Andrea Stroud and Ryland Stucke

4.1 Introduction

The rising global incidence and prevalence of type II diabetes (T2DM) has paralleled the rise in obesity. Projections suggest the prevalence of T2DM will reach 552 million by 2030, an increase of 150% from 2011 [1]. T2DM has significant impacts on morbidity, mortality, quality of life, and healthcare costs. It is the second leading cause of obesity related death, and the leading cause of obesity related disability [2, 3]. Estimates in the United States (US) predict nearly $500 billion in annual health care costs by 2030 for diabetes care [4].

Bariatric surgery is currently the most effective treatment for obesity [5]. In the early 1990s researchers began to recognize that bariatric surgery was also an effective treatment for diabetes [6, 7]. Approximately 90% of T2DM is attributable to excess weight [8], and multiple trials have now demonstrated the superiority of bariatric surgery compared to maximal medical and lifestyle management for treating T2DM [9–11]. Multiple observational studies have demonstrated a reduction in all-cause mortality following bariatric surgery, with a 92% decrease in diabetes related deaths [12–15]. Additionally, surgical treatment of T2DM with bariatric surgery is cost effective based on clinical data and economic modeling. The cost-benefit ratio improves over-time related to avoidance of incident co-morbid disease [16, 17].

Eligibility and insurance payment for bariatric surgery has followed the National Institutes of Health (NIH) guidelines and has been primarily based on body mass index (BMI). These guidelines were published in 1991 and have not been updated

A. Stroud (✉)
Bariatric Surgery, Oregon Health & Science University, Portland, OR, USA
e-mail: strouda@ohsu.edu

R. Stucke
General Surgery, Dartmouth-Hitchcock Medical Center, Lebanon, NH, USA

© Springer Nature Switzerland AG 2021
J. Alverdy, Y. Vigneswaran (eds.), *Difficult Decisions in Bariatric Surgery*,
Difficult Decisions in Surgery: An Evidence-Based Approach,
https://doi.org/10.1007/978-3-030-55329-6_4

Table 4.1 PICO table

P (Patients)	I (Interventions)	C (Comparator)	O (Outcomes)
Patients with diabetes and obesity	Bariatric surgery	Maximal medical or lifestyle intervention	Glycemic control, diabetes remission/resolution, morbidity, mortality, weight loss, cost

in nearly three decades, despite significant changes in the practice of bariatric surgery (i.e.: laparoscopy, change in procedures offered, bariatric accreditation) [18, 19]. Of all obesity-related comorbid illnesses, T2DM has the most evidence as an indication for bariatric surgery. In 2015, the Second Diabetes Surgery Summit (DSS-II) developed global consensus guidelines based on high-quality evidence. This multi-disciplinary group concluded that the indications for bariatric surgery should be revised to include T2DM as a primary indication for surgery. Additionally, the DSS-II found compelling evidence to recommend bariatric surgery to patients with class I obesity (BMI 30–34.9) and poorly controlled T2DM [20]. In this chapter, we review the data to support bariatric surgery as a treatment for diabetes in obese patients, and diabetic patients who would not traditionally qualify for bariatric surgery. We argue that bariatric surgery should be considered early in the treatment for pre-diabetes and diabetes, and should no longer be viewed as last resort therapy.

4.2 Search Strategy

A comprehensive search of MEDLINE (PubMed), EMBASE, and the Cochrane library databases was conducted for English language publications from 2009 to 2020, and included the following terms: diabetes AND gastric bypass (RYGB), jejunoileal bypass, duodenal switch (DS), gastric sleeve (SG), biliopancreatic diversion (BPD), bariatric surgery, metabolic surgery, obesity surgery, intestinal bypass, along with all relevant related keywords (Table 4.1). For comprehensiveness, we included evidence-based guidelines and practice recommendations from leading diabetes associations, some of which preformed independent systematic reviews. We also included papers of historical importance or commonly referenced landmark studies. Bibliographies were cross referenced to identify additional relevant articles. Recommendations were classified using the GRADE system. Endoscopic and device-based interventions were excluded from this analysis. Data for the adjustable gastric band (AGB) procedure is included, but is given limited attention as it has widely fallen out of favor in the modern era.

4.3 Results

4.3.1 Bariatric Surgery for Type 2 Diabetes

4.3.1.1 Procedure Specific Diabetes Remission Rates

High quality evidence has demosntrated that bariatric surgery is highly effective for the treatment of T2DM [6, 7, 21, 22]. Published T2DM remission rates following bariatric surgery range between 9 and 100% [23]. This reflects variability in how diabetes remission is defined between studies, as well as the heterogeneity of patient characteristics, procedures, and technique. A large volume of data exists describing the long-term anti-diabetic effectiveness of modern bariatric procedures. It is important to note that while "diabetes remission and/or resolution" is the primary endpoint in these studies, the definition to achieve this endpoint is not standardized. Variability exists in the cutoffs for glycated hemoglobin (A1C) and fasting plasma glucose (FPG), and how insulin and other anti-diabetic medications are considered when defining the primary endpoint. This is an important consideration that has clinical implications when discussing expected outcomes with diabetic patients contemplating bariatric surgery.

Long-term diabetes remission rates following RYGB are 29–77% [24–36] in studies reporting at least 5 years, and up to 27 years, of follow-up data. Heterogeneity of surgical technique, variation in the average pre-surgery BMI, and severity of pre-existing diabetes in these studies make direct comparison of reported remission rates challenging. Rates of long-term remission of T2DM are 20–100% following SG [37–47]. Existing data for DS and BPD are older and more limited, but reported rates of T2DM remission are 83–93% [48–50], and 98–100% [51, 52] respectively. Importantly, studies looking at BPD and DS have the longest follow-up period with data at 10–20 years out from surgery, and diabetes remission rates remain high despite these long follow-up intervals.

Madadi, et al. performed a systematic review and meta-analysis of T2DM remission following SG compared to RYGB and AGB. 35 studies were identified for analysis including 18,138 T2DM patients (2480 SG, 10597 RYGB, 5061 AGB). Meta-analysis demonstrated pooled remission rates of 56.29% after SG and 60.91% after RYGB, with an odds ratio for T2DM remission after SG of 0.71 when compared to RYGB at 1 year of follow up. Interestingly, no difference in remission rates could be demonstrated when looking at studies with more than 1 year of follow up. These data where obtained using the study specific remission criteria. When a standardized definition of T2DM remission was applied across studies, a trend towards improved remission with RYGB was observed, but was not statistically significant. Additional analyses demonstrated an odds ratio at 1 year (OR = 2.17) and > 1 year (OR = 3.16) favoring SG over AGB for T2DM remission [53].

4.3.1.2 Outcomes of Surgery Compared to Maximal Medical Treatment

Bariatric surgery has consistently demonstrated improved glycemic control when compared to maximal medical treatment based on a large body of high-quality data. Multiple meta-analyses were identified, published within the past 5 years, comparing bariatric surgery to medical management to achieve a desired glycemic endpoint (Table 4.2) [54–57]. Additionally, the DSS-II preformed a meta-analysis of high-quality primary evidence during guideline development [20]. Overall, these data demonstrate the superior effectiveness of bariatric surgery in the treatment of diabetes when compared to medical management.

Wu, et al. identified 8 RCTs for inclusion. Most were single-center, and almost none reported number of participating surgeons. Study follow-up ranged from

Table 4.2 Comparison of randomized controlled trials within last 5 years for surgical versus medical treatment in patients with type 2 diabetes

Author (year)	Country	Follow-up duration (year)	Glycemic endpoint	Arms (# patients)	Patients achieving endpoint (%)
Ikramuddin^ (2018) [77]	USA	5	A1C <7%, med use not specified	MM (56)	14
				RYGB (57)	55
Simonson (2018) [78]	USA	3	A1C <6.5%, FPG <126 mg/dL, on or off meds	MM (19)	0
				RYGB (19)	42
Schauer (2017) [26]	USA	5	A1C <6.0%, on or off meds	MM (38)	0
				SG (47)	22.4
				RYGB (49)	14.9
Cummings (2016) [79]	USA	1	A1C <6.0%, off meds	MM (17)	5.9
				RYGB (15)	60
Courcoulas^ (2015) [80]	USA	3	Remission: A1C <6.5%, FPG <125 mg/dL	MM (23)	0
			Resolution: A1C <5.7%, FPG <100 mg/dL, off meds	AGB (22)	29
				RYGB (24)	40
Mingrone (2015) [30]	Italy	5	A1C <6.5%, FPG <5.6 mmol/L, off meds	MM (20)	0
				BPD (20)	63
				RYGB (20)	37
Ding (2015) [81]	USA	1	A1C <6.5%, FPG < 7.0 mmol/L, on or off meds	MM (22)	23
				AGB (23)	33
Halperin (2014) [82]	USA	1	A1C <6.5%, FPG <126 mg/dL, med use not specified	MM (19)	16
				RYGB (19)	58
Wentworth^ (2014) [83]	Australia	5	FPG <7.0, 2hPG <11.1 mmol/L	MM (23)	9
				AGB (22)	23

Notes: Only the most recent data are included from each cohort if multiple publications exist. A number of trials included in the table included patient cohorts with a mean BMI < 35 mg/kg^2 and are designated by [^]

Legend: *FPG* fasting plasma glucose, *2hPG* Plasma glucose after 2 h 75 g glucose challenge, *MM* Medical management (as defined by the study), *AGB* Adjustable gastric band, *RYGB* Roux-en-Y gastric bypass, *SG* Sleeve gastrectomy, *BPD* Biliopancreatic diversion

1–5 years. 619 patient were included, with 341 in surgical treatment arms. All studies had T2DM remission as a primary endpoint, although this was variably defined in each study. Relative risk for T2DM remission was nearly six-fold higher after bariatric surgery compared to non-surgical arms. All eight studies reported change in A1C, with a mean difference of -1.29 favoring surgery. Subgroup analysis did not reveal a difference in T2DM remission rates comparing studies with 1–2 year and 3–5 year follow-up duration. Publication bias was suspected to be high based on qualitative analysis, funnel plots were not published. Heterogeneity was high for all endpoints [54].

Khorgami, et al. identified 7 RCTs excluding studies with less than 2y follow-up duration. This included 463 total patients with 236 patients in the surgical arms. Overall, T2DM remission (either partial or complete) was observed at a rate of 52.7% in surgical arms versus 3.5% in medical arms. Relative risk of remission by procedure was 15.2 for RYGB, 5.8 for AGB, and was unable to be obtained for BPD and SG as these procedures were only reported in single studies. The observed remission rates in the single studies were 95% for BPD and 24% for SG, respectively. This was in contrast to remission rates of 0% and 5% in each respective medical arm. Four studies included data at 5 years follow-up duration. Remission at 5 years was 27.5% in surgical arms, compared to 3.8% in medical arms. Publication bias was considered to be low-risk or unclear [55].

Yan, et al. used data sets from the same cohorts as the other studies described, but limited their comparison to RYGB arms against medical treatment. This included 6 RCTs with 204 patients in RYGB arms and 206 patients in medical arms. As previously described, definitions of glycemic endpoints were highly variable. 5 of 6 studies reported remission rates, which overall was 56.8% after RYGB compared to 0% with medical treatment. The mean A1C decreased by 1.25 points in the surgical arms compared to the medical arms [56].

The DSS-II performed a systematic review of high quality RCTs comparing surgical to non-surgical groups with a follow-up interval of 1–5 years. Surgery was nearly 8.5 times more likely to achieve the glycemic endpoint, as defined by each trail, compared to medical management. The observed mean A1C decreased by 1.5 points in the surgical arms compared to the medical arms. The DSS-II generated guidelines from this review based on clearly demonstrated superiority of bariatric surgery over medical management for 1–5 years of follow-up [20].

Favorable outcomes after bariatric surgery appear to occur rapidly in a weight independent fashion [58, 59]. Predictors of a more durable anti-diabetic response to bariatric surgery include, shorter duration of diabetes, no insulin requirement, and better preoperative glycemic control, possibly related to preservation of beta cell function [60–63]. Accurately predicting outcomes for diabetic patients undergoing bariatric surgery is of key importance to appropriate patient counseling. Data to support specific procedure selection is covered elsewhere.

4.3.1.3 The Role of BMI in Patient Selection

A reliance on BMI as the sole indication for bariatric surgery inadequately addresses the heterogeneity of patients with T2DM. BMI is not a reliable indicator of burden or severity of disease in T2DM patients [64]. A majority of patients with T2DM have a BMI <35, the traditional cut-off for inclusion in a bariatric program [65, 66]. The criteria for inclusion in US bariatric programs are based on NIH consensus data from nearly three decades ago [18, 19]. The current criteria limit insurance access for many patients who may benefit from surgical management of diabetes.

Multiple meta-analyses have demonstrated the favorable glycemic outcomes of patients undergoing bariatric surgery who do not meet standard NIH criteria for bariatric surgery (Table 4.3). Most recently, Rubio-Almanza, et al. preformed a meta-analysis of studies including T2DM patients undergoing bariatric surgery with a mean pre-operative BMI range of 23.1–29.26. This included a total of 1105 patients undergoing bariatric surgery (multiple procedure types). All studies were conducted outside of the US. The most commonly used definition of remission was patients with an A1C <6.0% and off all anti-diabetic medications. Remission rates varied between 0 and 90.2%, with an overall estimate of 43%. The highest remission rates were observed in laparoscopic one anastomosis gastric bypass or mini-bypass. Heterogeneity between studies was high, while potential for publication bias was low [67].

Muller-Stich, et al. preformed a meta-analysis comparing surgical versus medical treatment of T2DM in non-severely obese patients (BMI < 35). This included 818 bariatric surgery patients, and found on overall odds ratio of 14.1 favoring surgery compared to medical management for achieving diabetes remission. HbA1C decreased by a mean of 1.4 points [68].

Panunzi, et al. report on 94 studies including >94,000 patients undergoing bariatric surgery. A subset analysis was performed on 4944 T2DM patients comparing remission rates in patients with baseline BMI < 35 and > 35. Remission rates were 72% and 71% respectively and were not significantly different, despite having significantly greater reduction in post-operative BMI for the more obese group [69].

BMI criteria were developed from populations of European origin, but patients from diverse genetics backgrounds have differences in metabolic risks for any given BMI. Asians generally have a realtively elevated percentage of body fat, and risk of T2DM per given BMI, and data support a lower BMI cutoff for inclusion in a bariatric surgery program [70]. Additionally, equivalent incident rates of diabetes occur at a lower BMI in South Asian, Chinese, and black patients compared to white subjects [71]. Other genetically diverse populations are underrepresented in the existing literature.

A shift to using the term "metabolic surgery" more accurately reflects the important weight-independent metabolic changes that occur after surgery. The branding of a surgical program as "metabolic surgery" or "bariatric surgery" significantly influences the population of patients seeking surgery. Rubino, et al. found that when a program adopted the "metabolic surgery" label, it attracted older patients, more male patients, patients with lower BMI, and higher rates and severity of T2DM [72].

4.3.2   Bariatric Surgery for Type 1 Diabetes

The majority (90%) of the diabetes burden worldwide is attributable to T2DM, however, Type 1 diabetes T1DM is also on the rise. Increasingly, individuals with T1DM have obesity (~50%) [73, 74]. Fewer studies have focused on the effect of bariatric surgery on T1DM, but the existing studies point to a beneficial effect of bariatric surgery in patients T1DM and obesity.

Three systematic reviews evaluating the effect of bariatric surgery on T1DM were identified and results are summarized in Table 4.4. Ashrafian et al. found that

Table 4.3 Summary of recent meta-analyses for outcomes in patients with type 2 diabetes and body mass index < 35 undergoing bariatric surgery

Author (year)	Study design	Number of studies	Number of patients	Pre-operative BMI range (kg/m²)	Patients achieving glycemic endpoint (%)	Risk of bias	Heterogeneity
Rubio-Almanza (2019) [67]	Meta-analysis	26	1105	23.1–29	0–90.2 (mean 43)	Low	High
Huang (2018) [84]	Systematic review	21	921	22.3–30	13–90.2	N/A	N/A
Baskota (2015) [85]	Meta-analysis	10	290	(mean 26.6)	76.2	NR	High
Rao (2015) [86]	Meta-analysis	9	269	19.3–35	59.8	Low	High
Panunzi (2015) [69]	Meta-analysis	35ᵃ	1138	25.7–34.9	72	NR	High
Muller-Stich (2015) [68]	Meta-analysis	13	706	NR	27.8–90.3	None/low	NR
Parikh (2013) [87]	Meta-analysis	39	1389	(mean 30.5)	54.7	NR	NR

ᵃSubgroup analysis within larger study

BMI body mass index, *NR* not reported, *N/A* not applicable

Table 4.4 Summary of systematic reviews for outcomes of bariatric surgery in patients with type 1 diabetes

Author (year)	Study design	Number of studies	Number of patients	Quality of evidence	Summary of findings
Ashrafian (2016) [73]	Systematic review	27	142	Low	• Weight mean decrease in insulin requirement: 44.5 units, 95%CI 34.62–54.42, (p < 0.00001) • Weighted mean decrease in insulin requirement per kilogram: 0.037 units, 95%CI 0.172–0.443, (p < 0.00001) • Weighted mean decreased in AIC: 0.788%, 95%CI 0.334–1.24, (p < 0.001)
Chow (2016) [74]	Systematic review	13	86	Low	• Statistically significant reduction in BMI at 12 months and study endpoint • Weighted mean total daily insulin 98 ± 26 IU/d decreased to 36 ± 15 IU/d at 12 months (p < 0.00001) and 42 ± 11 IU/d at study endpoint (p < 0.00001) • Pre-operative weighted mean 8.46 ± 0.78%, decreased to 7.95 ± 0.55 at 12 months, (P = 0.01) and 8.13 ± 0.86% at study endpoint (p = 0.03)
Mahawar (2016) [75]	Systematic review	15	89	Low	• Total insulin requirement improved in almost all studies, requirement in units/kilogram/day improved in 8/15 studies • Glycemic control remained unaltered in most patients after surgery, improved in some, worsened in a few

95%CI 95% confidence interval, *A1C* hemoglobin A1C, *BMI* body mass index, *IU/d* international units per day bariatric surgery in obese T1DM patients was associated with a significant reduction in insulin requirement (−44.5 units per day), insulin requirement per kilogram (0.307), and A1C (0.788%). Surgery was also associated with a significant reduction in systolic and diastolic blood pressure and a significant, beneficial rise in HDL, outcomes that may influence long-term diabetes related microvascular complications. Heterogeneity within the included studies was high, and the overall quality of studies was low, as all were non-randomized, retrospective studies [73].

Chow et al. similarly reported significant improvements in total daily insulin use down by 62 units per day at 12 months and A1C decreased by 0.51 points at 12 months. The quality of included studies was low and heterogeneity between studies was high [74].

Finally, Mahawar et al. concluded that obese T1DM patients can expect significant weight loss, comorbidity resolution, and reduction in insulin dose with bariatric surgery. However, they concluded that surgery does not result in improved glycemic control in a significant proportion of patients [75].

T1DM results from an autoimmune destruction of the insulin-producing pancreatic beta cells. However, individuals with obesity and T1DM may suffer from both the pathophysiologic mechanisms of T1DM and T2DM [75, 76]. Patients with obesity and T1DM, potentially repesent a unique population for future research into mechanisms of diabetes improvement following bariatric surgery.

4.4   Recommendations Based on the Data

Recommendation	Quality of evidence	Strength of recommendation
1. T2DM is an indication for bariatric surgery in class II or III obesity.	High	Strong
2. Bariatric surgery should be recommended to patients with class II or III obesity and poor glycemic control.	High	Strong
3. Bariatric should be discussed early in the progression of disease for patients with T2DM.	Moderate	Conditional
4. For obese patients with T2DM, bariatric surgery is superior to medical management for long-term glycemic control.	High	Strong
5. Bariatric surgery is a durable treatment for T2DM, and remains superior to medical management for at least 5 years.	High	Strong
6. BMI is not a reliable indicator of disease severity or potential for metabolic benefit after bariatric surgery for diabetic patients.	Moderate	Moderate
7. NIH consensus criteria to qualify for bariatric scery should be updated to more accurately reflect existing data supporting metabolic benefits after bariatric surgery in diabetic patients.	High	Strong

(continued)

Recommendation	Quality of evidence	Strength of recommendation
8. Payer coverage for bariatric surgery should be evidence driven and should be updated from current standards to include T2DM as a primary indication for surgery. This will require a paradigm shift away from the sole use of BMI for patient selection.	NA	NA
9. Underrepresented racial and ethnic groups benefit from bariatric surgery at a lower BMI and are disadvantaged by current selection criteria.	Moderate	Moderate
10. Bariatric Surgery can improve glycemic control and medication requirements in patients with T1DM and obesity.	Low	Conditional
11. We propose using the name "metabolic surgery" to more accurately reflect the effect of these interventions.	NA	NA

4.5   A Personal View of the Data

Prevention and treatment of diabetes, a disease with significant impacts on quality of life, early mortality, and healthcare expenditure, is arguably the most important comorbid indication for bariatric surgery. Given the strength of the data to support bariatric surgery as a treatment for diabetes, surgery should be considered earlier in the treatment algorithm, and is superior to medical and intensive lifestyle management strategies alone. Nevertheless, the optimal management strategy for patients with diabetes is a multi-disciplinary approach that includes surgery, medications, and lifestyle interventions. Evidence suggests that the earlier surgeons can intervene on the disease, the better chance we have for "cure", suggesting that the greatest impact may be in the surgical treatment of patients with prediabetes and early onset diabetes. However, with the staggering statistical projections about the global burden of both diabetes and obesity, bariatric surgical resources cannot be expected to meet this demand. This highlights the importance of patient selection and resource management.

The evidence presented above argues for an update in the selection criteria and insurance payment for bariatric surgery. Movement away from BMI centric decision making, to a model which includes more patient specific factors, could improve overall effectiveness and outcomes of bariatric surgery. Finally, better understanding of the mechanisms of diabetes improvement after bariatric surgery is an important target for future research, and may lead to additional drug targets or less invasive endoscopic therapies.

References

1. Whiting DR, et al. IDF diabetes atlas: global estimates of the prevalence of diabetes for 2011 and 2030. Diabetes Res Clin Pract. 2011;94(3):311–21.

2. GBD 2015 Obesity Collaborators. Health effects of overweight and obesity in 195 countries over 25 years. N Engl J Med. 2017;377(1):13–27.
3. Zhou B, et al. Worldwide trends in diabetes since 1980: a pooled analysis of 751 population-based studies with 44 million participants. Lancet. 2016;387(10027):1513–30.
4. Zhang P, et al. Global healthcare expenditure on diabetes for 2010 and 2030. Diabetes Res Clin Pract. 2010;87(3):293–301.
5. Gloy VL, et al. Bariatric surgery versus non-surgical treatment for obesity: a systematic review and meta-analysis of randomised controlled trials. BMJ. 2013;347:f5934.
6. Pories WJ, et al. Is type II diabetes mellitus (NIDDM) a surgical disease? Ann Surg. 1992;215(6):633–43.
7. Pories WJ, et al. Who would have thought it? An operation proves to be the most effective therapy for adult-onset diabetes mellitus. Ann Surg. 1995;222(3):339–52.
8. Hossain P, Kawar B, El Nahas M. Obesity and diabetes in the developing world—a growing challenge. N Engl J Med. 2007;356(3):213–5.
9. Mingrone G, et al. Bariatric surgery versus conventional medical therapy for type 2 diabetes. N Engl J Med. 2012;366(17):1577–85.
10. Schauer PR, et al. Bariatric surgery versus intensive medical therapy in obese patients with diabetes. N Engl J Med. 2012;366(17):1567–76.
11. Courcoulas AP, et al. Surgical vs medical treatments for type 2 diabetes mellitus: a randomized clinical trial. JAMA Surg. 2014;149(7):707–15.
12. Adams TD, et al. Long-term mortality after gastric bypass surgery. N Engl J Med. 2007;357(8):753–61.
13. Schauer PR, et al. Clinical outcomes of metabolic surgery: efficacy of glycemic control, weight loss, and remission of diabetes. Diabetes Care. 2016;39(6):902–11.
14. Arterburn DE, et al. Association between bariatric surgery and long-term survival. JAMA. 2015;313(1):62–70.
15. Sjöström L, et al. Effects of bariatric surgery on mortality in Swedish obese subjects. N Engl J Med. 2007;357(8):741–52.
16. Wentworth JM, et al. Cost-effectiveness of gastric band surgery for overweight but not obese adults with type 2 diabetes in the US. J Diabetes Complicat. 2017;31(7):1139–44.
17. Gulliford MC, et al. Costs and outcomes of increasing access to bariatric surgery: cohort study and cost-effectiveness analysis using electronic health records. Value Health. 2017;20(1):85–92.
18. National Institutes of Health Consensus Development Panel. Gastrointestinal surgery for severe obesity. Ann Intern Med. 1991;115:956–61.
19. Cummings DE, Cohen RV. Beyond BMI: the need for new guidelines governing the use of bariatric and metabolic surgery. Lancet Diabetes Endocrinol. 2014;2(2):175–81.
20. Rubino F, et al. Metabolic surgery in the treatment algorithm for type 2 diabetes: a joint statement by international diabetes organizations. Obes Surg. 2017;27(1):2–21.
21. Sjöström L, et al. Lifestyle, diabetes, and cardiovascular risk factors 10 years after bariatric surgery. N Engl J Med. 2004;351(26):2683–93.
22. Colquitt JL, et al. Surgery for obesity. Cochrane Database Syst Rev. 2009;2
23. Azagury D, et al. ASMBS position statement on medium-and long-term durability of weight loss and diabetic outcomes after conventional stapled bariatric procedures. Surg Obes Relat Dis. 2018;14(10):1425–41.
24. Brethauer SA, et al. Can diabetes be surgically cured?: long-term metabolic effects of bariatric surgery in obese patients with type 2 diabetes mellitus. Ann Surg. 2013;258(4):628–37.
25. Arterburn DE, et al. A multisite study of long-term remission and relapse of type 2 diabetes mellitus following gastric bypass. Obes Surg. 2013;23(1):93–102.
26. Schauer PR, et al. Bariatric surgery versus intensive medical therapy for diabetes—5-year outcomes. N Engl J Med. 2017;376(7):641–51.
27. Adams TD, et al. Weight and metabolic outcomes 12 years after gastric bypass. N Engl J Med. 2017;377:1143–55.
28. Kothari SN, et al. Long-term (>10-year) outcomes after laparoscopic Roux-en-Y gastric bypass. Surg Obes Relat Dis. 2017;13(6):972–8.

29. Chen Y, et al. Gastric bypass surgery leads to long-term remission or improvement of type 2 diabetes and significant decrease of microvascular and macrovascular complications. Ann Surg. 2016;263(6):1138–42.
30. Mingrone G, et al. Bariatric–metabolic surgery versus conventional medical treatment in obese patients with type 2 diabetes: 5 year follow-up of an open-label, single-Centre, randomised controlled trial. Lancet. 2015;386(9997):964–73.
31. Obeid NR, et al. Long-term outcomes after Roux-en-Y gastric bypass: 10- to 13-year data. Surg Obes Relat Dis. 2016;12(1):11–20.
32. Pajecki D, et al. Bariatric surgery in the elderly: results of a mean follow-up of five years. Arquivos Brasileiros de Cirurgia Digestiva (São Paulo). 2015;28:15–8.
33. Aftab H, et al. Five-year outcome after gastric bypass for morbid obesity in a Norwegian cohort. Surg Obes Relat Dis. 2014;10(1):71–8.
34. Dogan K, et al. Long-term effects of laparoscopic Roux-en-Y gastric bypass on diabetes mellitus, hypertension and dyslipidaemia in morbidly obese patients. Obes Surg. 2014;24(11):1835–42.
35. Nergaard BJ, et al. Gastric bypass with long alimentary limb or long pancreato-biliary limb—long-term results on weight loss, resolution of co-morbidities and metabolic parameters. Obes Surg. 2014;24(10):1595–602.
36. Neto RML, et al. Comorbidities remission after Roux-en-Y gastric bypass for morbid obesity is sustained in a long-term follow-up and correlates with weight regain. Obes Surg. 2012;22(10):1580–5.
37. Noel P, et al. What are the long-term results 8 years after sleeve gastrectomy? Surg Obes Relat Dis. 2017;13(7):1110–5.
38. Aminian A, et al. Can sleeve gastrectomy "cure" diabetes? Long-term metabolic effects of sleeve gastrectomy in patients with type 2 diabetes. Ann Surg. 2016;264(4):674–81.
39. Aridi HD, et al. Long-term outcomes of laparoscopic sleeve gastrectomy: a Lebanese center experience. Surg Obes Relat Dis. 2016;12(9):1689–96.
40. Casella G, et al. Long-term results after laparoscopic sleeve gastrectomy in a large monocentric series. Surg Obes Relat Dis. 2016;12(4):757–62.
41. Ruiz-Tovar J, et al. Long-term weight and metabolic effects of laparoscopic sleeve gastrectomy calibrated with a 50-Fr Bougie. Obes Surg. 2016;26(1):32–7.
42. Alexandrou A, et al. Laparoscopic sleeve gastrectomy for morbid obesity: 5-year results. Am J Surg. 2015;209(2):230–4.
43. Golomb I, et al. Long-term metabolic effects of laparoscopic sleeve gastrectomy. JAMA Surg. 2015;150(11):1051–7.
44. Sieber P, et al. Five-year results of laparoscopic sleeve gastrectomy. Surg Obes Relat Dis. 2014;10(2):243–9.
45. Zhang Y, et al. A randomized clinical trial of laparoscopic Roux-en-Y gastric bypass and sleeve gastrectomy for the treatment of morbid obesity in China: a 5-year outcome. Obes Surg. 2014;24(10):1617–24.
46. Abbatini F, et al. Long-term remission of type 2 diabetes in morbidly obese patients after sleeve gastrectomy. Surg Obes Relat Dis. 2013;9(4):498–502.
47. Rawlins L, et al. Sleeve gastrectomy: 5-year outcomes of a single institution. Surg Obes Relat Dis. 2013;9(1):21–5.
48. Bolckmans R, Himpens J. Long-term (>10 yrs) outcome of the laparoscopic biliopancreatic diversion with duodenal switch. Ann Surg. 2016;264(6):1029–37.
49. Marceau P, et al. Long-term metabolic outcomes 5 to 20 years after biliopancreatic diversion. Obes Surg. 2015;25(9):1584–93.
50. Michaud A, et al. Biliopancreatic diversion with duodenal switch in the elderly: long-term results of a matched-control study. Obes Surg. 2016;26(2):350–60.
51. Larrad-Jiménez Á, et al. Short-, mid-and long-term results of Larrad biliopancreatic diversion. Obes Surg. 2007;17(2):202–10.
52. Marinari GM, et al. A 15-year evaluation of biliopancreatic diversion according to the bariatric analysis reporting outcome system (BAROS). Obes Surg. 2004;14(3):325–8.

53. Madadi F, et al. Remission of type 2 diabetes and sleeve gastrectomy in morbid obesity: a comparative systematic review and Meta-analysis. Obes Surg. 2019:1–11.
54. Wu G-Z, et al. Meta-analysis of bariatric surgery versus non-surgical treatment for type 2 diabetes mellitus. Oncotarget. 2016;7:87511.
55. Khorgami Z, et al. Outcomes of bariatric surgery versus medical management for type 2 diabetes mellitus: a meta-analysis of randomized controlled trials. Obes Surg. 2019;29(3):964–74.
56. Yan Y, et al. Roux-en-Y gastric bypass versus medical treatment for type 2 diabetes mellitus in obese patients: a systematic review and meta-analysis of randomized controlled trials. Medicine. 2016;95
57. Ribaric G, Buchwald JN, McGlennon TW. Diabetes and weight in comparative studies of bariatric surgery vs conventional medical therapy: a systematic review and meta-analysis. Obes Surg. 2014;24(3):437–55.
58. Rubino F, Marescaux J. Effect of duodenal–jejunal exclusion in a non-obese animal model of type 2 diabetes: a new perspective for an old disease. Ann Surg. 2004;239(1):1–11.
59. Cho YM. A gut feeling to cure diabetes: potential mechanisms of diabetes remission after bariatric surgery. Diabetes Metab J. 2014;38(6):406–15.
60. Nguyen KT, et al. Preserved insulin secretory capacity and weight loss are the predominant predictors of glycemic control in patients with type 2 diabetes randomized to Roux-en-Y gastric bypass. Diabetes. 2015;64(9):3104–10.
61. Lee W-J, et al. Predicting success of metabolic surgery: age, body mass index, C-peptide, and duration score. Surg Obes Relat Dis. 2013;9(3):379–84.
62. Still CD, et al. A probability score for preoperative prediction of type 2 diabetes remission following RYGB surgery. Lancet Diabetes Endocrinol. 2014;2:38.
63. Aminian A, et al. Individualized metabolic surgery score: procedure selection based on diabetes severity. Ann Surg. 2017;266(4):650–7.
64. Pories WJ, Dohm LG, Mansfield CJ. Beyond the BMI: the search for better guidelines for bariatric surgery. Obesity (Silver Spring). 2009;18(5):865–71.
65. Bays HE, et al. The relationship of body mass index to diabetes mellitus, hypertension and dyslipidaemia: comparison of data from two national surveys. Int J Clin Pract. 2007;61(5):737–47.
66. Inzucchi SE, et al. Management of hyperglycemia in type 2 diabetes, 2015: a patient-centered approach: update to a position statement of the American Diabetes Association and the European Association for the Study of Diabetes. Diabetes Care. 2015;38(1):140–9.
67. Rubio-Almanza M, et al. Does metabolic surgery lead to diabetes remission in patients with BMI< 30 kg/m 2?: a meta-analysis. Obes Surg. 2019;29(4):1105–16.
68. Müller-Stich BP, Senft JD, Warschkow R, et al. Surgical versus medical treatment of type 2 diabetes mellitus in nonseverely obese patients. Ann Surg. 2015;261(3):421–9.
69. Panunzi S, et al. Predictors of remission of diabetes mellitus in severely obese individuals undergoing bariatric surgery: do BMI or procedure choice matter? A meta-analysis. Ann Surg. 2015:459–67.
70. Kasama K, et al. IFSO-APC consensus statements 2011. Obes Surg. 2012;22(5):677–84.
71. Chiu M, Austin PC, Manuel DG, et al. Deriving ethnic-specific BMI cutoff points for assessing diabetes risk. Diabetes Care. 2011;34:1741–8.
72. Rubino F, et al. Bariatric, metabolic, and diabetes surgery: what's in a name? Ann Surg. 2014;259(1):117–22.
73. Ashrafian H, et al. Type 1 diabetes mellitus and bariatric surgery: a systematic review and meta-analysis. Obes Surg. 2016;26(8):1697–704.
74. Chow A, et al. A systematic review and meta-analysis of outcomes for type 1 diabetes after bariatric surgery. J Obes. 2016;
75. Mahawar KK, et al. Bariatric surgery in type 1 diabetes mellitus: a systematic review. Obes Surg. 2016;26(1):196–204.
76. Pozzilli P, et al. Obesity, autoimmunity, and double diabetes in youth. Diabetes Care. 2011;34(2):S166–70.

77. Ikramuddin S, et al. Lifestyle intervention and medical management with vs without Roux-en-Y gastric bypass and control of hemoglobin A1c, LDL cholesterol, and systolic blood pressure at 5 years in the diabetes surgery study. JAMA. 2018;319(3):266–78.

78. Simonson DC, et al. Clinical and patient-centered outcomes in obese patients with type 2 diabetes 3 years after randomization to Roux-en-Y gastric bypass surgery versus intensive lifestyle management: the SLIMM-T2D study. Diabetes Care. 2018;41(4):670–9.

79. Cummings DE, et al. Gastric bypass surgery vs intensive lifestyle and medical intervention for type 2 diabetes: the CROSSROADS randomised controlled trial. Diabetologia. 2016;59(5):945–53.

80. Courcoulas AP, et al. Three-year outcomes of bariatric surgery vs lifestyle intervention for type 2 diabetes mellitus treatment: a randomized clinical trial. JAMA Surg. 2015;150(10):931–40.

81. Ding S-A, et al. Adjustable gastric band surgery or medical management in patients with type 2 diabetes: a randomized clinical trial. J Clin Endocrinol Metabol. 2015;100(7):2546–56.

82. Halperin F, et al. Roux-en-Y gastric bypass surgery or lifestyle with intensive medical management in patients with type 2 diabetes: feasibility and 1-year results of a randomized clinical trial. JAMA Surg. 2014;149(7):716–26.

83. Wentworth JM, et al. Five-year outcomes of a randomized trial of gastric band surgery in overweight but not obese people with type 2 diabetes. Diabetes Care. 2017;40(4):e44–5.

84. Huang Z-P, et al. The effect of metabolic surgery on nonobese patients (BMI< 30 kg/m2) with type 2 diabetes: a systematic review. Surg Obes Relat Dis. 2018;14(6):810–20.

85. Baskota A, et al. Bariatric surgery for type 2 diabetes mellitus in patients with BMI< 30 kg/m2: a systematic review and meta-analysis. PloS One. 2015;10(7)

86. Rao W-S, et al. A meta-analysis of short-term outcomes of patients with type 2 diabetes mellitus and BMI≤ 35 kg/m 2 undergoing Roux-en-Y gastric bypass. World J Surg. 2015;39(1):223–30.

87. Parikh M, et al. Role of bariatric surgery as treatment for type 2 diabetes in patients who do not meet current NIH criteria: a systematic review and meta-analysis. J Am Coll Surg. 2013;217(3):527–32.

Bariatric Procedure Selection in Diabetics

5

Andrea Stroud and Ryland Stucke

5.1   Introduction

Bariatric surgery is the most effective treatment for obesity [1], and often results in Type 2 diabetes (T2DM) remission [2–10]. Of all obesity-related comorbid illnesses, T2DM has the most evidence as an indication for bariatric surgery. T2DM resolution following bariatric surgery likely involves multiple mechanisms, and has yet to be fully elucidated. Complex neuroendocrine and metabolic effects including reductions in glycated hemoglobin (A1C), and concomitant increases in circulating incretin concentrations, insulin sensitivity, and β-cell function have been described [11, 12]. Interestingly, these metabolic effects appear to have weight-independent effects on T2DM and begin to occur prior to discharge from the hospital [13, 14]. Several procedures exist in the modern era of bariatric surgery with important difference in anticipated weight loss, rates of diabetes resolution, and complications, including nutritional deficiencies. The role of the modern bariatric surgeon is to understand the nuances of existing surgical options and guide patients in individualized decision-making based on their unique characteristics and goals. In this chapter, we review existing evidence to guide procedure selection for diabetic patients seeking bariatric surgery.

A. Stroud (✉)
Bariatric Surgery, Oregon Health & Science University, Portland, OR, USA
e-mail: strouda@ohsu.edu

R. Stucke
General Surgery, Dartmouth-Hitchcock Medical Center, Lebanon, NH, USA

© Springer Nature Switzerland AG 2021
J. Alverdy, Y. Vigneswaran (eds.), *Difficult Decisions in Bariatric Surgery*,
Difficult Decisions in Surgery: An Evidence-Based Approach,
https://doi.org/10.1007/978-3-030-55329-6_5

5.2   Search Strategy

A comprehensive search of MEDLINE (PubMed), EMBASE, and the Cochrane library databases was conducted for English language publications from 2009 to 2020, and included the following terms: diabetes AND gastric bypass (RYGB), jejunoileal bypass, duodenal switch (DS), gastric sleeve (SG), biliopancreatic diversion (BPD), bariatric surgery, metabolic surgery, obesity surgery, intestinal bypass, along with all relevant related keywords (Table 5.1). We also included papers of historical importance or commonly referenced landmark studies. Bibliographies were cross-referenced to identify additional relevant articles. Recommendations were classified using the GRADE system. Endoscopic and device-based interventions were excluded from this analysis.

5.3   Results

5.3.1   Individualizing Procedure Choice for Diabetic Patients

In patients with obesity, bariatric surgery is superior to maximal lifestyle and medical management of T2DM [2–10]. In general, bariatric procedures that result in more weight lost and higher rates of diabetes remission also carry higher rates of post-procedural and nutritional complications. However, the data suggest a more nuanced appreciation of the various procedures and unique patient factors is required to make appropriate individualized decisions with patients. For diabetic patients, the most common primary goal in pursuing bariatric surgery is the resolution of diabetes [15]. Patient-centered decision-making should weigh the potential of metabolic improvements and diabetes resolution against post-operative and nutritional complications.

SG and RYGB currently make up >90% of primary bariatric procedures performed in the United States, with over half of all procedures being SG [16–18]. Emerging data from randomized controlled trials (RCT) suggests minimal differences in diabetic outcomes comparing RYGB to SG. Aminian, et al. identified four modern RCTs comparing diabetic endpoints in patients with T2DM undergoing RYGB versus SG. The individual studies had small sample size and taken together included 174 patients undergoing RYGB and 175 undergoing SG. Interestingly, no significant difference in diabetes remission was identified in any single study or in

Table 5.1 PICO table

P (Patients)	I (Interventions)	C (Comparator)	O (Outcomes)
Patients with diabetes and obesity	Bariatric surgery as a metabolic intervention	Outcomes of various operative approaches accounting for patient factors	Glycemic control, diabetes remission/resolution, morbidity, mortality, weight loss, cost

Table 5.2 RCTs comparing SG v RYGB (adapted from Aminian, et al. [19])

	RYGB			SG		
	Complete remission	Long-term remission		Complete remission	Long-term remission	
Author (year)	n with remission/n total cohort (%)	n with remission/n total cohort (%)	P value	n with remission/n total cohort (%)	n with remission/n total cohort (%)	P value
Schauer, et al. (2017) [37]	11/49 (22)	7/47 (15)	0.49	15/49 (31)	11/47 (23)	0.57
Salminen, et al. (2018) [41]	10/40 (25)	5/41 (12)	0.23	18/40 (45)	15/41 (37)	0.59
Peterli, et al. (2018) [42]	19/28 (68)	16/26 (62)	0.84	21/28 (75)	20/26 (77)	0.88
Ruiz-Trovar, et al. (2019) [43]	47/59 (79)	48/61 (77)	0.92	51/59 (86)	50/61 (82)	0.67
4 RCTs combined	87/176 (50)	76/175 (43)	0.31	105/176 (60)	96/175 (55)	0.42

pooled analysis (Table 5.2). Primary inclusion criteria in all trials was based on BMI. Thus, diabetic outcomes were secondary endpoints and data came from subgroup analyses. The sub-group analyses were not designed nor powered to detect a difference in diabetes remission between SG and RYGB in any of the individual RCTs. Aminian, et al. performed pooled analyses. *Complete remission* of T2DM (HbA1C < 6%, off diabetic medications) at 5 years was 50% after RYGB and 43% after SG (RR = 0.07, CI-0.2–0.15), while *long-term remission* (HbA1C < 6.5%, off diabetic medications) at 5 years of follow-up was 60% after RYGB and 55% after SG (RR 0.05, CI-0.04–0.14). Because the confidence interval crosses 0, the effect size of 7% for *complete remission* and 5% for *long-term remission* are not statistically significant. These RCT data are underpowered to make strong procedural recommendations regarding differences in diabetic outcomes. However, closely examining the confidence intervals, suggests that at a maximum RYGB might provide a relatively small advantage in complete remission of 15% [19].

The PCORnet Bariatric Study included a cohort of 9710 adults with T2DM who underwent bariatric surgery between 2010 and 2014 in the United States (US). In this unmatched surgical cohort, 64.2% underwent RYGB and 35.8% had SG, although pre-operative diabetes severity was similar between groups. The majority of diabetes remission occurred in the first 2 years following surgery. Patients who underwent RYGB had slightly higher T2DM remission rates compared to SG (HR 1.10 [95% CI, 1.04–1.16]). At each time point, there was higher T2DM remission following RYGB compared with SG, 59.2% vs 55.9% at 1 year, 84.3% vs 81.5% at 3 years, and 86.1% vs 83.5% at 5 years. The authors conclude that in a real world setting RYGB results in small, but improved long-term T2DM outcomes compared to SG [20].

Existing data for diabetes remission following RYGB and SG vary widely and depend on multiple factors including the severity and duration of pre-existing diabetes, as well as the study's definition of *resolution* and/or *remission*. Overall, studies consistently favor RYGB over SG for diabetic endpoints, but the differences are small. Existing data encompass only 5 years of follow-up, and longer-term data are needed, especially when considering possible differences in recidivism.

Duodenal switch (DS) comprises less than 1% of bariatric procedures performed in the US [16]. DS causes more pronounced post-operative metabolic changes and higher rates of immediate and delayed complications [21–25]. Long-term rates of diabetes remission following DS are 83–93%, higher than published rates in RYGB and SG [26–28]. No RCTs or prospective trials were identified comparing diabetic outcomes of DS versus RYGB and/or SG. However, limited retrospective data suggests higher rates of diabetes remission, lower HbA1C, and decreased need for anti-diabetic medications for DS compared to SG [22–26]. A systematic review performed by Buchwald, et al. in 2009 identified 103 treatment arms with 3188 patients measuring diabetic resolution. This study primarily identified single-arm series and only 1.6% of studies contributed class I evidence. However, in this analysis, DS demonstrated complete T2DM remission of 95% compared to 80% after RYGB. Rates of complications were not compared [21]. As minimally invasive techniques improve, more comparative data and risk/benefit analyses are needed to determine the role for DS in obese diabetic patients.

5.3.2   Use of Decision-Aid Tools for Procedure Selection

While there does not appear to be large differences in diabetic outcomes based on broad population data, patient specific factors are also important to consider when selecting an appropriate bariatric procedure. A shared decision-making model informs patients about anticipated benefits and complications, and elicits patient's preference and desires. Diabetic outcomes are dependent on pre-existing factors such as duration of disease, severity of insulin resistance, insulin use, and ability to achieve adequate glycemic control [29–32]. Several evidenced-based decision-aid tools now exist to support shared-decision making conversations. These tools take into account specific patient and procedure factors and can help with procedure selection for diabetic patients.

The ABCD [29] and DiaRem [30] scores are validated tools to predict remission of T2DM following RYGB at 12 and 14 months respectively. The ABCD score incorporates age, BMI, C-peptide levels, and duration of diabetes, whereas the DiaRem score incorporates use of insulin, age, HbA1C, and type of antidiabetic medications. These two scores have similar performance characteristics overall [32].

The Individualized Metabolic Surgery (IMS) score helps frame anticipated outcomes when considering RYGB versus SG operations for diabetic patients. This validated online calculator utilizes accessible patient information including, the number of pre-op T2DM medications, insulin use, and HbA1C, as well as duration of T2DM, to guide expectations for diabetes remission. The tool was developed from retrospective data of 659 patients undergoing RYGB or SG, and validated in 241 patients at a second center. Short- and long-term complication rates are not explicitly considered in this model. Follow-up data was captured out to 5 years. This tool divides patients into mild, moderate, and severe diabetic catagories, which corresponds to 15%, 51%, and 34% of the study population respectively. For patients with mild diabetes, RYGB and SG are both highly effective, but RYGB was significantly better at achieving diabetes resolution (92% vs. 74%, p = 0.04) and decreasing the need for diabetic medication at 5 years. Patients with moderate diabetes, which comprised 51% of the study cohort, experienced a significant and dramatic difference in remission rates at 5 years favoring RYGB over SG (60% v. 25%, p = <0.001). Additionally, RYGB patients with moderate T2DM were significantly more likely to achieve a HbA1C <7, take less anti-diabetic medications, or remain off all diabetic medications. The authors suggest a clear advantage of RYGB over SG for moderate diabetics. In patients with severe diabetes there was no difference in rates of diabetes remission (12% in both SG and RYGB groups). However, the validation cohort of severe diabetics did demonstrate a difference in remission rates of 8% in the RYGB arm versus 3% in the SG arm. Given that SG has potentially less post-operative and nutritional complications, the authors favor SG in severe diabetics, and argue this avoids the slightly increased risk of complications associated with RYGB [31]. More data are needed to understand the true difference in diabetes remission rates in severe diabetics.

While rates of diabetes remission is an important factor to consider when counseling bariatric patient on procedure choice, other factors such as weight loss, risk profile of post-operative and nutritional complications, and options for revision surgery are important to consider. Additionally, co-morbid conditions such as gastroesophageal reflux or Barrett's esophagus, inflammatory bowel disease, abdominal hernias, and psychiatric disease may influence procedure selection.

5.3.3 Recidivism and Incident Diabetes

It is important to recognize that 35–50% of patients who achieve remission of T2DM following bariatric surgery experience recurrence within 5 years [33–35]. In the PCORnet Bariatric Study, T2DM relapse rate was lower for RYGB than SG (HR 0.75 [95% CI, 0.67–0.84)]. The proportion of patients who experienced diabetes recidivism after RYGB was lower at each time point compared to SG, (8.4% vs 11% at 1 year, 21.2 vs 27.2% at 3 years, and 33.1% vs 41.6% at 5 years) [20]. However, with or without relapse, patients who undergo surgery maintain substantial improvement in glycemic control from baseline for at least 5–15 years [36]. Predictors of a more durable anti-diabetic response to bariatric surgery include, shorter duration of diabetes, no insulin requirement, and better preoperative glycemic control, possibly related to preservation of beta cell function [34, 35, 37, 38]. The Individualized Diabetes Relapse (IDR) score has been developed to calculate the risk of diabetes relapse in patients who have experienced early remission [39]. These data are not yet robust enough to inform procedure selection, but may become important as more long-term data are reported.

Metabolic surgery may additionally have a role in the prevention of diabetes in obese, at-risk patients. The Swedish Obese Subjects (SOS) trial is the largest and longest multi-center prospective bariatric trial and includes secondary diabetic endpoints. Recruitment occurred from 1987 to 2001 with 20 years of follow-up data, and included 1658 surgical patients (311 underwent gastric banding, 1140 underwent vertical banded gastroplasty, and 207 underwent RYGB), matched with 1771 obese controls. In the post-surgical arm, T2DM developed with an incidence rate of 6.8 cases per 1000 person-years versus 28.4 cases per 1000 person-years in controls, representing a nearly 80% risk reduction of incident diabetes following bariatric surgery. Assessment of incident diabetes in at-risk obese patients following bariatric surgery is an important outcome to consider in future bariatric studies [40].

5.4   Recommendations Based on the Data

1. Sleeve gastrectomy and Roux-en-Y gastric bypass are both effective procedures to induce remission of T2DM.	High	Strong
2. Roux-en-Y gastric bypass and sleeve gastrectomy have similar rates of diabetes remission over 5 years of follow-up.	High	Strong
3. Individual patient factors are important for appropriate procedure selection.	High	Strong
4. Patients with moderate diabetes have superior outcomes after RYGB compared to SG.	Moderate	Moderate
5. DS leads to increased rates of T2DM remission and complications compared to RYGB and SG.	Low	Weak
6. Despite rates of recidivism, diabetic patients still have significant benefit compared to baseline following bariatric surgery, and recidivism should not be considered a "failure".	Moderate	Moderate

5.5   A Personal View of the Data

It is well established that bariatric surgery is superior to the best medical management for the treatment of T2DM. As surgeons, we must help guide our patients to an optimal outcome using the best available evidence. Currently, we can be confident that the majority of patients with T2DM will experience diabetes remission after bariatric surgery. However, it is important to acknowledge a moderate rate of long-term relapse.

Procedure selection involves understanding individual patients' priorities and goals, as well as comorbidities and prior surgery that may influence surgical decision-making. If diabetes resolution is the highest priority to the patient, RYGB will offer superior results to SG. This relationship is most pronounced in those with moderate disease. The metabolic benefits of RYGB to patients with mild or severe disease is more controversial. The use of the IMS online prediction tool can help guide preoperative discussions with diabetic patients. Of note, minimally invasive variations of the duodenal switch are increasingly performed in the US and may offer another strong anti-diabetic operation, but high quality comparative studies are needed.

Moderate rates of long-term relapse of T2DM exist. However, these cases should not be considered a failure as patients still have improved long-term outcomes despite recidivism. In a patient-centered shared-decision making model, patient specific factors and preferences should be accounted for, including thoughtful discussions of risks and benefits, in order to guide procedure selection.

References

1. Gloy VL, et al. Bariatric surgery versus non-surgical treatment for obesity: a systematic review and meta-analysis of randomised controlled trials. BMJ. 2013;347:f5934.
2. Mingrone G, et al. Bariatric surgery versus conventional medical therapy for type 2 diabetes. N Engl J Med. 2012;366(17):1577–85.
3. Schauer PR, et al. Bariatric surgery versus intensive medical therapy in obese patients with diabetes. N Engl J Med. 2012;366(17):1567–76.
4. Ikramuddin S, et al. Lifestyle intervention and medical management with vs without Roux-en-Y gastric bypass and control of hemoglobin A1c, LDL cholesterol, and systolic blood pressure at 5 years in the diabetes surgery study. JAMA. 2018;319(3):266–78.
5. Simonson DC, et al. Clinical and patient-centered outcomes in obese patients with type 2 diabetes 3 years after randomization to Roux-en-Y gastric bypass surgery versus intensive lifestyle management: the SLIMM-T2D study. Diabetes Care. 2018;41(4):670–9.
6. Cummings DE, et al. Gastric bypass surgery vs intensive lifestyle and medical intervention for type 2 diabetes: the CROSSROADS randomised controlled trial. Diabetologia. 2016;59(5):945–53.
7. Courcoulas AP, et al. Three-year outcomes of bariatric surgery vs lifestyle intervention for type 2 diabetes mellitus treatment: a randomized clinical trial. JAMA Surg. 2015;150(10):931–40.
8. Ding S-A, et al. Adjustable gastric band surgery or medical management in patients with type 2 diabetes: a randomized clinical trial. J Clin Endocrinol Metabol. 2015;100(7):2546–56.
9. Halperin F, et al. Roux-en-Y gastric bypass surgery or lifestyle with intensive medical management in patients with type 2 diabetes: feasibility and 1-year results of a randomized clinical trial. JAMA Surg. 2014;149(7):716–26.
10. Wentworth JM, et al. Five-year outcomes of a randomized trial of gastric band surgery in overweight but not obese people with type 2 diabetes. Diabetes Care. 2017;40(4):e44–5.
11. Kashyap SR, et al. Metabolic effects of bariatric surgery in patients with moderate obesity and type 2 diabetes: analysis of a randomized control trial comparing surgery with intensive medical treatment. Diabetes Care. 2013;36(8):2175–82.
12. Batterham RL, Cummings DE. Mechanisms of diabetes improvement following bariatric/metabolic surgery. Diabetes Care. 2016;39(6):893–901.
13. Rubino F, Marescaux J. Effect of duodenal–jejunal exclusion in a non-obese animal model of type 2 diabetes: a new perspective for an old disease. Ann Surg. 2004;239(1):1–11.
14. Cho YM. A gut feeling to cure diabetes: potential mechanisms of diabetes remission after bariatric surgery. Diabetes Metab J. 2014;38(6):406–15.
15. Weinstein AL, Marascalchi BJ, Spiegel MA, et al. Patient preferences and bariatric surgery procedure selection; the need for shared decision-making. Obes Surg. 2014;24:1933–9. https://doi.org/10.1007/s11695-014-1270-6.

16. English WJ, et al. American Society for Metabolic and Bariatric Surgery estimation of metabolic and bariatric procedures performed in the United States in 2016. Surg Obes Relat Dis. 2018;14(3):259–63.
17. Khorgami Z, et al. Trends in utilization of bariatric surgery, 2010-2014: sleeve gastrectomy dominates. Surg Obes Relat Dis. 2017;13(5):774–8.
18. Kizy S, et al. National trends in bariatric surgery 2012–2015: demographics, procedure selection, readmissions, and cost. Obes Surg. 2017;27(11):2933–9.
19. Aminian A. Bariatric procedure selection in patients with type 2 diabetes: choice between Roux-en-Y gastric bypass or sleeve gastrectomy. Surg Obes Relat Dis. 2020;16(2):332–9.
20. McTigue KM, Wellman R, Nauman E, et al. Comparing the 5-year diabetes outcomes of sleeve gastrectomy and gastric bypass: the national patient-centered clinical research network (PCORNet) Bariatric study. JAMA Surg. 2020 Mar 4:e200087.
21. Buchwald H, et al. Weight and type 2 diabetes after bariatric surgery: systematic review and meta-analysis. Am J Med. 2009;122(3):248–56.
22. Skogar ML, Sundbom M. Weight loss and effect on co-morbidities in the long-term after duodenal switch and gastric bypass: a population-based cohort study. Surg Obes Relat Dis. 2020;16(1):17–23.
23. Nelson DW, Blair KS, Martin MJ. Analysis of obesity-related outcomes and bariatric failure rates with the duodenal switch vs gastric bypass for morbid obesity. Arch Surg. 2012;147(9):847–54.
24. Dorman RB, et al. Case-matched outcomes in bariatric surgery for treatment of type 2 diabetes in the morbidly obese patient. Ann Surg. 2012;255(2):287–93.
25. Dorman RB, et al. Benefits and complications of the duodenal switch/biliopancreatic diversion compared to the Roux-en-Y gastric bypass. Surgery. 2012;152(4):758–67.
26. Bolckmans R, Himpens J. Long-term (> 10 yrs) outcome of the laparoscopic biliopancreatic diversion with duodenal switch. Ann Surg. 2016;264(6):1029–37.
27. Marceau P, et al. Long-term metabolic outcomes 5 to 20 years after biliopancreatic diversion. Obes Surg. 2015;25(9):1584–93.
28. Michaud A, et al. Biliopancreatic diversion with duodenal switch in the elderly: long-term results of a matched-control study. Obes Surg. 2016;26(2):350–60.
29. Lee W-J, et al. Predicting success of metabolic surgery: age, body mass index, C-peptide, and duration score. Surg Obes Relat Dis. 2013;9(3):379–84.
30. Still CD, et al. A probability score for preoperative prediction of type 2 diabetes remission following RYGB surgery. Lancet Diabetes Endocrinol. 2014;2(1):38.
31. Aminian A, et al. Individualized metabolic surgery score: procedure selection based on diabetes severity. Ann Surg. 2017;266(4):650–7.
32. Lee W-J, et al. Preoperative prediction of type 2 diabetes remission after gastric bypass surgery: a comparison of DiaRem scores and ABCD scores. Obes Surg. 2016;26(10):2418–24.
33. Sjöström L, et al. Association of bariatric surgery with long-term remission of type 2 diabetes and with microvascular and macrovascular complications. JAMA. 2014;311(22):2297–304.
34. Brethauer SA, et al. Can diabetes be surgically cured?: long-term metabolic effects of bariatric surgery in obese patients with type 2 diabetes mellitus. Ann Surg. 2013;258(4):628–37.
35. Arterburn DE, et al. A multisite study of long-term remission and relapse of type 2 diabetes mellitus following gastric bypass. Obes Surg. 2013;23(1):93–102.
36. Sjöström L, et al. Lifestyle, diabetes, and cardiovascular risk factors 10 years after bariatric surgery. N Engl J Med. 2004;351(26):2683–93.
37. Schauer PR, et al. Bariatric surgery versus intensive medical therapy for diabetes—5-year outcomes. N Engl J Med. 2017;376(7):641–51.
38. Nguyen KT, et al. Preserved insulin secretory capacity and weight loss are the predominant predictors of glycemic control in patients with type 2 diabetes randomized to Roux-en-Y gastric bypass. Diabetes. 2015;64(9):3104–10.
39. Aminian A, et al. Late relapse of diabetes after bariatric surgery: not rare, but not a failure. Diabetes Care. 2020;43(3):534–40.

40. Carlsson LMS, et al. Bariatric surgery and prevention of type 2 diabetes in Swedish obese subjects. N Engl J Med. 2012;367(8):695–704.
41. Salminen P, et al. Effect of laparoscopic sleeve gastrectomy vs laparoscopic Roux-en-Y gastric bypass on weight loss at 5 years among patients with morbid obesity: the SLEEVEPASS randomized clinical trial. JAMA. 2018;319(3):241–54.
42. Peterli R, et al. Effect of laparoscopic sleeve gastrectomy vs laparoscopic Roux-en-Y gastric bypass on weight loss in patients with morbid obesity: the SM-BOSS randomized clinical trial. JAMA. 2018;319(3):255–65.
43. Ruiz-Tovar J, et al. Long-term follow-up after sleeve gastrectomy versus Roux-en-Y gastric bypass versus one-anastomosis gastric bypass: a prospective randomized comparative study of weight loss and remission of comorbidities. Surg Endosc. 2019;33(2):401–10.

Should Patients with Obesity Hypoventilation Syndrome Undergo Bariatric Surgery

6

Maximiliano Tamae-Kakazu

6.1   Introduction

Obesity hypoventilation syndrome (OHS) is characterized by the presence of obesity, defined as body mass index (BMI) $\geq$ 30 kg/m^2, sleep-disordered breathing (SDB) and chronic daytime hypoventilation (PaCO2 > 45 mmHg) in the absence of other known causes of hypercapnia [1]. Most of the patients with OHS have severe obesity [1] and have severe obstructive sleep apnea (OSA) [2]. As the prevalence of obesity increases [3–5], the prevalence of OHS is likely to increase. Patients with OHS have a higher risk of cardiovascular morbidity [6] and death [7, 8]. If untreated, it can progress to significant adverse outcomes.

Although obesity is an important factor in the development of OHS, the main treatment strategy is treating SDB with positive airway pressure (PAP) therapy during sleep. Yet despite PAP treatment, multiple studies have shown that cardio-metabolic risk factors of severe obesity persist [9–11] and morbidity and mortality remain high in patients with OHS [12–14].

Weight loss can have an impact in SDB and the morbidity and mortality associated with obesity. However as we know lifestyle interventions can lead to temporary weight loss in patients with obesity without improving long-term cardiovascular outcomes because the weight loss is often regained [15, 16]. Bariatric surgery is the best current treatment for durable weight loss that can produce improvements in cardio-metabolic outcomes. Clinical trials of sleeve gastrectomy or gastric bypass surgery have reported significant improvements in metabolic, cardiovascular morbidities and reductions in all-cause and cardiovascular mortality [21–27]. However, most studies excluded patients with OHS or simply did not assess whether the

M. Tamae-Kakazu (✉)
Division of Pulmonary, Critical Care and Sleep Medicine, Spectrum Health – Michigan State University College of Human Medicine, Grand Rapids, MI, USA
e-mail: Maximiliano.TamaeKakazu@spectrumhealth.org

© Springer Nature Switzerland AG 2021   49
J. Alverdy, Y. Vigneswaran (eds.), *Difficult Decisions in Bariatric Surgery*,
Difficult Decisions in Surgery: An Evidence-Based Approach,
https://doi.org/10.1007/978-3-030-55329-6_6

enrolled patients had OHS, it is unclear whether bariatric surgery could provide the same benefit in patients with OHS compared to other interventions.

6.2 Search Strategy

The population, intervention, comparator, outcome (PICO) format was used to address the following question: "Should patients with obesity hypoventilation syndrome undergo bariatric surgery".

A literature search of English language publications from 1974 to March 2019 for Embase and from 1946 to March 2019 for Medline were used to identify polished data on bariatric surgery in patients with obesity hypoventilation syndrome. Terms used in the search were "exp obesity hypoventilation syndrome/", "obesity hypoventilation.mp", "Pickwick", "OHS", "hypox$.mp", "hypercapni$.mp","hypoventilat$.mp", "ex Respiratory failure.mp", "(obes$ or overweight).mp. or body mass index.tw. or bmi.ti.", "((sleep or apn?ea? or OSA or OSAHS) and (obese or obesity or overweight)).ti", "sleep apnea, obstructive/or Sleep Apnea Syndromes/", "OSAHS.ti,ab,kw,kf. or osa.ti.", "((sleep or obstructive) adj2 (apn?ea? or hypopn?ea?)).ti,ab,kw,kf.", "paco2.tw", "((serum or plasma) adj3 (bicarb$ or hco3$)).tw.". Due to the low numbers of high evidence studies, case series with more than 20 patients were included. We assessed the risk of bias in the included studies using the Cochrane risk of bias tool for randomized controlled trials and the Newcastle-Ottawa scale for comparative non-randomized studies and single arm studies.

6.3 Results

There were two randomized control studies including patients with OHS and four non-randomized studies without comparator (case series of at least 20 patients with OHS) selected for final analysis. These studies used current weight loss interventions or surgical approaches in bariatric surgery and had relevant data or outcomes of interest.

One randomized controlled trial in patients with OHS compared 17 patients allocated to an exercise and nutrition rehabilitation program in addition to noninvasive ventilation (NIV) with 20 patients allocated to standard weight loss counseling in addition to NIV. The primary outcome was weight change at 12 months. Secondary outcomes were anthropometric and body composition, gas exchange, exercise capacity with 6-min walk test, muscle mass and strength, health related quality of life, and NIV adherence. The mean difference from baseline of 140 kg was 11.8 kg lower in the weight loss program at 3 months (95% CI 22.1 lower to 0.63 higher). The rehabilitation program improved 6-min walk distance, and dyspnea based on MRC breathlessness scale at 3 months. The mean difference in the 6-min walk test was 29.3 m higher (95% CI 0.7 lower to 18 higher). These interventions did not show any significant difference in weight loss at 12 months (mean difference-9.4 kg 95% CI-23.5–4.6 kg) [27].

One randomized controlled trial compared 33 patients allocated to intensive nutritional care (INC) with 30 patients who underwent laparoscopic adjustable gastric banding (LAGB). OHS was present in 42% of the intensive nutritional care and 39% of the LAGB groups. The primary outcome was weaning from NIV at 1 and 3 years based on improvements in apnea-hypopnea index (AHI) or PaCO2. Secondary outcomes were weight loss, BMI, AHI, and excessive body weight loss. The baseline mean weight was 130 kg. After 1 year the mean weight was 115.5 kg in the LAGB group compared to 116.4 kg patients in the INC group, resulting in an excess weight loss of 15% for the INC and 33% for the LAGB. At 3 years the mean weight was 117.4 kg in the LAGB group and 121.1 kg in the INC group with an excess weight loss of 8% in the INC group and 27% in the LAGB group. At baseline the AHI between groups did not have any significant difference. After 1 year the INC group had a reduction of 9% in AHI, and the LAGB had a 44% reduction in AHI. However, there was no significant difference in AHI between INC and LAGB at 1 year. There was no significant difference in improvement of OHS (based on PaCO2). Few patients required gastric and repositioning due to dysphagia, change of reservoir location and gastric band replacement. No nutritional deficiency was observed. Five patients reported gastric band removal after RCT because of gastric band slippage, gastric ulcer, gastric cancer (7 years after surgery) [28].

There were five case series that reported a cohort of more than 20 patients with OHS undergoing bariatric surgery.

A prospective cohort between 2000 and 2007 included 102 patients with weight between 105 and 199 kg and BMI between 35 and 70.9 who underwent derivative biliodigestive surgery (biliopancreatic diversion with duodenal switch) for treatment of morbid obesity. The mean excess weight loss ranged between 45% and 64% at 3–5 years. This study reported improvement or resolution of OSA and OHS in 94 patients (92.2% of the cohort). There were 16 patients with OHS included in this study and all of them had resolution of OHS 5–7 years after bariatric surgery. This study did not characterize the weight loss in the OHS group. In the short term postoperative period 1.9% of the patients developed pulmonary embolism, 1.9% developed transient hypoxemia, and 3.9% developed phlebitis. The most common complications in the long term were iron deficiency, diarrhea, foul-smelling, potassium deficiency, fatigue and proctitis. Specific long term-post-operative complications in the first 2 years after surgery were abdominal abscess (1.9%), gastroduodenal reflux (3.9%), and incisional hernia (5.9%). In summary, no serious intra- or postoperative complications were observed, except for two cases of pulmonary embolism in two super-obese young women with no significant co-morbidities, despite physical and medical prophylaxis. There was no mention whether these patients' pulmonary embolism had OHS [29].

The other four publications were performed by the same author in the same institution. One of these observational studies included a cohort of 30 patients with OHS that underwent gastric bypass. Sleep apnea syndrome was present in 19 patients. The outcomes were AHI, pulmonary function, and blood gases. The patient had an average weight loss of 50 kg (95% CI 39–60) from baseline of 155 kg at 2 years. This study showed resolution of OHS in 25 patients (86.2%) at 2 years [30].

Two observational studies compared the PaO2 and PaCO2 in patients with OHS before gastric bypass and between 3 and 9 months after the procedure, resulting in a mean increase in PaO2 of 15 mmHg (95% CI 9–21) [30] and 19 mmHg higher (11–27) [31] with a mean reduction in PaCO2 of 10 mmHg (95% CI 7–13) [30] and 10 mmHg (6–14) [31] respectively. One study reported the death of 1 patient died of peritonitis from gastric leak resulting in a mortality of 3% [30] and adverse events in one-fifth of the patients. The other study reported one death out 26 patients from occluded tracheostomy (inserted for severe OHS) [31].

On observational study included 26 patients with OHS, 17 of them with sleep apnea syndrome. Hemodynamic evaluation with pulmonary catheter was performed in 18 of the patients before and after gastric bypass surgery and there was a significant decrease in their pulmonary artery pressure from 36 mmHg to 23 mmHg, and reduction in wedge pressure from 17 mmHg to 12 mmHg [31].

One observational study reported 61 patients with OHS that underwent gastric bypass. The mean weight at baseline was 163 kg with an excess weight loss of 45 ± 34% after the procedure. The arterial blood gas at baseline showed a mean PaO2 of 53 ± 10 mmHg and a mean PaCO2 of 53 ± 9 mmHg. One year after the procedure, the blood gas was revaluated in 31 patients showing a mean PaO2 of 73 ± 15 mmHg and a mean PaCO2 of 44 ± 8 mmHg [32]. The mortality rate in patients with OHS was 4% compared with 0.7% for the entire series of patients undergoing gastric bypass.

An observational cohort of 64 patients with morbid obesity and venous stasis disease included 19 patients with OHS. The mean weight at baseline for the entire cohort was 179 ± 39 kg and 3.9 ± 4 year after gastric bypass surgery there was a mean weight reduction of 62 ± 33 kg. The patients with OHS had resolution of this comorbidity after bariatric surgery. This report was part of a larger cohort of 1976 patients with morbid obesity whom underwent gastric bypass and adverse events were reported from the total group with distinction based on the presence of venous stasis, but not OHS. Fatal pulmonary embolism occurred in 0.2–4%, incisional hernia in 26–38%, leak/peritonitis/death 0.5–3%, surgical death 0.8–8%, major wound infection in 4–8%, minor wound infection in 9–10%, stable line disruption in 1.5–3%, marginal ulcer in 16–13%, stomal stenosis in 16–12%, small bowel obstruction in 4–5% depending the presence of venous stasis disease or not respectively [33].

One observation study included a cohort of 16 patients with OHS whom underwent biliopancreatic diversion with duodenal switch. All the 16 patients resolved their OHS 5–7 years after bariatric surgery [29]. This study reported no significant complications in the short term post-operative period except for pulmonary embolism in 1.9% of the cases and transient hypoxemia in 1.9% of the cases.

Study	Intervention	Weight baseline	Weight at time of follow up	Outcome	At baseline	At follow up	Time of follow up	Study type (quality of evidence)
Mandal (2018) [27]	Standard of care	141.2 ± 30.7 kg	−3 ± 6.2 kg	6MWT	165 (100–288) m	20 (0–90) m	3 months	Randomized controlled study (very low)
	Standard of care plus rehabilitation	139.3 ± 28.8 kg	−9.6 ± 6.7 kg	6MWT	200 (100–320) m	60 (20–190) m		
Feigel-Guiller (2015) [28]	Intensive nutritional care	123 ± 25.1 kg	116.4 ± 28.2 kg	AHI	47.9 ± 25.3	43.4 ± 25	1 year	Randomized controlled study (very low)
	Laparoscopic adjustable gastric banding	135 ± 25.3 kg	115.5 ± 21.8 kg	AHI	56.2 ± 25.7	31.5 ± 22.2		
Sugerman (1986) [30]	Gastric surgery	155 ± 44 kg	−50 ± 29 kg	$PaCO_2$	51 ± 7 mmHg	41 ± 4 mmHg	3 to 5 months	Retrospective cohort (very low)
				AHI	44 ± 15	8 ± 11		
Sugerman (1988) [31]	Gastric surgery	224 ± 59%IBW	167 ± 57%IBW	PaO_2	50 ± 10 mmHg	69 ± 14 mmHg	3 to 9 months	Retrospective cohort (very low)
				$PaCO_2$	52 ± 7 mmHg	42 ± 4 mmHg		
				PAP	36 ± 14 mmHg	23 ± 7 mmHg		
				PAOP	17 ± 7 mmHg	12 ± 6 mmHg		
Sugerman (1992) [32]	Gastric surgery	163 ± 39 kg	113 ± 30 kg	PaO_2	53 ± 10 mmHg	73 ± 15 mmHg	1 year	Retrospective cohort (very low)
				$PacCO_2$	53 ± 9 mmHg	44 ± 8 mmHg		
Sugerman (2001) [33]	Gastric surgery	179 ± 39 kg	−62 ± 33 kg	Patients with OHS	19	100% resolution	3.9 ± 4 year	Retrospective cohort (very low)
DeCesare (2014) [29]	Derivative biliodigestive surgery	105 to 199 kg	−35 to −60.8 kg	OHS	16	100% resolution	2 years	Retrospective cohort (very low)

6.4   Conclusions

In this systematic review of weight loss interventions in patients with OHS two randomized controlled studies and five observational studies were included. The weight loss interventions reported in these studies were bariatric surgery, intensive nutritional care and a hybrid inpatient-outpatient motivation, exercise and nutrition rehabilitation program.

The effect of the weight loss interventions in OHS is likely related with the degree or efficiency of weight loss. The studies that reported patients undergoing gastric bypass had an excess weight loss of at least 40–55% resulting in improvement or resolution in OHS, oxygenation, hypercapnia, and apnea index [30–33].

One study reported patients who underwent bilio-intestinal diversion with an excess weight loss of 45–64% with resolution of OHS that was present in 15% of the patients [29].

The study comparing intensive nutritional care and LAGB resulted in excess weight loss of 15% and 33% respectively at 1 year, with improvement in AHI compared to baseline. However, this excessive weight loss was not significant to produce resolution of OSA or OHS and wean from NIV therapy. However, one of the studies by Sugerman [32] showed a normalization of $PaCO2$ with a weight loss of 30%.

This percentage of weight loss is more likely to be achieved with weight loss surgery, suggesting a role of bariatric surgery in patients with OHS.

The data reported on adverse events is limited and most of these studies included cohort with the procedure performed 30 years ago. The morbidity and mortality outcomes with bariatric surgery have improved since then. Identification of patients with OHS that will benefit from bariatric surgery with a reasonable risk or to determine if there is any additional risk in patients with OHS undergoing bariatric surgery require further studies.

The strength of this systematic review is that we looked at studies that included patients with OHS. The limitations of the study are that some of the studies did not include exclusively OHS patients, many of the cohorts had the surgical procedure decades ago, and the quality of the evidence is very low. We excluded studies that we were not able to separate patients with COPD or other cause of hypercapnia to minimize confounders, but still the quality of the data is very low. The most recent cohort with bariatric surgery included the study reporting biliopancreatic diversion with duodenal switch [29] that was performed between 2000 and 2007.

Based on the lack of good evidence and the limited literature available, bariatric surgery should be offered when estimated benefit outweighs the risk.

6.5   A Personal View to the Data

Bariatric surgery is more likely to achieve an effective and sustained weight loss in the long term to produce improvement or resolution of OHS, improvement in gas exchange and potential cardiovascular benefits. Bariatric surgery has become a safe surgical procedure in patients with morbid obesity. However, the evidence of safety in OHS are limited. Further studies are needed to determine the safety of bariatric surgery in OHS.

6.6 Recommendations

Bariatric surgery should be offered in individual cases after evaluation of benefits and risks.

Special consideration for bariatric surgery should be made when considering a weight loss of 30% or more.

References

1. Mokhlesi B, Kryger MH, Grunstein RR. Assessment and management of patients with obesity hypoventilation syndrome. Proc Am Thorac Soc. 2008;5:218–25.
2. Masa JF, Corral J, Alonso ML, Ordax E, Troncoso MF, Gonzalez M, et al. Spanish sleep network. Efficacy of different treatment alternatives for obesity hypoventilation syndrome: Pickwick study. Am J Respir Crit Care Med. 2015;192:86–95.
3. Hales CM, Fryar CD, Carroll MD, Freedman DS, Ogden CL. Trends in obesity and severe obesity prevalence in US youth and adults by sex and age, 2007-2008 to 2015-2016. JAMA. 2018;19(16):1723–5.
4. Flegal KM, Kruszon-Moran D, Carroll MD, Fryar CD, Ogden CL. Trends in obesity among adults in the United States, 2005 to 2014. JAMA. 2016;315(21):2284–91.
5. Ng M, Fleming T, Robinson M, et al. Global, regional, and national prevalence of overweight and obesity in children and adults during 1980–2013: a systematic analysis for the global burden of disease study 2013. Lancet. 2014;384:766–81.
6. Borel JC, Burel B, Tamisier R, Dias-Domingos S, Baguet JP, Levy P, Pepin JL. Comorbidities and mortality in hypercapnic obese under domiciliary noninvasive ventilation. PLoS One. 2013;8:e52006.
7. Nowbar S, Burkart KM, Gonzales R, Fedorowicz A, Gozansky WS, Gaudio JC, Taylor MR, Zwillich CW. Obesity-associated hypoventilation in hospitalized patients: prevalence, effects, and outcome. Am J Med. 2004;116:1–7.
8. Ojeda Castillejo E, de Lucas RP, Lopez Martin S, Resano Barrios P, Rodríguez P, Morán Caicedo L, et al. Noninvasive mechanical ventilation in patients with obesity hypoventilation syndrome: long-term outcome and prognostic factors. Arch Bronconeumol. 2015;51:61–8.
9. Masa JF, Corral J, Alonso ML, Ordax E, Troncoso MF, Gonzalez M, Lopez-Martínez S, Marin JM, Marti S, Díaz-Cambriles T, Chiner E, Aizpuru F, Egea C. Efficacy of different treatment for obesity hypoventilation syndrome. Pickwick study. Am J Respir Crit Care Med. 2015;192:86–95.
10. Borel JC, Tamisier R, Gonzalez-Bermejo J, Baguet JP, Monneret D, Arnol N, Roux-Lombard P, Wuyam B, Levy P, Pépin JL. Noninvasive ventilation in mild obesity hypoventilation syndrome: a randomized controlled trial. Chest. 2012;141:692–702.
11. Howard ME, Piper AJ, Stevens B, Holland AE, Yee BJ, Dabscheck E, Mortimer D, Burge AT, Flunt D, Buchan C, Rautela L, Sheers N, Hillman D, Berlowitz DJ. A randomised controlled trial of CPAP versus non-invasive ventilation for initial treatment of obesity hypoventilation syndrome. Thorax. 2017;72:437–44.
12. Castro-Añón O, Pérez de Llano LA, De la Fuente Sánchez S, Golpe R, Méndez Marote L, Castro-Castro J, González Quintela A. Obesity-hypoventilation syndrome: increased risk of death over sleep apnea syndrome. PLoS One. 2015;10(2):e0117808.

13. Masa JF, Mokhlesi B, Benítez I, Gomez de Terreros FJ, Sánchez-Quiroga MÁ, Romero A, Caballero-Eraso C, Terán-Santos J, Alonso-Álvarez ML, Troncoso MF, González M, López-Martín S, Marin JM, Martí S, Díaz-Cambriles T, Chiner E, Egea C, Barca J, Vázquez-Polo FJ, Negrín MA, Martel-Escobar M, Barbe F, Corral J. Long-term clinical effectiveness of continuous positive airway pressure therapy versus non-invasive ventilation therapy in patients with obesity hypoventilation syndrome: a multicentre, open-label, randomized controlled trial. Lancet. 2019;27(393):1721–32.
14. Bouloukaki I, Mermigkis C, Michelakis S, Moniaki V, Mauroudi E, Tzanakis N, Schiza SE. The association between adherence to positive airway pressure therapy and long-term outcomes in patients with obesity hypoventilation syndrome: a prospective observational study. J Clin Sleep Med. 2018;14:1539–50.
15. Look AHEAD Research Group. Cardiovascular effects of intensive lifestyle intervention in type 2 diabetes. N Engl J Med. 2013;369:145–54.
16. Diabetes Prevention Program Outcomes Study Research Group. Long-term effects of the diabetes prevention program interventions on cardiovascular risk factors: a report from the DPP Oucomes study. Diabet Med. 2013;30:46–55.
17. Fisher BL, Schauer P. Medical and surgical options in the treatment of severe obesity. Am J Surg. 2002;184(6B):9S–16S.
18. Ponce J, DeMaria EJ, Nguyen NT, Hutter M, Sudan R, Morton JM. American Society for Metabolic and Bariatric Surgery estimation of bariatric surgery procedures in 2015 and surgeon workforce in the United States. Surg Obes Relat Dis. 2016;12:1637–9.
19. Esteban Varela J, Nguyen NT. Laparoscopic sleeve gastrectomy leads the U.S. utilization of bariatric surgery at academic medical centers. Surg Obes Relat Dis. 2015;11:987–90.
20. Chang SH, Stoll CR, Song J, Varela JE, Eagon CJ, Colditz GA. The effectiveness and risks of bariatric surgery. JAMA Surg. 2014;149:275–87.
21. Carlsson LM, Peltonen M, Ahlin S, Anveden Å, Bouchard C, Carlsson B, Jacobson P, Lönroth H, Maglio C, Näslund I, Pirazzi C, Romeo S, Sjöholm K, Sjöström E, Wedel H, Svensson PA, Sjöström L. Bariatric surgery and prevention of type 2 diabetes in Swedish obese subjects. N Engl J Med. 2012;367:695–704.
22. Sjostrom L, Peltonen M, Jacobson P, Ahlin S, Andersson-Assarsson J, Anveden Å, Bouchard C, Carlsson B, Karason K, Lönroth H, Näslund I, Sjöström E, Taube M, Wedel H, Svensson PA, Sjöholm K, Carlsson LM. Association of bariatric surgery with long-term remission of type 2 diabetes and with microvascular and macrovascular complications. JAMA. 2014;311:2297–304.
23. Schauer PR, Schauer PR, Bhatt DL, Kirwan JP, Wolski K, Aminian A, Brethauer SA, Navaneethan SD, Singh RP, Pothier CE, Nissen SE, Kashyap SR. Bariatric surgery versus intensive medical therapy for diabetes—5-year outcomes. N Engl J Med. 2017;376:641–51.
24. Sjostrom L, Lindroos AK, Peltonen M, Torgerson J, Bouchard C, Carlsson B, Dahlgren S, Larsson B, Narbro K, Sjöström CD, Sullivan M, Wedel H. Lifestyle, diabetes, and cardiovascular risk factors 10 years after bariatric surgery. N Engl J Med. 2004;351:2683–93.
25. Sjostrom L, , Narbro K, Sjöström CD, Karason K, Larsson B, Wedel H, Lystig T, Sullivan M, Bouchard C, Carlsson B, Bengtsson C, Dahlgren S, Gummesson A, Jacobson P, Karlsson J, Lindroos AK, Lönroth H, Näslund I, Olbers T, Stenlöf K, Torgerson J, Agren G, Carlsson LM. Effects of bariatric surgery on mortality in Swedish obese subjects. N Engl J Med 2007;357:741–752.
26. Sjostrom L, Peltonen M, Jacobson P, Sjöström CD, Karason K, Wedel H, Ahlin S, Anveden Å, Bengtsson C, Bergmark G, Bouchard C, Carlsson B, Dahlgren S, Karlsson J, Lindroos AK, Lönroth H, Narbro K, Näslund I, Olbers T, Svensson PA, Carlsson LM. Bariatric surgery and long-term cardiovascular events. JAMA. 2012;307:56–65.
27. Mandal S, Suh ES, Harding R, Vaughan-France A, Ramsay M, Connolly B, Bear DE, MacLaughlin H, Greenwood SA, Polkey MI, Elliott M, Chen T, Douiri A, Moxham J, Murphy PB, Hart N. Nutrition and exercise rehabilitation in obesity hypoventilation syndrome (NERO): a pilot randomised controlled trial. Thorax. 2018;73(1):62–9.

28. Feigel-Guiller B, Drui D, Dimet J, Zair Y, Le Bras M, Fuertes-Zamorano N, Cariou B, Letessier EE, Nobecourt-Dupuy E, Krempf M. Laparoscopic gastric banding in obese patients with sleep apnea: a 3-year controlled study and follow-up after 10 years. Obes Surg. 2015;25(10):1886–92.
29. De Cesare A, Cangemi B, Fiori E, Bononi M, Cangemi R, Basso L. Early and long-term clinical outcomes of bilio-intestinal diversion in morbidly obese patients. Surg Today. 2014;44(8):1424–33.
30. Sugerman HJ, Fairman RP, Baron PL, Wentus JA. Gastric surgery for respiratory insufficiency of obesity. Chest. 1986;90(1):81–6.
31. Sugerman HJ, Baron PL, Fairman RP, Evans CR, Vetrovec GW. Hemodynamic dysfunction in obesity hypoventilation syndrome and the effects of treatment with surgically induced weight loss. Ann Surg. 1988;207(5):604–13.
32. Sugerman HJ, Fairman RP, Sood RK, Engle K, Wolfe L, Kellum JM. Long-term effects of gastric surgery for treating respiratory insufficiency of obesity. Am J Clin Nutr. 1992;55(2 Suppl):597S–601S.
33. Sugerman HJ, Sugerman EL, Wolfe L, Kellum JM Jr, Schweitzer MA, DeMaria EJ. Risks and benefits of gastric bypass in morbidly obese patients with severe venous stasis disease. Ann Surg. 2001;234(1):41–6.

Bariatric Surgery in Heart Failure

7

Mark Belkin and John Blair

7.1 Introduction

Over 6.2 million adults are diagnosed with heart failure (HF), per the most recent National Health and Nutrition Examination Survey (NHANES) report. The prevalence of this disease is estimated to eclipse 8 million adults by the year 2030. Similarly, obesity rates continue to rise, with 39.6% of United States (US) adults diagnosed with obesity (body mass index (BMI) $\geq$ 30 kg/m^2) per the 2015–2016 NHANES data, an increase from 37.7% in 2013–2014. Rates of morbid obesity (BMI $\geq$ 40 kg/m^2) remained stable, though significantly elevated, at 7.7% according to these two reports [1].

Obesity is associated with an increased risk of cardiovascular disease, including HF, coronary artery disease (CAD), and stroke [1]. However, obesity has the strongest association with HF, specifically. Obesity is associated with an almost four-fold (HR 3.73) increase in development of HF in patients with BMI $\geq$ 35 kg/m^2, compared to a two-fold increase in risk of CAD and stroke [2]. Earlier studies noted an "obesity paradox," in which more patients with obesity had a lower all-cause mortality [3–5]. However, further research has shown that this is likely due to lead-time bias: patients with obesity develop cardiovascular disease earlier in life than patients without obesity, and therefore appear to have reduced mortality as they live longer from the time of disease diagnosis [6]. Importantly, this "obesity paradox" does not apply to cardiovascular morbidity, including HF. In fact, BMI is directly related to the risk of incident HF, with increasing risk associated with rising BMI in middle aged men and women: HR 1.23–1.37 for overweight individuals (BMI 25–29.9 kg/m^2), HR 1.95–2.28 for patients with oesity (BMI 30–39.9 kg/m^2), and HR 4.32–5.26 for patients with morbid obesity (BMI $\geq$ 40 kg/m^2) [6]. While obesity confers a

M. Belkin · J. Blair (✉)
Department of Medicine, Section of Cardiology, University of Chicago, Chicago, IL, USA
e-mail: jblair2@medicine.bsd.uchicago.edu

© Springer Nature Switzerland AG 2021
J. Alverdy, Y. Vigneswaran (eds.), *Difficult Decisions in Bariatric Surgery*,
Difficult Decisions in Surgery: An Evidence-Based Approach,
https://doi.org/10.1007/978-3-030-55329-6_7

higher risk of development of both HF with preserved ejection fraction (HFpEF) as well as HF with reduced ejection fraction (HFrEF), there is a higher risk of HFpEF than HFrEF development for each standard deviation increase in BMI. Interestingly, while obesity in men carry an increased risk of both phenotypes of HF, obesity in women only have an increased risk of development of HFpEF, and not HFrEF [7].

Bariatric surgery has become an accepted therapy for morbidly obesity (BMI $\geq$ 40 kg/m^2) without concomitant disease, as well as obesity (BMI $\geq$ 35 kg/m^2) with significant co-morbidities, including cardiovascular risk factors, though not HF specifically [8]. In this chapter, we discuss the effect of bariatric surgery on the incidence of new-onset HF in morbidly obesity, as well as its role in the treatment of known HF. Finally, we will address the unique surgical challenges associated with bariatric surgery in patients with known HF.

7.2 Search Strategy

We aim to assess and review the published data regarding the effect of bariatric surgery on HF outcomes in morbidly obesity, when compared to optimal medical therapy (see Table 7.1). We included the following terms in our search of the PubMed database: "Heart Failure" AND "Bariatric Surgery" OR "Gastric Banding" OR "Gastric Bypass" OR "Gastroduodenal Bypass" OR "Laparoscopic Gastric Bypass" OR "Laparoscopic Gastroduodenal Bypass" OR "Laparoscopic Roux-en-Y Gastric Bypass" OR "Roux-en-Y Gastric Bypass" OR "Sleeve Gastrectomy" OR "surgical weight loss." Search limits included English language, clinical trials, controlled clinical trials, meta-analyses, observational studies, randomized controlled trials, and systemic reviews. The database was searched from inception through December 3, 2019.

7.2.1 Bariatric Surgery Improves Cardiac Function

While there are no trials evaluating bariatric surgery with heart failure incidence as the primary outcome, studies assessing serum biomarkers, invasive hemodynamics, and cardiac function have been completed in this population. First, bariatric surgery is associated with a decrease in Cardiac Troponin-I, an indicator of subclinical myocardial injury, and an increase in N-terminal pro-brain natriuretic peptide, when

Table 7.1 PICO

P (Patients)	I (Intervention)	C (Comparator)	O (Outcomes)
Patients with morbid obesity	Bariatric surgery	Optimal medical therapy	Incidence of new onset heart failure, heart failure hospitalization, cardiovascular mortality, surgical complications

compared to non-surgical weight management [9, 10]. Second, bariatric surgery has been shown to improve the cardiac hemodynamics of obese patients. In a systematic review and meta-analysis of studies evaluating invasive hemodynamics before and after weight loss intervention, three of nine included studies used bariatric surgery as the form of weight loss. The median weight loss of 43 kg in the analysis was associated with significant reduction in heart rate and blood pressure, as well as a significant decrease in invasively measured right atrial pressure, mean pulmonary artery pressure, and pulmonary capillary wedge pressure at both rest and exercise [11].

Additionally, bariatric surgery has been associated with improvements in cardiac structure and function. Two recent systematic reviews and meta-analyses evaluated multiple echocardiographic indicators of cardiac structure and function. These studies showed that weight loss following bariatric surgery led to significant reductions in left ventricular mass index, left ventricular end-diastolic volume, and left atrial size. Furthermore, they noted a significant improvement in left ventricular ejection fraction (LVEF) and echocardiographic indices of diastolic function [12, 13].

7.2.2   Bariatric Surgery Decreases Incidence of Heart Failure

Bariatric surgery has been associated with a decreased incidence of HF. A recent Swedish registry-based study analyzed over 47,000 adult, obese patients to assess the effect of bariatric surgery on incidence of HF. Approximately half of the population underwent bariatric surgery, including gastric banding, vertical banded gastroplasty, and gastroduodenal bypass. There was a five-fold increase in the risk of HF incidence in the non-surgical group when compared to the surgical group, 6.9/1000 person-years compared to 1.0/1000 person-years, respectively. Bariatric surgery conferred a 63% reduction in risk of HF after adjustment for HF risk factors (HR 0.37, 95% CI 0.30–0.46). This reduced risk was significant across age, sex, and co-morbidities, including diabetes, hypertension, and CAD [14]. A separate Swedish registry noted a similar significant risk reduction in incident heart failure following gastric bypass surgery (HR 0.54, 95% CI 0.35–0.82), over a median 4.1 years of follow-up. This risk reduction was in the setting of an additional 22.6 kg weight loss after 2-year follow-up in the surgical cohort compared to the lifestyle modification cohort [15].

7.2.3   Bariatric Surgery Reduces Morbidity and Improves Cardiac Function in Heart Failure Patients

There are no randomized control trials evaluating bariatric surgery versus placebo in patients with HF. However, there are multiple, small observational studies indicating bariatric surgery is associated with an improvement in HF symptoms and functional status, as well as a decrease in HF hospitalization [16–20].

HF symptoms and functional status have been shown to improve with bariatric surgery in HF patients. In a small retrospective review of 12 morbidly obese patients with HFrEF undergoing bariatric surgery, New York Heart Association (NYHA) functional class improved significantly in the surgical group, 2.9 ± 0.7 to 2.3 ± 0.5 ($p = 0.02$), and worsened significantly in the control group, 2.4 ± 0.7 to 3.3 ± 0.9 ($p = 0.02$) [16]. Similar improvement in NYHA functional class was noted among 14 patients with morbid obesity that underwent bariatric surgery, including laparoscopic and open Roux-en-Y gastric bypass, sleeve gastrectomy, and laparoscopic gastric banding. At baseline, 43%, 43%, and 14% of patients had NYHA class II, III, and IV functional status, respectively. Post-operatively, this improved to 86%, 14%, and 0%, respectively [18]. In another small retrospective study, 13 patients with HFrEF underwent bariatric surgery and six received non-operative weight management, after which surgery was associated with improved symptoms. Over 4.3 ± 2.7 years of follow-up, the surgical patients had improved dyspnea on exertion and lower extremity edema when compared to the non-surgical controls [17].

These data also indicate an improvement in LVEF in HF patients following bariatric surgery. In the retrospective study by Ramani et al., baseline LVEF increased significantly in the surgical group, from $21.7 \pm 6.5\%$ to $35 \pm 14.8\%$ ($p = 0.005$), but not in the ten matched control non-surgical patients, LVEF $23.5 \pm 6.7\%$ to $28.5 \pm 14.0\%$ ($p = 0.25$) [16]. McCloskey et al. reported similar improvement in LVEF, from $23 \pm 2\%$ to $32 \pm 4\%$ in HF patients with morbid obesity following bariatric surgery [18]. Finally, this improvement in LVEF was also seen in a larger retrospective study of 42 patients with obesity and LVEF <50% in which bariatric surgery was associated with a significant increase in LVEF ($5.1 \pm 8.3\%$, $p = 0.0005$). Comparatively, a matched cohort of HF patients with obesity that did not undergo bariatric surgery had a non-significant improvement in LVEF ($3.4 \pm 10.5\%$, $p = 0.056$) [19].

HF hospitalizations are one of the major sources of morbidity for HF patients [1]. Importantly, bariatric surgery has been associated with reduced HF hospitalizations in this population. In the study by McCloskey et al., five of the 14 patients were hospitalized for a HF exacerbation in the 6 months prior to surgery, while none were hospitalized in the 6 months following surgery [18]. Furthermore, in their retrospective case series, Ramani et al. showed a significant reduction in HF hospitalizations in the first year following bariatric surgery when compared to the control group (0.4 ± 0.8 vs 2.4 ± 2.6, $p = 0.04$) [16]. Finally, a large, retrospective case series of 524 HF patients that underwent bariatric surgery indicated a non-significant reduction in emergency department visits for HF exacerbations in the first 12 months following surgery when compared to the 12 months prior to surgery (15.3% to 12%, $p = 0.052$). However, there was a significant reduction during the following year (post-operative months 13–24), with a reduction from 15.3% to 9.9%, adjusted OR 0.57, $p = 0.003$) [21]. While there are no prospective studies evaluating the effects of bariatric surgery on HF, the published data indicate positive effects on cardiac function, patient symptoms, and heart failure hospitalizations.

7.2.4   Heart Failure Patients Are Not at Increased Risk for Major Bariatric Surgical Complications

Non-cardiac surgery in HF patients is associated with an increased risk of re-hospitalization and mortality [22]. However, the limited published data regarding bariatric surgery in this specific population suggests its relative safety. In a cohort of 14 patients with average BMI 50.8 ± 2.04 kg/m^2 and LVEF $23 \pm 2\%$, bariatric surgery, including laparoscopic and open Roux-en-Y gastric bypass, sleeve gastrectomy, and laparoscopic gastric banding, surgical complications included one patient with pulmonary edema, one patient with hypotension, and two patients with acute renal injury. There were no incidences of peri-operative myocardial infarction or mortality [18]. Similar data were noted in a retrospective evaluation for 32 patients with diagnosed HF prior to Roux-en-Y gastric bypass surgery. Again, there were no incidences of peri-operative myocardial infarction or mortality. However, one patient was re-admitted on post-operative day (POD) #3 for gastrointestinal bleeding in the setting of a supratherapeutic INR related to warfarin used. The patient died of an anoxic brain injury on POD #6 [23]. A larger retrospective study of 2630 obese patients, of which 42 had an LVEF <50%, indicated significantly more post-operative HF exacerbations and post-operative myocardial infarctions, although numerically these were small numbers; there were only four HF exacerbations and one post-operative myocardial infarction among the 42 patients with reduced EF. Notably, there were no differences between the groups in intensive care unit stay, hospital stay, 30-day mortality, or 12-month mortality [19]. In fact, reported average length of stay post-operatively was 3 days, consistent with the literature in obese patients without HF [18, 23–25].

It is important to note that these are limited data, and many of these patients were aggressively optimized for surgery. For instance, in the case series by Ramani et al., seven of the 12 patients were admitted prior to surgery for invasive hemodynamic assessment and optimization. Additionally, all 12 patients spent the first post-operative day in the cardiac intensive care unit for monitoring [16]. There are limited data reported on peri-operative management of HF patients for bariatric surgery specifically, however it is important to follow established guidelines for pre-operative and peri-operative management of patients with HF undergoing non-cardiac surgery [22].

7.3   Recommendations Based on Data

The published data suggest that cardiac function and the incidence of HF are reduced in morbidly obese patients following bariatric surgery. There are a lack of prospective, randomized trials, and therefore, these data should be categorized as moderate quality, with a low risk of bias due to the large number of patients included without significant heterogeneity in results. Additionally, the published data indicate that bariatric surgery is associated with improved morbidity and cardiac

Table 7.2 Evidence and recommendations

Supposed advantage of bariatric surgery	Grade of evidence	Recommendation	Strength of recommendation
Reduction in risk of incident HF	Moderate quality	Bariatric surgery likely reduces the risk of incidence of HF in the morbidly obese patients without a prior diagnosis of HF	Strong
Improvement in cardiac function for patients with HF	Weak quality	Bariatric surgery may improve cardiac function in morbidly obese patients regardless of prior HF diagnosis	Weak
Improvement in functional status for patients with HF	Weak quality	Bariatric surgery may improve functional status in morbidly obese patients with prior history of HF	Weak
Reduction in HF hospitalization	Weak quality	Bariatric surgery may reduce frequency of HF hospitalizations in patients with prior history of HF	Weak
Reduction in cardiovascular mortality for HF or non-HF patients	NA	There are no reliable published data addressing cardiovascular mortality in morbidly obese patients following bariatric surgery	NA
Bariatric surgery is safe in HF patients	Weak quality	Limited data suggest bariatric surgery is safe in HF patients when pre-operative and peri-operative care is provided per the ACC/AHA guidelines for non-cardiac surgery [22].	Weak

function in patients with morbidly obesity and HF. However, these small, observational studies should be categorized as low quality with a high risk of bias due to the limited numbers of patients included. However, the consistency across these studies indicate higher likelihood of a true association between bariatric surgery and these positive outcomes (Table 7.2).

7.4 Personal View of the Data

HF is an increasingly common worldwide disease, as is obesity. These two diseases are intertwined, as the risk of HF development is increased in patients with obesity, while obesity also worsens morbidity amongst HF patients. The significant weight loss associated with bariatric surgery, when compared to usual care, has shown positive effects in the cardiovascular health of patients both with and without HF. These positive effects are apparent from improvements in baseline cardiac function and hemodynamics, to clinical outcomes such as functional status and HF hospitalization. While to date there are limited data on this specific population undergoing bariatric surgery, in aggregate, bariatric surgery appears to improve HF-related outcomes for patients with morbidly obesity and without known HF, as well as improve cardiovascular outcomes for patients with morbidly obesity and HF. We anticipate that further studies in this field will reinforce the signal for positive outcomes.

References

1. Benjamin EJ, Muntner P, Alonso A, Bittencourt MS, Callaway CW, Carson AP, et al. Heart disease and stroke Statistics-2019 update: a report from the American Heart Association. Circulation. 2019;139(10):e56–e528. https://doi.org/10.1161/CIR.0000000000000659.
2. Ndumele CE, Matsushita K, Lazo M, Bello N, Blumenthal RS, Gerstenblith G, et al. Obesity and subtypes of incident cardiovascular disease. J Am Heart Assoc. 2016;5(8):e003921. https://doi.org/10.1161/JAHA.116.003921.
3. Horwich TB, Fonarow GC, Hamilton MA, MacLellan WR, Woo MA, Tillisch JH. The relationship between obesity and mortality in patients with heart failure. J Am Coll Cardiol. 2001;38(3):789–95. https://doi.org/10.1016/s0735-1097(01)01448-6.
4. Lavie CJ, Osman AF, Milani RV, Mehra MR. Body composition and prognosis in chronic systolic heart failure: the obesity paradox. Am J Cardiol. 2003;91(7):891–4. https://doi.org/10.1016/s0002-9149(03)00031-6.
5. Clark AL, Chyu J, Horwich TB. The obesity paradox in men versus women with systolic heart failure. Am J Cardiol. 2012;110(1):77–82. https://doi.org/10.1016/j.amjcard.2012.02.050.
6. Khan SS, Ning H, Wilkins JT, Allen N, Carnethon M, Berry JD, et al. Association of body mass index with lifetime risk of cardiovascular disease and compression of morbidity. JAMA Cardiol. 2018;3(4):280–7. https://doi.org/10.1001/jamacardio.2018.0022.
7. Savji N, Meijers WC, Bartz TM, Bhambhani V, Cushman M, Nayor M, et al. The association of obesity and cardiometabolic traits with incident HFpEF and HFrEF. JACC Heart Fail. 2018;6(8):701–9. https://doi.org/10.1016/j.jchf.2018.05.018.
8. Mechanick JI, Youdim A, Jones DB, Garvey WT, Hurley DL, McMahon MM, et al. Clinical practice guidelines for the perioperative nutritional, metabolic, and nonsurgical support of the bariatric surgery patient—2013 update: cosponsored by American Association of Clinical Endocrinologists, the Obesity Society, and American Society for Metabolic & Bariatric Surgery. Obesity (Silver Spring). 2013;21(Suppl 1):S1–27. https://doi.org/10.1002/oby.20461.
9. Lyngbakken MN, Omland T, Nordstrand N, Norseth J, Hjelmesaeth J, Hofso D. Effect of weight loss on subclinical myocardial injury: a clinical trial comparing gastric bypass surgery and intensive lifestyle intervention. Eur J Prev Cardiol. 2016;23(8):874–80. https://doi.org/10.1177/2047487315618796.
10. Gabrielsen AM, Omland T, Brokner M, Fredheim JM, Jordan J, Lehmann S, et al. The effect of surgical and non-surgical weight loss on N-terminal pro-B-type natriuretic peptide and its relation to obstructive sleep apnea and pulmonary function. BMC Res Notes. 2016;9(1):440. https://doi.org/10.1186/s13104-016-2241-x.
11. Reddy YNV, Anantha-Narayanan M, Obokata M, Koepp KE, Erwin P, Carter RE, et al. Hemodynamic effects of weight loss in obesity: a systematic review and meta-analysis. JACC Heart Fail. 2019;7(8):678–87. https://doi.org/10.1016/j.jchf.2019.04.019.
12. Mahajan R, Stokes M, Elliott A, Munawar DA, Khokhar KB, Thiyagarajah A, et al. Complex interaction of obesity, intentional weight loss and heart failure: a systematic review and meta-analysis. Heart. 2019; https://doi.org/10.1136/heartjnl-2019-314770.
13. Aggarwal R, Harling L, Efthimiou E, Darzi A, Athanasiou T, Ashrafian H. The effects of bariatric surgery on cardiac structure and function: a systematic review of cardiac imaging outcomes. Obes Surg. 2016;26(5):1030–40. https://doi.org/10.1007/s11695-015-1866-5.
14. Persson CE, Bjorck L, Lagergren J, Lappas G, Giang KW, Rosengren A. Risk of heart failure in obese patients with and without bariatric surgery in Sweden—a registry-based study. J Card Fail. 2017;23(7):530–7. https://doi.org/10.1016/j.cardfail.2017.05.005.
15. Sundstrom J, Bruze G, Ottosson J, Marcus C, Naslund I, Neovius M. Weight loss and heart failure: a nationwide study of gastric bypass surgery versus intensive lifestyle treatment. Circulation. 2017;135(17):1577–85. https://doi.org/10.1161/CIRCULATIONAHA.116.025629.
16. Ramani GV, McCloskey C, Ramanathan RC, Mathier MA. Safety and efficacy of bariatric surgery in morbidly obese patients with severe systolic heart failure. Clin Cardiol. 2008;31(11):516–20. https://doi.org/10.1002/clc.20315.

17. Miranda WR, Batsis JA, Sarr MG, Collazo-Clavell ML, Clark MM, Somers VK, et al. Impact of bariatric surgery on quality of life, functional capacity, and symptoms in patients with heart failure. Obes Surg. 2013;23(7):1011–5. https://doi.org/10.1007/s11695-013-0953-8.
18. McCloskey CA, Ramani GV, Mathier MA, Schauer PR, Eid GM, Mattar SG, et al. Bariatric surgery improves cardiac function in morbidly obese patients with severe cardiomyopathy. Surg Obes Relat Dis. 2007;3(5):503–7. https://doi.org/10.1016/j.soard.2007.05.006.
19. Vest AR, Patel P, Schauer PR, Satava ME, Cavalcante JL, Brethauer S, et al. Clinical and echocardiographic outcomes after bariatric surgery in obese patients with left ventricular systolic dysfunction. Circ Heart Fail. 2016;9(3):e002260. https://doi.org/10.1161/CIRCHEARTFAILURE.115.002260.
20. McDowell K, Petrie MC, Raihan NA, Logue J. Effects of intentional weight loss in patients with obesity and heart failure: a systematic review. Obes Rev. 2018;19(9):1189–204. https://doi.org/10.1111/obr.12707.
21. Shimada YJ, Tsugawa Y, Brown DF, Hasegawa K. Bariatric surgery and emergency department visits and hospitalizations for heart failure exacerbation: population-based, self-controlled series. J Am Coll Cardiol. 2016;67(8):895–903. https://doi.org/10.1016/j.jacc.2015.12.016.
22. Fleisher LA, Fleischmann KE, Auerbach AD, Barnason SA, Beckman JA, Bozkurt B, et al. ACC/AHA guideline on perioperative cardiovascular evaluation and management of patients undergoing noncardiac surgery: a report of the American College of Cardiology/American Heart Association task force on practice guidelines. J Am Coll Cardiol. 2014;64(22):e77–137. https://doi.org/10.1016/j.jacc.2014.07.944.
23. Alsabrook GD, Goodman HR, Alexander JW. Gastric bypass for morbidly obese patients with established cardiac disease. Obes Surg. 2006;16(10):1272–7. https://doi.org/10.1381/096089206778663779.
24. Samuel I, Mason EE, Renquist KE, Huang YH, Zimmerman MB, Jamal M. Bariatric surgery trends: an 18-year report from the international bariatric surgery registry. Am J Surg. 2006;192(5):657–62. https://doi.org/10.1016/j.amjsurg.2006.07.006.
25. Stenberg E, Szabo E, Agren G, Naslund E, Boman L, Bylund A, et al. Early complications after laparoscopic gastric bypass surgery: results from the Scandinavian Obesity Surgery Registry. Ann Surg. 2014;260(6):1040–7. https://doi.org/10.1097/SLA.0000000000000431.

Bariatric Surgery in Those with Coronary Artery Disease

8

Nathan W. Kong and John E. A. Blair

8.1 Introduction

Bariatric surgery is well known to have a robust and sustained effect on weight loss [1–4]. With weight loss comes many of the downstream benefits on cardiovascular disease including reduction in diabetes, hypertension, and major atherosclerotic coronary events [5–8]. The patient population requiring bariatric surgery (BMI $\geq$ 40 or $\geq$35 with a co-morbid condition) are also at high risk for already having coronary artery disease (CAD). In patients with established coronary artery disease, do the long-term benefits of bariatric surgery outweigh the potential risks of surgery?

8.2 Search Strategy

A literature search of English language publications from 2000 to 2019 was used to identify published data on the outcomes of bariatric surgery on patients with known or suspected coronary artery disease. Databases searched were PubMed, Embase, and Cochrane Central. The terms used in the search were "coronary artery disease," "myocardial ischemia," "coronary atherosclerosis," "coronary obstructive disease," "coronary angiogram," "left heart catheterization," "revascularization" AND "gastric bypass," "Roux-en-Y gastric bypass," "Greenville gastric bypass," "gastroileal bypass," "gastrojejunostomy." (Table 8.1).

N. W. Kong · J. E. A. Blair (✉)
Department of Medicine, Section of Cardiology, University of Chicago, Chicago, IL, USA
e-mail: jblair2@medicine.bsd.uchicago.edu

© Springer Nature Switzerland AG 2021
J. Alverdy, Y. Vigneswaran (eds.), *Difficult Decisions in Bariatric Surgery*,
Difficult Decisions in Surgery: An Evidence-Based Approach,
https://doi.org/10.1007/978-3-030-55329-6_8

Table 8.1 PICO

P (Patients)	I (Intervention)	C (Comparator)	O (Outcomes)
Patients with morbid obesity	Bariatric surgery	Optimal medical therapy	Mortality, long term cardiovascular events, ED visits, hospitalizations, perioperative cardiovascular events

8.3   Results

8.3.1   Prevalence

The 2018 Heart Disease and Stroke Statistics Update published by the American Heart Association estimated that amongst US adults ≥20 years of age, the prevalence of coronary heart disease is 7.4% for males and 5.3% for females with a slightly greater prevalence of males (55%) [9]. Amongst younger patients, the bariatric surgery population, the rates are even lower, 0.6% and 0.7% for men and women, respectively, aged 20–39.

While patients undergoing bariatric surgery are generally younger, they have significant risk factors for coronary artery disease including obesity and higher rates of dyslipidemia, hypertension, diabetes, and obstructive sleep apnea [7]. In a large meta-analysis of over 22,000 patients, it was found that 7% of patients who underwent bariatric surgery carried a diagnosis of coronary artery disease at the time diagnosis [1]. It should be noted that the average age was 39 years old and 72.6% of patients were female.

In a 2014 update to the above meta-analysis, it was found that 7.15% of 26,000 patients who underwent bariatric surgery had cardiovascular disease at the time of surgery. Again, the study had a young age (mean = 44.6 years old) and had significantly more females at 78.9%. Results from these large patient samples support the idea that bariatric surgery candidates are at increased risk of coronary artery disease as compared to the general population.

8.3.2   Benefits

Bariatric surgery is known to result in significant weight loss in individuals over time [1, 2, 4]. In fact, bariatric surgery as compared to non-surgical treatments for obesity provides and greater and more sustained weight loss [10]. This weight reduction has significant cardiovascular benefits. A prospective study from Sweden which recruited over 2000 patients and followed them for a mean of 15 years found that bariatric surgery when compared to no surgery reduced the number of cardiovascular deaths (adjusted hazard ratio 0.47, 95% confidence interval 0.26–0.76, $p = 0.002$) and cardiovascular events (adjusted hazard ratio 0.76, 95% confidence interval 0.54–0.83, $p < 0.001$) [11]. A larger, retrospective study of nearly 10,000 patients, found that gastric bypass surgery reduced all-cause mortality by 40% and coronary artery disease mortality by 56% over their 7 year follow-up period [12].

While data exists for the effects of bariatric surgery on cardiovascular disease, there is limited data on the effects of surgery on patients with known coronary artery disease. In a large meta-analysis of over 22,000 patients, only 8.5% of the studied patients were in trials which even commented on the diagnosis of coronary artery disease prior to surgery [1].

Our review of the literature revealed only two studies which examined the benefits and risks of bariatric surgery on patients with known obstructive coronary artery disease. The first was a 2005 retrospective cohort study of 567 patients who underwent bariatric surgery at the Mayo Clinic from 1995 to 2002 [13]. Fifty two (9.2%) of these patients had clinical CAD as defined by history, >30% stenosis on angiogram in at least 1 major coronary artery, or inducible ischemia on stress testing. Six of the 52 patients with CAD had stress testing before and after surgery. Of these six patients, four experienced reduction in the extent and severity of their reversible ischemic segments on imaging [13]. Due to the small number of patients who received pre- and post-operative stress testing as well as the lack of comparison group in the non-coronary artery disease patients, no statistical testing was done for these results.

A more recent study, published in 2018, was a self-controlled case series which examined patient hospitalizations in a number of common cardiovascular diseases, including coronary artery disease, before and after bariatric surgery [14]. They found that the number of emergency department visits and/or unplanned hospitalizations in the coronary artery disease group decreased significantly in the 2 years following surgery (adjusted odds ratio 0.51, 95% confidence interval 0.40–0.65, $p < 0.001$) [14].

8.3.3 Risks

While there are potential benefits of bariatric surgery for those with coronary artery disease, there are significant risks of surgery in this patient population (Table 8.2). The risk of major atherosclerotic coronary events after non-cardiac surgeries is directly tied to prior coronary events. A study from 1990 demonstrated that postoperative myocardial infarction (MI) rates was inversely proportional to time between prior MI and non-cardiac operations [15]. However, in reviewing the literature on baritric surgeries, there were only a few studies which examined the risks of baritatric surgery in patients with coronary artery disease.

In the 2005 Mayo Clinic study mentioned previously, it was found that patients with CAD trended towards higher rates of cardiovascular complications as compared to patients without CAD after a mean follow-up of 2.5 years ($p = 0.06$). No relationship existed for non-cardiovascular complications ($p = 0.90$) [13].

In 2007, a retrospective case study of a single surgeon's experience on 1000 open gastric bypass surgeries, it was found that the presence of CAD (defined by prior

Table 8.2 Benefit/risks of bariatric surgery in patients with coronary artery disease

Author (year)	N (% of total)	Study Type	Benefit Finding	Risk Finding	Quality
Lopez-Jimenez et al. [13]	52 (9.3%)	Retrospective	Four patients had improvement of reversible ischemia on imaging	Cardiovascular complications: 5.8% in CAD group vs 1.4% in non-CAD group (p = 0.06)	Low
Shimada et al. [14]	360 (3.2%)	Case control	Decreased number of unplanned ED visits (aOR 0.42 [0.32–0.54] at 1 year, 0.51 [0.40–0.65] at 2 years)	None	Moderate
Flancbaum and Belsley [16]	55 (5.5%)	Retrospective	None	7.5× relative risk of all-cause mortality if they had angiographic evidence of CAD	Low

N number of studied patients with coronary artery disease; *CAD* coronary artery disease; *ED* emergency department; *aOR* adjusted odds ratio

history) resulted in a 7.5 times greater relative risk of all-cause mortality following surgery [16]. This was largely driven by a subset of males with angiographically demonstrated CAD who had a 30 times greater likelihood of death. Interestingly, CAD was not a predictor of mortality in women. However this study was of open bariatric surgeries, which is much different from the common practice of current bariatric surgeons with the wide use of minimally invasive techniques. Additionally these retrospective studies are extremely prone to bias as evidenced by the Lopez-Jimenez et al. study which found that the group who had coronary artery disease at the time of surgery were significantly older than the non-CAD group (51.2 vs. 44.3 years old, p < 0.001).

8.3.4 Conclusion

It is clear from review of the literature that the potential benefits and risks of bariatric surgery in patients with coronary artery disease is an area that would benefit from further study. The lack of data in this area is likely compounded by the fact that only 7% of bariatric patients have coronary artery disease prior to surgery. Thus, in asymptomatic, younger individuals, the yield for universal angiographic or stress test screening of coronary artery disease is unlikely to be beneficial or cost-effective.

The robust weight loss from bariatric surgery has clearly established benefits in preventing cardiovascular pathologies, such as coronary artery disease, in a population that is high risk [11, 12]. However, no study has definitively shown that bariatric surgery reduces further cardiovascular disease in patients with already established coronary artery disease. The study conducted by Lopez-Jimenez et al., suggested that bariatric surgery may benefit those with coronary disease as they found a reduction in reversible ischemia observed on stress testing in 4 of their patients. Whether this finding is translatable to a larger population or even clinically relevant is largely unknown.

There remains an increased risk of morbidity and mortality for patients with established coronary artery disease undergoing bariatric surgery. The 2014 American College of Cardiology (ACC) and American Heart Association (AHA) guidelines on perioperative cardiovascular management recommend at least 1 full year between receiving drug-eluting stents and elective non-cardiac surgery, and at least 30 days after receiving bare-metal stents [17]. In review of the literature, it was found that retrospective studies observed increased mortality in patients with angiographically proven CAD [16]. Thus, we recommend following the 2014 ACC/AHA guidelines to establish the timing of elective bariatric surgery and to have a personalized discussion with the patient regarding the risks and benefits of surgery.

8.4 Recommendations

- In individuals with established coronary artery disease (confirmed with stress testing or with angiographic evidence), we recommend an individualized approach weighing the risks and benefits of bariatric surgery as there appears to be long term benefit for reduced events related to cardiovascular disease after surgery (Evidence quality low, moderate recommendation).
- Angiographic screening for obstructive coronary disease can be considered in individuals without symptoms if they are older than 40 years old, have multiple cardiovascular risk factors, or have previously established coronary artery disease (Evidence quality low, moderate recommendation)

8.5 Personal View of Data

It is clear in the literature that in patients with morbid obesity, bariatric surgery is associated with reduced rates of myocardial infarction and cardiovascular-related mortality. The difficulty in selecting patients for bariatric surgery exists in the paradox that those patients who are at greatest potential to receive this benefit (i.e. those with the highest cardiovascular risk or with established coronary artery disease), may also be the most likely to develop cardiovascular complications perioperatively. Fortunately, the actual rate of coronary artery disease and cardiovascular events following bariatric surgery is low, likely due to the relatively young age at the time of surgery. Given these findings, we do not recommend deviation from the established perioperative guidelines for non-cardiac surgery. However, when addressing risk for asymptomatic prospective bariatric surgery patients, those older than 40 years of age, those with a high burden of cardiovascular risk factors, and especially in those with established coronary artery disease, we recommend a low threshold for screening for obstructive coronary disease. Dobutamine stress echocardiography has been determined to reliably produce high-quality diagnostic images in a population that is difficult to image due to various potential artifacts in nuclear scintigraphy [18].

References

1. Buchwald H, Avidor Y, Braunwald E, et al. Bariatric surgery: a systematic review and meta-analysis. JAMA. 2004;292(14):1724–37.
2. Garb J, Welch G, Zagarins S, Kuhn J, Romanelli J. Bariatric surgery for the treatment of morbid obesity: a meta-analysis of weight loss outcomes for laparoscopic adjustable gastric banding and laparoscopic gastric bypass. Obes Surg. 2009;19(10):1447–55.
3. Logue J, Murray HM, Welsh P, et al. Obesity is associated with fatal coronary heart disease independently of traditional risk factors and deprivation. Heart. 2011;97(7):564–8.
4. Maggard MA, Shugarman LR, Suttorp M, et al. Meta-analysis: surgical treatment of obesity. Ann Intern Med. 2005;142(7):547–59.
5. Christou NV, Sampalis JS, Liberman M, et al. Surgery decreases long-term mortality, morbidity, and health care use in morbidly obese patients. Ann Surg. 2004;240(3):416–24.
6. MacDonald KG Jr, Long SD, Swanson MS, et al. The gastric bypass operation reduces the progression and mortality of non-insulin-dependent diabetes mellitus. J Gastrointest Surg. 1997;1(3):213–20. discussion 220
7. Sjostrom L, Lindroos AK, Peltonen M, et al. Lifestyle, diabetes, and cardiovascular risk factors 10 years after bariatric surgery. N Engl J Med. 2004;351(26):2683–93.
8. Sugerman HJ, Wolfe LG, Sica DA, Clore JN. Diabetes and hypertension in severe obesity and effects of gastric bypass-induced weight loss. Ann Surg. 2003;237(6):751–8.
9. Benjamin EJ, Virani SS, Callaway CW, et al. Heart disease and stroke statistics-2018 update: a report from the American Heart Association. Circulation. 2018;137(12):e67–e492.
10. Gloy VL, Briel M, Bhatt DL, et al. Bariatric surgery versus non-surgical treatment for obesity: a systematic review and meta-analysis of randomised controlled trials. BMJ. 2013;347:f5934.
11. Sjöström L, Peltonen M, Jacobson P, et al. Bariatric surgery and long-term cardiovascular events. JAMA. 2012;307(1):56–65.
12. Adams TD, Gress RE, Smith SC, et al. Long-term mortality after gastric bypass surgery. N Engl J Med. 2007;357(8):753–61.
13. Lopez-Jimenez F, Bhatia S, Collazo-Clavell ML, Sarr MG, Somers VK. Safety and efficacy of bariatric surgery in patients with coronary artery disease. Mayo Clin Proc. 2005;80(9):1157–62.
14. Shimada YJ, Gibo K, Tsugawa Y, et al. Bariatric surgery is associated with lower risk of acute care use for cardiovascular disease in obese adults. Cardiovasc Res. 2018;115(4):800–6.
15. Shah KB, Kleinman BS, Rao TL, Jacobs HK, Mestan K, Schaafsma M. Angina and other risk factors in patients with cardiac diseases undergoing noncardiac operations. Anesth Analg. 1990;70(3):240–7.

16. Flancbaum L, Belsley S. Factors affecting morbidity and mortality of Roux-en-Y gastric bypass for clinically severe obesity: an analysis of 1,000 consecutive open cases by a single surgeon. J Gastrointest Surg. 2007;11(4):500–7.
17. Fleisher LA, Fleischmann KE, Auerbach AD, et al. ACC/AHA guideline on perioperative cardiovascular evaluation and management of patients undergoing noncardiac surgery: executive summary. Circulation. 2014;130(24):2215–45.
18. Lerakis S, Kalogeropoulos AP, El-Chami MF, et al. Transthoracic dobutamine stress echocardiography in patients undergoing bariatric surgery. Obes Surg. 2007;17(11):1475–81.

What Are the Nutritional "Red Flags" to Look Out for Prior to Bariatric Surgery?

9

Jessica Schultz

9.1 Introduction

Bariatric surgery is a tool to help assist a patient in achieving weight loss; however, without the proper motivation, knowledge, and ongoing support, patients are at risk for failure following a given procedure. It is important for a registered dietitian, specializing in bariatric surgery, to complete a comprehensive nutritional assessment on each patient prior to surgery to ensure the patient has the proper motivation, nutrition knowledge, and continued support to be successful following their weight loss surgery. A systematic identification and nutritional evaluation by a bariatric dietitian can identify specific "red flags" that might trigger further investigation and dietary and/or lifestyle modifications prior to the patient undergoing bariatric surgery.

9.2 Search Strategy

A comprehensive literature search was conducted to obtain relevant data surrounding patients diet behaviors and nutritional knowledge prior to elective bariatric surgery. This was an English literature search between the publication years of 2015–2019. Specific terms used within this search included "nutrient deficiencies prior to bariatric surgery", "postoperative nutritional outcomes in bariatric surgery", "supervised weight loss program" "preoperative weight loss", "nutrition knowledge and bariatric outcomes", "nutrition before bariatric surgery", "morbid obesity",

J. Schultz (✉)
The Center for the Surgical Treatment of Obesity, University of Chicago Medicine,
Chicago, IL, USA
e-mail: Jessica.Schultz@uchospitals.edu

© Springer Nature Switzerland AG 2021
J. Alverdy, Y. Vigneswaran (eds.), *Difficult Decisions in Bariatric Surgery*,
Difficult Decisions in Surgery: An Evidence-Based Approach,
https://doi.org/10.1007/978-3-030-55329-6_9

"nutritional status", "micronutrient deficiencies" "vitamin D". Databases searched included Ebsco Host, PebMed, and google scholar. A total of seven articles were reviewed and included.

9.3   Results

9.3.1   Insurance Mandated Supervised Weight Loss

It is apparent that not every patient interested in bariatric surgery, is considered an ideal candidate from a nutritional standpoint. This statement can be further broken down to state that nutrition knowledge, nutritional motivation including eating behaviors, exercise behaviors and or ability to exercise, and key support systems all play a role in a patient's overall success or failure following bariatric surgery. Many private and non-private insurance companies require patients to complete a series of 3–6 months of supervised weight loss as a nutritional requirement prior to their elective bariatric surgery. This requirement evidently can delay a patient's surgery up to 6 months and also has been shown to increase surgical dropout [1, p. 874]. While many patients may be disappointed by this insurance requirement, this can be viewed as an opportunity to improve one's lifestyle behaviors in the months preceding their surgery. This opportunity may potentially serve as a method to increase the patient's likelihood of long term weight loss and maintenance of weight loss following bariatric surgery.

9.3.1.1 Obesity Related Micronutrient Deficiencies
While it is well known that weight loss surgery may increase ones risk for micronutrient deficiencies, especially for those patients undergoing malabsorptive procedures [2, p. 645], obesity related nutritional deficiencies should not be overlooked in the preoperative patient. Excessive calorie intake of low nutrient dense foods such as diets high in refined carbohydrates and high fat can greatly increase the risk of one or multiple micronutrient deficiencies in pre-operative patients. It is important to properly screen pre-operative patients for diet behaviors which would mimic these deficiencies. Patients living in a food desert with limited access to fresh foods are also at higher risk for micronutrient deficiencies given the poor nutritional make up of highly processed foods. A skilled dietitian should thoroughly examine a patient's daily food intake and eating behaviors at their initial bariatric evaluation in order to assess which patients may be at increased risk.

In a large cross-sectional, retrospective study conducted by Krzizek and colleagues, a total of 1732 Caucasian patients, majority women at 77.3%, with mean BMI of 44+ −9 kg, and a mean age of 40+ −12 years were assessed and counseled by a skilled dietitian prior to possible weight loss surgery. Laboratory levels of vitamin A, vitamin E, vitamin b12, folic acid, 25OH vitamin D, hemoglobin, ferritin, and PTH levels were collected and assessed. A total of 63.2% of patients had a folic acid deficiency, 5.1% vitamin b12 deficiency, 97.5% had a 25OH vitamin D deficiency, and 30.2% of patients had an elevated parathyroid hormone level. A total of

9.6% of patients had an iron deficiency and 6.2% of patients had a vitamin A deficiency. The patients were also categorized into three groups based on BMI which demonstrated that the group with the highest BMI had an increased prevalence of folic acid deficiency, 25OH vitamin D deficiency and subsequently higher levels of parathyroid hormone. The results of this large cross-sectional, retrospective study show that pre-operative micronutrient screening is warranted in this population given the high prevalence of deficiencies, especially 25OH vitamin D [2, p. 646].

In another study conducted by Sanchez and colleagues, multiple micronutrient deficiencies were observed in obese Chilean women prior to bariatric surgery. Of the most common deficiencies noted, 71.7% of the women were deficient in 25OH vitamin D, 66% had an elevated parathyroid hormone level, and 12.6% had low plasma iron levels [3, p. 365]. In a study by Porat and colleagues, they examined 19 patients' micronutrient levels prior to a sleeve gastrectomy. Of these pre-operative patients, 44% were deficient in iron, 11.5% with anemia, 46% with a folic acid deficiency, 7.7% with a vitamin b12 deficiency, 96.2% with a vitamin D deficiency, and 52% with an elevated parathyroid hormone level [4, p. 1140].

9.3.1.2 Increasing Patients Nutrition Knowledge

It is known that many insurance providers mandate that patients complete a series of supervised weight loss visits prior to bariatric surgery, however increased nutrition knowledge gained from these sessions may be much less than expected. Depending on the content and method of the supervised weight loss visit and the comprehensiveness of the dietitian and patient discussion, there may be significant variability regarding the nutrition knowledge gained and hence the benefit conferred. Sherf-Degan and colleagues studied the effect of pre-surgery information via an online lecture and how it impacted the nutrition knowledge and anxiety among bariatric surgery candidates. This study was an interventional non-randomized controlled trial including a total of 200 bariatric surgery candidates. The first 100 candidates were assigned to the control group while the last 100 candidates were assigned to the intervention group. The intervention group watched a 15 min online lecture 1–2 weeks prior to surgery. All of the participants completed a bariatric surgery nutrition knowledge and the state-trait anxiety intervention questionnaires at the pre bariatric surgery committee and again at the pre-surgery clinic. The results of this study show there was an increase in both state-trait anxiety scores as well as nutrition knowledge scores, however, nutrition knowledge scores were significantly higher in the intervention group. This shows that a comprehensive, short, online lecture improves nutrition knowledge in the pre-operative patient [5]. With the increased use of smartphones and ever evolving phone applications, Mundi and colleagues studies the feasibility of smartphone-based education in pre-operative patients. Within this study, participants seeking bariatric surgery were provided a smartphone application which included education modules complete with follow up assessments to gauge mastery of topics discussed. Of the 30 subjects enrolled, 20 completed the study. A total of 70.9% of the education modules were completed and 30.7% of the assessments were answered. The participants were highly satisfied with the application and the ease of fitting it into their daily routine and felt that it not only helped with increased weight loss, but also was helpful in preparing them for surgery [6]. This begs the question whether all bariatric programs should follow the same comprehensive pre-operative nutrition education based on current guidelines set by the American Society of Metabolic and Bariatric Surgery.

9.4   Recommendations Based on the Data

Many insurance companies will continue to require pre-surgical supervised weight loss prior to bariatric surgery, and this should be viewed as an optimal nutrition opportunity for individual patients. During the months of supervised weight loss a patient should work closely with a highly skilled registered dietitian who specializes in the care of obesity and bariatric surgery. The literature shows there is a high prevalence of micronutrient deficiencies associated with obesity, specifically 25OH vitamin D, folic acid, and iron deficiency [2, p. 646]. Vitamin and mineral supplementation is required after all bariatric surgeries, however if deficiencies are not identified prior to surgery, this will incur increased dosages of postoperative vitamin and mineral supplements and may put the patient at higher risk for side effects related to these deficiencies. With adherence to vitamin and mineral supplementation already a post-operative concern [7, p. 417], adding additional supplementation to a patient's daily regimen is not ideal. Therefore, pre-operative screening for vitamin and mineral deficiencies prior to surgery is essential and appropriate micronutrient repletion by a bariatric dietitian should follow. While pre-operative weight loss is not always a requirement prior to surgery, it should be mandated that patients show that they are capable of making the necessary diet and lifestyle changes prior to surgery. This can be done by completing supplementary nutrition education visits following the bariatric evaluation as deemed necessary by the registered dietitian based on patients current behaviors and or lack of sufficient nutrition knowledge. Diet and lifestyle behavior improvement should also be documented during patients' insurance required supervised weight loss visits. These visits should be completed with a weight management dietitian specializing in bariatric surgery.

9.5   A Personal View of the Data

In my 7 years working within the bariatric clinic at The University of Chicago Medicine, we have always assessed patients' nutrition knowledge and diet behaviors through a comprehensive nutrition evaluation completed the same day the patient comes into clinic seeking bariatric surgery. Both I and the other dietitian working within our multidisciplinary bariatric surgery clinic are solely weight management dietitians specializing in the care of bariatric patients. Our approach to insurance mandated supervised weight loss requirements include a series of comprehensive nutrition education classes both offered in group sessions as well as individual sessions as deemed necessary based on each patient's needs. Within these teaching sessions, a series of six nutrition focused classes lead by a bariatric dietitian for 30–60 min is completed once per month. Each patient is required to be weighed in at the start of each session and is also required to completed individual specific, measurable, attainable, realistic, and timely (SMART) goals to best prepare the patient for life long diet and behavior practices after surgery. Within our clinic, I believe that these classes have shown to improve patient's nutrition knowledge leading into their surgery. I have personally noticed that those patients that have improved nutrition knowledge before surgery tend to show improved success with the necessary diet and lifestyle changes required for weight loss and maintenance of weight loss after bariatric surgery. We hope to specifically examine outcomes correlated to the successful completion of our comprehensive supervised weight loss classes in the future.

In early 2019, we began drawing 25OH vitamin D levels on patients at the beginning of their 3 or 6 months of supervised weight loss in our individual nutrition clinics. The prevalence of vitamin D deficiencies seen pre-operatively in our patients was dramatic. Instead of waiting until the patients pre-operative lab draw 1–2 weeks prior to surgery to detect a deficiency, we are now identifying this early on in an effort to replete and normalize levels prior to surgery. Not only are we observing very good patient adherence, but also this approach is helping us decrease the need for high doses of vitamin D3 post-operatively. We plan to implement additional vitamin and mineral screening at initial supervised weight loss visits with the expectation of identifying and correcting vitamin and mineral deficiencies related to the obesity disorder itself prior to surgery.

The use of smart phone applications to track macronutrient intake such as that with My Fitness Pal application has been a popular way for patient to tally their protein and carbohydrate intake both pre-operatively and post-operatively. Another phone application which has been helpful for our patients is Medisafe. Medisafe allows patients to input their individual vitamin and mineral regimens into a schedule within the application. The patient's phone will alert them when it is time to take a certain vitamin. This not only helps with adherence to vitamin regimen, but it also helps the patient to remember to not take certain vitamins with others for best absorption. For example, a patient should not pair their calcium with iron given a large dose of calcium can decrease the body's absorption of iron. While we are not currently using a phone application for nutrition education purposes, this is clearly something we will explore in the future.

References

1. Love MK, Mehaffey JH, Safavian D, Schirmer B, Malin KS, Hallowell PT, Kirby LJ. Bariatric surgery insurance requirements independently predict surgery dropout. Surg Obes Relat Dis. 2017;13:871–6.
2. Krzizek CE, Brix MJ, Herz TC, Kopp PH, Schernthaner HG, Shcernthaner G, Ludvik B. Prevalence of micronutrient deficiency in patients with morbid obesity before bariatric surgery. Obes Surg. 2018;28:643–8.

3. Sanchez A, Rojas P, Basfi-Fer K, Carrasco F, Inostroza J, Codoceo J, Valencia A, Papapietro K, Csendes A, Ruz M. Micronutrient deficiencies in morbidly obese women prior to bariatric surgery. Obes Surg. 2016;26(2):361–8.
4. Porat BT, Elazary R, Goldenshluger A, Dagan SS, Mintz MY, Weiss R. Nutritional deficiencies four years after laparoscopic sleeve gastrectomy-are supplements required for a lifetime? Surg Obes Relat Dis. 2017;13(7):1138–44.
5. Sherf-Dagan S, Hod K, Mardy-Tilbor L, Gilksman S, Ben-Porat T, Sakran N, Zelber-Sagi S, Goitein D, Raziel A. The effect of pre-surgery information online lecture on nutrition knowledge and anxiety among bariatric surgery candidates. Obes Surg. 2018;28(7):1876–85.
6. Mundi SM, Lorentz AP, Grothe K, Kellogg AT, Collazo-Clavell LM. Feasibility of smartphone-based education modules and ecological momentary assessment/intervention in pre-bariatric surgery patients. Obes Surg. 2015;25(10):1875–81.
7. Sunil S, Santiago AV, Gougeon L, Warwick K, Okrainc A, Hawa R, Sockalingam S. Predictors of vitamin adherence after bariatric surgery. Obes Surg. 2017;27(2):416–23.

Are There Psychiatric Diagnoses That Preclude Safe Bariatric Surgery?

10

Emily R. Fink and Leslie J. Heinberg

10.1 Introduction

Bariatric surgery candidates demonstrate a greater lifetime prevalence of psychiatric diagnoses as compared to the general population and non-treatment seeking patients with severe obesity [1]. Although there is evidence that some mental health conditions (e.g., depression, binge-eating disorder) initially attenuate following surgery [2–4], a growing consensus warns of the risk for long-term psychiatric complications primarily in the realms of suicide/self-harm and alcohol/substance use disorders [5–7]. Given that psychological factors may affect the safety and outcomes of bariatric procedures by impacting adjustment, adherence, and medical comorbidities, clinical practice guidelines recommend psychological evaluation of surgical candidates before and after surgery [8]. This chapter examines psychological diagnoses and factors demonstrated to increase risk for postoperative complications.

10.2 Search Strategy

A systematic internet search of three bibliographic databases (Academic Search Complete, Medline, and Psychological and Behavioral Sciences Collection) was used to identify English language primary research published electronically or in

E. R. Fink
Cleveland Clinic Bariatric & Metabolic Institute, Cleveland, OH, USA
e-mail: finke3@ccf.org

L. J. Heinberg (✉)
Cleveland Clinic Bariatric & Metabolic Institute, Cleveland, OH, USA

Cleveland Clinic Lerner College of Medicine of Case Western Reserve University, Cleveland, OH, USA
e-mail: heinbel@ccf.org

© Springer Nature Switzerland AG 2021
J. Alverdy, Y. Vigneswaran (eds.), *Difficult Decisions in Bariatric Surgery*,
Difficult Decisions in Surgery: An Evidence-Based Approach,
https://doi.org/10.1007/978-3-030-55329-6_10

Table 10.1 PICO

Patients	Patients with a history of Major Depressive Disorder, Anxiety Disorder, Schizophrenia Spectrum Disorder, Bipolar Disorder, Alcohol Use Disorder, Substance Use Disorder
Intervention	Bariatric surgery
Comparator	Patients without a psychiatric history
Outcomes	Post-surgical readmission, medical complication or mortality; Post-surgical suicidal ideation/self-harm, ED visit for suicidal ideation/self-harm, psychiatric hospitalization or completed suicide; Post-surgical substance abuse or opioid use

print from 2014 to 2019 (Table 10.1). Terms used in the search were "depression," "bipolar," "anxiety," "PTSD," "post-traumatic stress disorder," "schizophrenia," "psychosis," "personality disorder," "axis II," "suicide," "suicidality," "cognitive impairment," "intellectual disability," "ADHD," "attention-deficit/hyperactivity disorder," "anorexia," "bulimia," "alcohol," "smoking," "tobacco," "substance abuse," "drug use" AND "bariatric surgery," "obesity surgery," "gastric bypass," "sleeve gastrectomy," "vertical banded gastroplasty" AND "complications," "adverse events," "mortality." For inclusion, we required that studies report associations between preoperative psychiatric diagnoses/self-harm events/substance use behaviors and bariatric surgery complications (i.e., mortality, morbidity, readmission, ED visit, psychiatric hospitalization, suicidality/self-harm, substance use) in the main aims or abstract of the article. Additional exclusionary criteria included dissertations, master's theses, qualitative studies, animal studies, pilot studies, case reports, research specific to body contouring or plastic surgery, and studies with less than 150 participants. Given the limited research meeting our criteria addressing Attention-Deficit/Hyperactivity Disorder (ADHD), Post-Traumatic Stress Disorder (PSTD), Intellectual Disability/Mild or Moderate Cognitive Impairment, Anorexia Nervosa, Bulimia Nervosa, and Personality Disorders, these diagnoses were not included in our analysis. Research involving smoking was identified by our search given relevance to substance use behaviors. However, Tobacco Use Disorder was exluded from our analysis as it is addressed in another chapter. A total of 28 studies meeting our criteria were classified according to the GRADE system.

10.3   Major Depressive Disorder (MDD)

Eight identified studies examined relationships between preoperative depression symptoms (including suicidality) and postoperative psychological complications. A 2018 prospective study of 284 bariatric patients from the Toronto Bari-Psych Cohort [9], identified lifetime suicidal ideation as the strongest predictor of post-surgical suicidal ideation in both univariate (ß = −2.47; 95%CI [0.03–0.25]; $p < 0.01$) and multivariate analyses (ß = −1.92; SE = 1.33; $p < 0.01$). This same study found that a past diagnosis of MDD significantly predicted post-surgical suicidal ideation in univariate analyses (ß = −1.34; 95%CI [0.09–0.74]; $p = 0.01$), but this relationship was not maintained in multivariate analyses. Similar results were obtained by a second study identifying history of self-harm as predicting post-surgical suicidality in both univariate and multivariate models [10] and a third study demonstrating antidepressant use as a risk factor for post-surgical suicide attempt (AHR 2.41; 95%CI [1.89–3.06]) [11]. Though a fourth study [12] indicated that lifetime and recent history of suicidality and pre-surgery antidepressant use increased risk for post-surgical self-harm or suicidal ideation, this research retrospectively assessed pre-surgical suicidal ideation and reported missing data specific to suicidality. In a fifth study involving gastric bypass (GB) patients, those who received an ICD code for depression from inpatient or outpatient services within 2 years of surgery had over a 50-fold higher risk for post-surgical hospitalization for depression compared to those without a history of mood disorders [13]. Hazard ratio for psychiatric hospitalization for self-harm following surgery was likewise greater in those with a self-harm history. A pair of retrospective cohort studies utilizing data from the Western Australian Department of Health Data Linkage Unit records identified pre-surgical psychiatric hospitalization due to mood disorders as a risk factor for post-surgical hospitalization due to deliberate self-harm [14] and pre-surgical emergency room visit for suicidality, psychiatric hospitalization for deliberate self-harm, and psychiatric hospitalization for mood disorders as risk factors for postoperative ED visit for self-harm or suicidal ideation [15]. Lastly, a study found that a majority of self-harm events were committed by patients with depression diagnoses [16]. Given the relative consistency of findings across studies, there is evidence to suggest that preoperative depression involving self-harm or psychopharmacological treatment increases risk for post-surgical depression involving suicidality.

Interestingly, the relationship between depression and postoperative morbidity was mixed. One study identified preoperative depression as a significant risk factor for all-cause hospital readmission [17], while a second demonstrated associations between depression and early readmission that trended towards but did not reach statistical significance [18]. A third and fourth identified increased odds of readmission/post-surgical hospital days in those diagnosed with Major Depression or Bipolar Disorder [19] and severe depression or anxiety [20] respectively, but did not identify unique risks conferred by specific diagnoses. A fifth found no difference in pre-surgical depression between cohorts experiencing vs. not experiencing surgical complications, but excluded patients with a history of significant psychiatric concerns [21]. This is likely to be a limitation throughout the literature as those with severe psychiatric illness are less likely to progress to surgery. Though no significant relationship between baseline depression score and 30-day adverse events was identified in a sixth study [22], increased risk for short-term adverse events was found in those prescribed antidepressant medication (AOR = 1.76; 95%CI [1.02–3.04]; $p = .04$); mild to severe depression scores on a common screener also increased risk (AOR = 1.77; 95%CI [1.03–3.05]; $p = .04$), as compared to minimal depression scores, suggesting that severity of psychopathology should be considered in addition to presence of negative affect. Relationships between pre-surgical depression and post-surgical substance use were inconsistent [23–25]. As there was inconsistent evidence regarding depression-related risk for post-surgical mortality or the link between depression and postoperative opioid use [26–29] conclusions cannot be made regarding these relationships.

10.4 Anxiety Disorder

Three studies published data regarding potential relationships between anxiety and post-surgical suicidality. A nationwide study of 8966 bariatric patients matched with non-surgical controls with obesity [11] identified pre-surgical anxiolytic treatment as a significant risk factor for post-surgical suicide attempt (AHR 3.37; 95%CI [2.62–4.31]), while a second identified history of hospitalization for neurotic disorder as a risk factor for postoperative psychiatric hospitalization for mood or neurotic disorder, but not self-harm [14]. A third study identified high prevalence of anxiety disorders in patients exhibiting pre-and postoperative self-harm events [16]. Given risks for bias related to assessment of anxiety, no evidence-based recommendations regarding these associations can be made.

Seven studies examining relationships between anxiety and post-surgical complications were likewise inconclusive. A retrospective study of 354 patients undergoing bariatric surgery demonstrated increased prevalence of 30-day readmission in those diagnosed with anxiety, as compared to controls (10.1% vs 3.7%, $p < .05$) [18]. A second study found that those with severe depression or anxiety were less likely to have zero hospital days at all post-surgical time points or ED visits at 1 and 2 year follow-ups [20], but did not identify risk specific to anxiety. Though 2 other studies found little evidence of pre-surgical anxiety-related risk for adverse events or readmission [19, 21], methodological limitations may account for absence of findings in one of these studies [21]. Findings regarding relationships between anxiety and post-surgical alcohol abuse/opioid use were inconsistent [23, 28, 29].

10.5 Bipolar Disorder and Schizophrenia Spectrum Disorder

Four studies in our analysis examined associations between serious mental illness (SMI) and post-surgical readmission. History of psychosis was identified as a risk factor for readmission following surgery (OR = 1.7; 95%CI [1.4–2.2]; $p < .001$) in a database of 22,139 bariatric patients [17]. A retrospective study of 354 patients similarly demonstrated increased prevalence of 30-day readmission in those diagnosed with bipolar disorder, as compared to those without a psychiatric history (45.5% vs 3.7%, $p < .05$) [18]. Two other studies identified groups of psychiatric diagnoses including SMI as contributing to risk for readmission, but did not document influences unique to specific diagnoses; the first identified that patients diagnosed with either Major Depressive Disorder or Bipolar Disorder had 46% greater odds of 30 day readmission ($p < .005$) as compared to those without these disorders [19]. In a similar fashion, a 2017 multi-site study [20] identified that those diagnosed with Bipolar Disorder, Schizophrenia or psychosis were less likely to have zero hospital days or ED visits at 1 and 2 year follow-up. Taken together, Bipolar

Disorder and Schizophrenia Spectrum Disorders are likely to be risk factors for readmission, potentially due to the negative impact on adherence behaviors. However, given the assessment of psychopathology in the current research, there are limited conclusions that can be drawn regarding the post-surgical impact of specific disorders.

One study, limited by poor follow-up, identified new persistent opioid users to be more likely to be diagnosed with Bipolar Disorder [29], while another demonstrated risk for anastomotic ulceration in those with a history of psychosis [30]. In the absence of corroborating evidence, no recommendations can be made regarding these specific associations.

10.6 Alcohol Use

Although previous literature has documented elevated rates of alcohol misuse in bariatric populations [6], few published studies meeting our criteria examined psychiatric characteristics that increase risk for postoperative substance abuse. In a multisite prospective study (LABS-2) [24], pre-surgical consumption of alcohol was found to increase risk for post-surgical AUD as compared to no alcohol consumption; hazard ratios were greater in those reporting alcohol consumption $\geq 2\times$/week (AHR 12.68; 95% [8.34–19.26]) rather than drinking $<2\times$/week (AHR 2.96; 95% [2.17–4.03]), suggesting that risk for AUD increases with greater preoperative frequency of use. Pre-surgical AUD also increased risk for post-surgical substance abuse treatment. However, this study did not assess lifetime history of AUD; given this limitation, it is unclear the extent to which post-surgical AUD in this study reflected development of new abuse behaviors or AUD relapse. This finding was supported by another study indicating decreased odds for postoperative AUD in patients without baseline AUD or alcohol consumption [25]. Current guidelines recommend elimination of alcohol consumption following surgery in high risk groups [8]. In light of evidence suggesting high rates of new onset alcohol abuse in post-surgical bariatric populations [6], accurate prediction of surgical candidates at risk for post-surgical AUD remains a domain requiring further research.

Two other studies identified high prevalence of preoperative alcohol misuse in bariatric surgery patients who later developed AUD [23, 31]; however, as one of these studies also utilized the LABS-2 cohort, similarities in findings may be attributable to overlap in participants. Inconsistent findings with regard to the potential impact of alcohol misuse on mortality [26, 32, 33], precludes conclusions regarding these relationships.

10.7 Drug Abuse and Opioid Use

Few identified studies examined associations between pre-surgical substance use and post-surgical complications. One study of 22,139 patients followed by the New York State Planning and Research Cooperative System, identified nonspecific substance abuse history as increasing risk for post-surgical readmission (OR = 2.0; 95%CI [1.1–3.5]; p = .022) [17]. A second study identified drug abuse as increasing likelihood for perforated ulceration (OR = 5.05; 95%CI [1.85–11.19]; p = .0003) [34], while a third, fourth and fifth provided preliminary evidence with regard to relationships between substance abuse and postoperative self-harm/suicidality [10, 15, 35]. In an examination of 157,559 GB patients, substance abuse was not significantly related to 30-day mortality [26]. Although several of these studies controlled for potential confounds, the majority failed to specify the type of substance abused prior to surgery or the manner by which this abuse was assessed. Given the imprecision of assessment of substance use, limited conclusions can be made regarding such associations.

With regard to post-surgical substance use, one study identified pre-surgical opioid use as a risk factor for new persistent opioid use, such that increasing days' supply magnified this risk (1–29 days OR = 1.89; 95%CI [1.24–2.88]; 30–59 days OR = 6.91; 95 %CI [4.16–11.47]; 60–89 days OR = 13.23; 95%CI [7.03–24.91]; 90–119 days OR = 14.29; 95%CI [6.94–29.42]) as compared with no use [28]. In other studies, no evidence of relationships were found between pre-surgical illicit drug use/abuse and post-surgical opioid use [29, 36], AUD [24] or substance abuse treatment [24].

10.8 Unspecified Psychiatric History

Two studies identified increased risk for postoperative self-harm associated with history of unspecified psychiatric diagnosis or service utilization [10, 12]. A third examining 2 Swedish cohorts with matched controls, [35] found evidence for increased risk for suicidality in surgery patients with and without a psychiatric history in one cohort, as compared to non-surgical controls; in the other cohort, patients without a psychiatric history experienced increased risk. Though this suggests that selection bias or the surgical procedure itself contributes to risk for postoperative self-harm, this study was limited by exclusion criteria involving certain psychiatric disorders and inconsistent assessment of psychiatric history across cohorts. Another study evaluated impact of multiple psychiatric diagnoses on likelihood of readmission [19], demonstrating that odds for post-surgical hospital care rose as the number of mental health diagnoses increased. Patients diagnosed with 1 psychiatric disorder possessed 31% greater odds for readmission (OR = 1.31; 95%CI [1.13–1.51]) compared to those without comorbidities, while patients diagnosed with 3 or more conditions possessed 59% greater odds (OR = 1.59; 95%CI [1.19–2.13]).

10.9 Conclusions and Recommendations

Pre-surgical depression involving self-harm, psychiatric hospitalization or antidepressant use increases risk for post-surgical suicidality; individuals reporting such a history should be monitored following surgery and may benefit from ongoing

Table 10.2 Evidence and recommendations regarding associations between preoperative psychiatric diagnoses and postoperative outcomes

Preoperative diagnosis	Association	Grade of evidence	Recommendation	Strength of recommendation
Major Depressive Disorder	Postoperative self-harm/ suicidality/ hospitalization for depression	Low	Monitor patients with a lifetime history of depression involving suicidality, psychiatric hospitalization, or antidepressant use for psychological complications during postoperative recovery.	Weak
SMI	Readmission	Very Low	Monitor patients with a lifetime history of Bipolar Disorder or Schizophrenia Spectrum Disorder following surgery.	Weak
Alcohol Use Disorder	Postoperative substance use	Very Low	Patients with a history of AUD should be provided psychoeducation on risk for post-surgical alcohol abuse and be monitored for relapse following surgery.	Weak

SMI Serious mental illness, *AUD* Alcohol use disorder

treatment to reduce risk of psychiatric complications (Table 10.2). Though limited, preliminary evidence suggests relationships between SMI and post-surgical service utilization. Individuals diagnosed with Bipolar Disorder or Schizophrenia Spectrum Disorders should be monitored for psychological complications that may negatively impact adherence after surgery. Patients with a history of alcohol use disorder should be provided psychoeducation on risk for relapse following surgery and may benefit from ongoing post-surgical monitoring. There is currently inadequate evidence for post-surgical risk associated with anxiety and substance use disorders although best practice would suggest the importance of stability prior to surgery and ongoing assessment and treatment.

10.10   Personal View of the Data

Bariatric surgery patients are more psychiatrically vulnerable than non-treatment seeking patients with severe obesity or the general population and psychiatric complications of suicide, self-harm and substance use disorders are of great concern. Our knowledge of outcomes is based on patients who were deemed psychiatrically stable and appropriate for surgery. The strength of the preceding associations may be greater if psychological evaluation and treatment were not a standard component of pre-surgical preparation. In making determinations about psychological candidacy for surgery, the risks of psychiatric complications must be balanced with the myriad of health and quality of life benefits resulting from bariatric procedures. However, the preceding summary highlights the importance of ongoing monitoring and treatment of patients at higher risk rather than only utilizing psychological services preoperatively.

Recommendation Summary

1. Patients with a lifetime history of depression involving suicidality, psychiatric hospitalization, or antidepressant use should be monitored for psychological complications during postoperative recovery (Evidence quality low; weak recommendation).
2. Those diagnosed with Bipolar Disorder or Schizophrenia Spectrum Disorder should be monitored following surgery, with attention to psychological complications that might negatively impact adherence (Evidence quality very low; weak recommendation).
3. Patients with a history of alcohol use disorder should be monitored for alcohol misuse following surgery and may benefit from psychoeducation and/or relapse prevention treatment (Evidence quality very low; weak recommendation).

References

1. Mitchell JE, Selzer F, Kalarchian MA, Devlin MJ, Strain GW, Elder KA, et al. Psychopathology before surgery in the longitudinal assessment of bariatric surgery-3 (LABS-3) psychosocial study. Surg Obes Relat Dis. 2012;8(5):533–41. https://doi.org/10.1016/j.soard.2012.07.001.
2. de Zwaan M, Enderle J, Wagner S, Mühlhans B, Ditzen B, Gefeller O, et al. Anxiety and depression in bariatric surgery patients: a prospective, follow-up study using structured clinical interviews. J Affect Disord. 2011;133(1-2):61–8. https://doi.org/10.1016/j.jad.2011.03.025.
3. Karlsson J, Taft C, Rydén A, Sjöström L, Sullivan M. Ten-year trends in health-related quality of life after surgical and conventional treatment for severe obesity: the SOS intervention study. Int J Obes. 2007;31(8):1248–61. https://doi.org/10.1038/sj.ijo.0803573.
4. Nasirzadeh Y, Kantarovich K, Wnuk S, Okrainec A, Cassin SE, Hawa R, et al. Binge eating, loss of control over eating, emotional eating, and night eating after bariatric surgery: results from the Toronto Bari-PSYCH Cohort Study. Obes Surg. 2018;28(7):2032–9. https://doi.org/10.1007/s11695-018-3137-8.
5. Tindle HA, Omalu B, Courcoulas A, Marcus M, Hammers J, Kuller LH. Risk of suicide after long-term follow-up from bariatric surgery. Am J Med. 2010a;123(11):1036–42. https://doi.org/10.1016/j.amjmed.2010.06.016.
6. King WC, Chen JY, Mitchell JE, Kalarchian MA, Steffen KJ, Engel SG, et al. Prevalence of alcohol use disorders before and after bariatric surgery. JAMA. 2012;307(23):2516–25. https://doi.org/10.1001/jama.2012.6147.
7. Conason A, Teixeira J, Hsu CH, Puma L, Knafo D, Geliebter A. Substance use following bariatric weight loss surgery. JAMA Surg. 2013;148(2):145–50. https://doi.org/10.1001/2013.jamasurg.265.
8. Mechanick JI, Apovian C, Brethauer S, Garvey WT, Joffe AM, Kim J, et al. Clinical practice guidelines for the perioperative nutrition, metabolic, and nonsurgical support of patients undergoing bariatric procedures–2019 update: cosponsored by American Association of Clinical Endocrinologists/American College of Endocrinology, The Obesity Society, American Society for Metabolic & Bariatric Surgery, Obesity Medicine Association, and American Society

of Anesthesiologists. Surg Obes Relat Dis. 2019 Nov 4 [cited 2019 Dec 30]. https://doi.org/10.1016/j.soard.2019.10.025. [Epub ahead of print].

9. Wnuk S, Parvez N, Hawa R, Sockalingam S. Predictors of suicidal ideation one-year post-bariatric surgery: results from the Toronto Bari-Psych Cohort Study. Gen Hosp Psychiatry. 2018 Nov 26 [cited 2019 Dec 30]. https://doi.org/10.1016/j.genhosppsych.2018.11.007. [Epub ahead of print].

10. Konttinen H, Sjöholm K, Jacobson P, Svensson PA, Carlsson LMS, Peltonen M. Prediction of suicide and nonfatal self-harm after bariatric surgery: a risk score based on sociodemographic factors, lifestyle behavior, and mental health: a nonrandomized controlled trial. Ann Surg. 2019 Dec 10 [cited 2019 Dec 30]. https://doi.org/10.1097/SLA.0000000000003742. [Epub ahead of print].

11. Thereaux J, Lesuffleur T, Czernichow S, Basdevant A, Msika S, Nocca D, et al. Long-term adverse events after sleeve gastrectomy or gastric bypass: a 7-year nationwide, observational, population-based, cohort study. Lancet Diabetes Endocrinol. 2019;7(10):786–95. https://doi.org/10.1016/S2213-8587(19)30191-3.

12. Gordon KH, King WC, White GE, Belle SH, Courcoulas AP, Ebel FE, et al. A longitudinal examination of suicide-related thoughts and behaviors among bariatric surgery patients. Surg Obes Relat Dis. 2019;15(2):269–78. https://doi.org/10.1016/j.soard.2018.12.001.

13. Lagerros YT, Brandt L, Hedberg J, Sundbom M, Bodén R. Suicide, self-harm, and depression after gastric bypass surgery: a nationwide cohort study. Ann Surg. 2017;265(2):235–43. https://doi.org/10.1097/SLA.0000000000001884.

14. Morgan DJ, Ho KM. Incidence and risk factors for deliberate self-harm, mental illness, and suicide following bariatric surgery: a state-wide population-based linked-data cohort study. Ann Surg. 2017;265(2):244–52. https://doi.org/10.1097/SLA.0000000000001891.

15. Morgan DJ, Ho KM, Platell C. Incidence and determinants of mental health service use after bariatric surgery. JAMA Psychiat. 2019 Sept 25 [cited 2019 Dec 30]. https://doi.org/10.1001/jamapsychiatry.2019.2741. [Epub ahead of print].

16. Bhatti JA, Nathens AB, Thiruchelvam D, Grantcharov T, Goldstein BI, Redelmeier DA. Self-harm emergencies after bariatric surgery: a population-based cohort study. JAMA Surg. 2016;151(3):226–32. https://doi.org/10.1001/jamasurg.2015.3414.

17. Telem DA, Talamini M, Gesten F, Patterson W, Peoples B, Gracia G, et al. Hospital admissions greater than 30 days following bariatric surgery: patient and procedure matter. Surg Endosc. 2015;29(6):1310–5. https://doi.org/10.1007/s00464-014-3834-x.

18. Jalilvand A, Dewire J, Detty A, Needleman B, Noria S. Baseline psychiatric diagnoses are associated with early readmissions and long hospital length of stay after bariatric surgery. Surg Endosc. 2019;33(5):1661–6. https://doi.org/10.1007/s00464-018-6459-7.

19. Litz M, Rigby A, Rogers AM, Leslie DL, Hollenbeak CS. The impact of mental health disorders on 30-day readmission after bariatric surgery. Surg Obes Relat Dis. 2018;14(3):325–31. https://doi.org/10.1016/j.soard.2017.11.030.

20. Fisher D, Coleman KJ, Arterburn DE, Fischer H, Yamamoto A, Young DR, et al. Mental illness in bariatric surgery: a cohort study from the PORTAL network. Obesity (Silver Spring). 2017;25(5):850–6. https://doi.org/10.1002/oby.21814.

21. Ho K, Hawa R, Wnuk S, Okrainec A, Jackson T, Sockalingam S. The psychosocial effects of perioperative complications after bariatric surgery. Psychosomatics. 2018;59(5):452–63. https://doi.org/10.1016/j.psym.2018.03.005.

22. Mitchell JE, King WC, Chen JY, Devlin MJ, Flum D, Garcia L, et al. Course of depressive symptoms and treatment in the longitudinal assessment of bariatric surgery (LABS-2) study. Obesity (Silver Spring). 2014;22(8):1799–806. https://doi.org/10.1002/oby.20738.

23. Mitchell JE, Steffen K, Engel S, King WC, Chen JY, Winters K, et al. Addictive disorders after Roux-en-Y gastric bypass. Surg Obes Relat Dis. 2015;11(4):897–905. https://doi.org/10.1016/j.soard.2014.10.026.

24. King WC, Chen JY, Courcoulas AP, Dakin GF, Engel SG, Flum DR, et al. Alcohol and other substance use after bariatric surgery: prospective evidence from a U.S. multicenter cohort study. Surg Obes Relat Dis. 2017;13(8):1392–402. https://doi.org/10.1016/j.soard.2017.03.021.

25. Ibrahim N, Alameddine M, Brennan J, Sessine M, Holliday C, Ghaferi, AA. New onset alcohol use disorder following bariatric surgery. Surg Endosc. 2019;33(8):2521–30. https://doi.org/10.1007/s00464-018-6545-x.
26. Benotti P, Wood GC, Winegar DA, Petrick AT, Still CD, Argyropoulos G, Gerhard GS. Risk factors associated with mortality after Roux-en-Y gastric bypass surgery. Ann Surg. 2014;259(1):123–30. https://doi.org/10.1097/SLA.0b013e31828a0ee4.
27. Sakran N, Sherf-Dagan S, Blumenfeld O, Romano-Zelekha O, Raziel A, Keren D, et al. Incidence and risk factors for mortality following bariatric surgery: a nationwide registry study. Obes Surg. 2018;28(9):2661–9. https://doi.org/10.1007/s11695-018-3212-1.
28. Raebel MA, Newcomer SR, Bayliss EA, Boudreau D, DeBar L, Elliott TE, et al. Chronic opioid use emerging after bariatric surgery. Pharmacoepidemiol Drug Saf. 2014;23(12):1247–57. https://doi.org/10.1002/pds.3625.
29. Smith ME, Lee JS, Bonham A, Varban OA, Finks JF, Carlin AM, et al. Effect of new persistent opioid use on physiologic and psychologic outcomes following bariatric surgery. Surg Endosc. 2019;33(8):2649–56. https://doi.org/10.1007/s00464-018-6542-0.
30. Spaniolas K, Yang J, Crowley S, Yin D, Docimo S, Bates AT, et al. Association of long-term anastomotic ulceration after Roux-en-Y gastric bypass with tobacco smoking. JAMA Surg. 2018;153(9):862–4. https://doi.org/10.1001/jamasurg.2018.1616.
31. Cuellar-Barboza AB, Frye MA, Grothe K, Prieto ML, Schneekloth TD, Loukianova LL, et al. Change in consumption patterns for treatment-seeking patients with alcohol use disorder post-bariatric surgery. J Psychosom Res. 2015;78(3):199–204. https://doi.org/10.1016/j.jpsychores.2014.06.019.
32. Weiss AC, Parina R, Horgan S, Talamini M, Chang DC, Sandler B. Quality and safety in obesity surgery-15 years of Roux-en-Y gastric bypass outcomes from a longitudinal database. Surg Obes Relat Dis. 2016;12(1):33–40. https://doi.org/10.1016/j.soard.2015.04.018.
33. Gribsholt SB, Thomsen RW, Svensson E, Richelsen B. Overall and cause-specific mortality after Roux-en-Y gastric bypass surgery: a nationwide cohort study. Surg Obes Relat Dis. 2017;13(4):581–7. https://doi.org/10.1016/j.soard.2016.10.007.
34. Altieri MS, Pryor A, Yang J, Yin D, Docimo S, Bates A, et al. The natural history of perforated marginal ulcers after gastric bypass surgery. Surg Endosc. 2018;32(3):1215–22. https://doi.org/10.1007/s00464-017-5794-4.
35. Neovius M, Bruze G, Jacobson P, Sjöholm K, Johansson K, Granath F, et al. Risk of suicide and non-fatal self-harm after bariatric surgery: results from two matched cohort studies. Lancet Diabetes Endocrinol. 2018;6(3):197–207. https://doi.org/10.1016/S2213-8587(17)30437-0.
36. King WC, Chen JY, Belle SH, Courcoulas AP, Dakin GF, Flum DR, et al. Use of prescribed opioids before and after bariatric surgery: prospective evidence from a U.S. multicenter cohort study. Surg Obes Relat Dis. 2017;13(8):1337–46. https://doi.org/10.1016/j.soard.2017.04.003.

Does Weight Loss Prior to Surgery Accurately Predict Success Following Bariatric Surgery?

11

Maria E. Linnaus and Tammy Lyn Kindel

11.1 Introduction

Preoperative weight loss (PWL) or supervised medical weight management in the setting of bariatric surgery has been a strongly debated topic since many insurance companies have mandated it as a requirement for reimbursement for bariatric surgery. It is the position of the American Society for Metabolic and Bariatric Surgery (ASMBS) that while PWL may be beneficial from a technical standpoint, it should not be a requirement for surgery and certainly should not limit access to vital life-saving surgical options [1]. There have also been studies demonstrating great heterogeneity in the ability of severely obese patients to lose weight even when mandatory diets are prescribed preoperatively [2, 3]. The data regarding mandatory preoperative weight loss have historically been weak and few high-level studies exist to characterize the role of PWL. The aim of this review is to evaluate the most current literature regarding PWL (defined as weight loss which is required and mandated before bariatric surgery will be scheduled) to determine its necessity in improving surgical outcomes, specifically:

1. Does PWL improve the success of bariatric surgery on metabolic disease resolution?
2. Does PWL improve the success of bariatric surgery on weight loss?
3. Does PWL improve the success of bariatric surgery on post-operative 30-day morbidity?

M. E. Linnaus · T. L. Kindel (✉)
Department of Surgery, Medical College of Wisconsin, Wauwatosa, WI, USA
e-mail: tkindel@mcw.edu

© Springer Nature Switzerland AG 2021
J. Alverdy, Y. Vigneswaran (eds.), *Difficult Decisions in Bariatric Surgery*,
Difficult Decisions in Surgery: An Evidence-Based Approach,
https://doi.org/10.1007/978-3-030-55329-6_11

11.2   Methods/Search Strategy

A literature review was performed in three databases, Ovid Medline, Scopus and Web of Science on all journal articles referring to PWL before bariatric surgeries excluding lap-Band and vertical banded gastroplasty from 2004–2019. The search was performed on November 13, 2019. Terms utilized for the search included "bariatric surgery," "stomach stapling," "metabolic surgery," "gastric bypass," "sleeve gastrectomy," "gastroplast" "gastroplasty," "jejunoileal bypass," AND "weight loss," "diet," "caloric restriction," "reducing diet" AND "preoperative period" or "preoperat" or "preoperative care." A total of 643 articles were identified. Articles were excluded if they were not in the English language, if full-text article was not available, or if they were in adolescent bariatric surgery. Case reports and case series were also excluded. Of the 643 articles screened, 151 were selected to be reviewed based on applicability to the topic of PWL in the setting of bariatric surgery. Articles exclusive to a very low-calorie diet used immediately preceding surgery for the purpose of decreasing liver volume were excluded. Of these, an additional 15 articles (including 2 randomized controlled trials) were previously included in three systematic reviews or meta-analyses and therefore were excluded from individual review. A systematic review was excluded due to inclusion of all surgical procedures rather than solely bariatric procedures [4]. The references in this review were screened for any additional articles that may have been missed during database search or manual exclusion. A total of 13 articles remained for evaluation (Table 11.1). There were 0 additional randomized controlled trials outside of the systematic reviews, 2 position statements based on expert opinion, 3 systematic reviews/meta-analyses, 3 retrospective large database reviews, and 5 retrospective studies that were identified for final analysis. Using the GRADE methodology, the data were critically reviewed and summative points described.

11.3   Impact of Preoperative Weight Loss on Postoperative Metabolic Outcomes

Bariatric surgery is known to have a positive effect on metabolic disease, inducing remission of diabetes, hypertension, hyperlipidemia and obstructive sleep apnea. Two-thirds of patients will experience resolution in at least one of their comorbidities at 1 year postoperatively from bariatric surgery [5]. Very few studies have addressed the impact of PWL on metabolic disease outcomes and resolution of comorbidities.

Including commonly performed procedures such as the gastric bypass, duodenal switch and sleeve gastrectomy, there is a paucity of literature evaluating the effect of PWL on obesity-associated comorbid disease resolution. A single institution retrospective review found that there was no difference in comorbidity resolution for those patients who underwent mandated PWL [6]. In fact, the group that underwent mandated PWL were less likely to resolve obstructive sleep apnea when compared to the non-PWL group [6]. Not only does there not appear to be a benefit on

Table 11.1 Pre-operative weight loss studies included for review to create consensus recommendation

Author (year)	N	%EWL	Complication rate	Comorbidity resolution	Study type (quality)
Monfared (2019)	776	ND	NA	ND	Retrospective cohort (low)
Livhits (2009)	3403	Pos	NA	NA	Systematic review (moderate)
Cassie (2011)	6686	ND	Pos	NA	Systematic review (moderate)
Kadeli (2012)	2254	ND	NA	NA	Systematic review (moderate)
Gerber (2016)	9570	Pos	NA	NA	Retrospective database (low)
Chinaka (2019)	155	ND	NA	NA	Retrospective cohort (low)
Krimpuri (2018)	218	ND	NA	NA	Retrospective cohort (low)
Parmar (2018)	192	ND	ND	NA	Retrospective cohort (low)
Steinbeisser (2017)	204	Pos	NA	NA	Retrospective cohort (low)
Anderin (2015)	22,327	NA	Pos	NA	Retrospective database (low)
Tewksbury (2019)	394,016	ND—at 30 days	Neg	NA	Retrospective database (low)

Pos PWL had a positive effect, *Neg* PWL had a negative effect, *ND* PWL made no difference, *NA* not assessed

co-morbidity resolution but also mandated PWL results in higher attrition and detrimental progression of comorbid conditions while awaiting surgical treatment of obesity [1, 7]. Due to a lack of evidence-based support of PWL, it is the position of the ASMBS that mandated PWL deters patients from receiving potentially life-saving therapies [1].

There is a paucity of low quality evidence studying the impact of PWL on comorbidity resolution. Expert opinion and consensus guidelines advocate against mandatory use of PWL for comorbidity resolution as it may lead to progression of comorbid conditions while awaiting surgical intervention.

11.4 Impact of Preoperative Weight Loss on Postoperative Weight Loss

Weight loss outcomes have been a focus of the literature surrounding PWL in bariatric surgery. Even with this, there are still only a few studies addressing this question. One of the largest systematic reviews and meta-analyses found a significant correlation between PWL and postoperative excess weight loss (EWL) at

1 year when data were pooled [8]. This data showing favorable outcomes for EWL assessed weight loss from the initial encounter rather than from the time of surgery. Another systematic review and meta-analysis found no difference in EWL at 1 year postoperatively when data were pooled [9]. At 2 years postoperatively, the EWL was significantly higher in the group that did not have PWL [9]. Similar to the Livhits et al. review, there was significant heterogeneity among the studies, specifically regarding the time period defined as PWL as the time point used for the initial weight (initial consult compared to day of surgery). In this review, there were 9 articles that reported a positive effect of PWL on postoperative weight loss while 15 demonstrated no significant difference. Yet another systematic review by Kadeli et al. found that losing weight prior to surgery contributes to more overall weight loss but that there is no significant difference in percent EWL postoperatively [10].

A large database study out of the Scandinavian Obesity Registry contrasts these findings [11]. Patients were classified into quartiles by their PWL. They demonstrated that patients achieving the 75th percentile (greater than 8.6%) for weight change preoperatively had 15% increased weight loss at 1-year postoperatively compared to those patients who achieved the 25th percentile [11]. However, it should be noted that those included in the 75th percentile started at the highest BMI with a median of 49 while the 25th percentile ranged as low as 33 for starting BMI [11].

There are a few retrospective studies that found no impact of PWL on postoperative weight loss. In a single institution retrospective review, patients without a weight loss goal prior to surgery compared to those with a weight loss goal demonstrated equal change in BMI 4 years out from surgery [6]. However, 1-year follow-up data were not expressed [6]. In a 10-year longitudinal retrospective cohort study, patients were categorized into two groups: able to achieve target 5% weight loss preoperatively or unable to achieve target 5% weight loss preoperatively [12]. They demonstrated that nearly one-fourth of patients were unable to achieve the 5% target. The study then compared the two groups and analyzed the postoperative weight loss results. They found that there was no significant difference in weight loss at 1 year between the two groups [12]. Another review found on univariate analysis that PWL was a significant predictor of 1-year weight loss outcomes [13]. However, on multivariate analysis there was no significant difference and therefore the authors concluded that demographics play a significant role [13]. Another review exclusive to sleeve gastrectomy found that PWL was not associated with significantly different PWL at 1 year [14]. Conversely, another retrospective review found that patients undergoing sleeve gastrectomy lost 7% more of the excess body weight when they were able to achieve 5% or greater PWL [15].

The data are conflicting regarding the efficacy of PWL on 1-year postoperative weight loss outcomes. There are a few low-quality studies which support the use of PWL for 1 year weight loss outcomes. More randomized trials are needed to confirm or dispute the efficacy of PWL on postoperative weight loss outcomes.

11.5 Impact of Preoperative Weight Loss on 30-Day Morbidity

One of the biggest cited reasons for mandatory PWL, particularly in the very high BMI population, is a decrease in technical difficulties during the operation and increased perioperative safety. However, despite this adage, few high-level studies are available to support this. In a systematic review, operative times were noted to be shortened for those patients undergoing PWL but the clinical significance of this is unknown and the data had significant heterogeneity [9]. The majority of studies included in this review reported no difference in complication rates after bariatric surgery; however, when data were pooled, a small decrease in the complication rate after PWL was noted as compared to those patients who did not undergo PWL ($18.8\% \pm 10.6\%$ vs. $21.4\% \pm 13.1\%$, $p = 0.02$) [9]. Complications were not further delineated. A large database study out of the Scandinavian Obesity Registry reported a decrease in anastomotic leak in patients who were in the 75th percentile of PWL, correlating to a greater than 7% weight loss preoperatively [16]. Additionally, they reported a decreased risk of deep space infections/abscess and minor wound infections for patients achieving 50th to 75th percentile weight loss preoperatively [16]. Although conversion to an open procedure is rare, patients with PWL have a lower risk of requiring conversion to an open operation when compared to those with minimal PWL [16]. Because of this, the authors strongly advocate for use of PWL [16].

Another systematic review and meta-analysis supports the finding of shorter operative time in the PWL groups by nearly 25 min [8] as compared to 12.5 min in the other systematic review [9]. Significant differences were reportedly not found in studies assessing complications rates between PWL and those without PWL and there may be evidence citing an increase in complication rate amongst patients who had PWL [8].

In another analysis, reintervention was utilized as a surrogate marker of morbidity between sleeve and gastric bypass patients [6]. No difference was noted between those with PWL and without PWL [6]. A large cohort study from the MBSAQIP demonstrated that PWL increased the risk of surgical site infection and urinary tract infection [17]. Preoperative weight loss was defined as a change in the highest weight and BMI within 1 year of surgery compared to the immediate preoperative BMI [17]. There were no other differences in 30 day postoperative morbidity reported [17].

Low level evidence (retrospective cohort studies) suggest PWL decrease operative times but this may be negated by an increase in post-operative complications. Higher level evidence including systematic reviews and meta-analyses which include randomized controlled trials fail to demonstrate a benefit to PWL in decreasing 30 day morbidity. Additional randomized controlled trials are needed to determine the benefit of PWL on postoperative morbidity.

11.6 Recommendations

- Preoperative medical weight loss is not recommended to improve post-operative weight loss, metabolic disease, or decrease surgical morbidity (Evidence quality low; weak recommendation)

11.7 Personal View of the Literature

Through this literature review, it is apparent that there is great variability in the definitions of PWL and this can contribute to inconsistent results within the literature. The natural history of dieting attempts for patients with severe obesity is that of obesity resistance and recidivism due not to lack of will power and compliance, but to complex counter-regulatory mechanisms against weight loss in the obese state including decreased satiety, enhanced hunger and depressed metabolism. As the satiety and metabolism mechanisms initiated by bariatric surgery counter those found with dieting (and thus lead to the success of the surgery), physiologically it does not make sense to mandate a patient once again undergo a medical weight loss attempt, instead of moving them forward once they have been educated and medically prepared for surgery. Further, as bariatric surgery transitions from weight loss focused to metabolic disease focused, it is imperative not to impede a patient's ability to undergo medically necessary metabolic surgery due to failed PWL with arbitrary weight loss goals. Metabolic surgery in its current state, without PWL, is exceptionally safe and is the most efficacious treatment of obesity-associated comorbidities. At best, PWL, if documented in prospective, balanced studies to enhance metabolic disease outcomes, could be encouraged to maximize metabolic responsiveness, but never mandated.

References

1. Kim JJ, Rogers AM, Ballem N, Schirmer B. American Society for M, Bariatric Surgery Clinical Issues C. ASMBS updated position statement on insurance mandated preoperative weight loss requirements. Surg Obes Relat Dis. 2016;12(5):955–9.
2. Keith CJ Jr, Goss LE, Blackledge CD, Stahl RD, Grams J. Insurance-mandated preoperative diet and outcomes after bariatric surgery. Surg Obes Relat Dis. 2018;14(5):631–6.
3. Schneider A, Hutcheon DA, Hale A, Ewing JA, Miller M, Scott JD. Postoperative outcomes in bariatric surgical patients participating in an insurance-mandated preoperative weight management program. Surg Obes Relat Dis. 2018;14(5):623–30.
4. Roman M, Monaghan A, Serraino GF, et al. Meta-analysis of the influence of lifestyle changes for preoperative weight loss on surgical outcomes. Br J Surg. 2019;106(3):181–9.
5. Conaty EA, Bonamici NJ, Gitelis ME, et al. Efficacy of a required preoperative weight loss program for patients undergoing bariatric surgery. J Gastrointest Surg. 2016;20(4):667–73.
6. Monfared S, Athanasiadis DI, Furiya A, et al. Do mandated weight loss goals prior to bariatric surgery improve postoperative outcomes? Obes Surg. 2019;09:09.
7. Brethauer S. ASMBS Position Statement on Preoperative Supervised Weight Loss Requirements. Surg Obes Relat Dis. 2011;7(3):257–60.

8. Livhits M, Mercado C, Yermilov I, et al. Does weight loss immediately before bariatric surgery improve outcomes: a systematic review. Surg Obes Relat Dis. 2009;5(6):713–21.
9. Cassie S, Menezes C, Birch DW, Shi X, Karmali S. Effect of preoperative weight loss in bariatric surgical patients: a systematic review. Surg Obes Relat Dis. 2011;7(6):760–7; discussion 767.
10. Kadeli DK, Sczepaniak JP, Kumar K, Youssef C, Mahdavi A, Owens M. The effect of preoperative weight loss before gastric bypass: a systematic review. J Obes. 2012;2012:867540.
11. Gerber P, Anderin C, Gustafsson UO, Thorell A. Weight loss before gastric bypass and postoperative weight change: data from the Scandinavian Obesity Registry (SOReg). Surg Obes Relat Dis. 2016;12(3):556–62.
12. Chinaka U, Fultang J, Ali A. Does preoperative weight loss predict significant postoperative weight loss among patients who underwent laparoscopic sleeve gastrectomy? Cureus. 2019;11(10).
13. Krimpuri RD, Yokley JM, Seeholzer EL, Horwath EL, Thomas CL, Bardaro SJ. Qualifying for bariatric surgery: is preoperative weight loss a reliable predictor of postoperative weight loss? Surg Obes Relat Dis. 2018;14(1):60–4.
14. Parmar AD, Drosdeck JM, Mattar SG, Spight D, Husain FA. Impact of preoperative weight loss on postoperative weight loss after sleeve gastrectomy. Bariatric Surg Pract Patient Care. 2018;13(2):69–74.
15. Steinbeisser M, McCracken J, Kharbutli B. Laparoscopic sleeve gastrectomy: preoperative weight loss and other factors as predictors of postoperative success. Obes Surg. 2017;27(6):1508–13.
16. Anderin C, Gustafsson UO, Heijbel N, Thorell A. Weight loss before bariatric surgery and postoperative complications: data from the Scandinavian Obesity Registry (SOReg). Ann Surg. 2015;261(5):909–13.
17. Tewksbury C, Crowley N, Parrott JM, et al. Weight loss prior to bariatric surgery and 30-day mortality, readmission, reoperation, and intervention: an MBSAQIP analysis of 349,016 cases. Obes Surg. 2019;21:21.

Optimization Prior to Knee and Hip Arthroplasty as an Indication for Bariatric Surgery

Alexander S. McLawhorn and David C. Landy

12.1 Introduction

Symptomatic osteoarthritis (OA) of the knee affects roughly 15% of United States population over 60 years of age [1] and is strongly associated with obesity where a 5 kg/m^2 change in BMI predicts a 35% increased risk OA [2]. For many patients, OA symptoms can significantly limit their activity and quality of life [3, 4]. A recent study found that over 10% of patients of waiting for a total joint arthroplasty in the United Kingdom had a health state described as worse than death using the EuroQol five-dimension general health questionnaire [5]. While non-operative management strategies including physical therapy, assist devices, bracing, oral medications, and injections can help limit the symptoms of osteoarthritis, joint replacement known as arthroplasty is the only treatment which addresses the underlying pathology and remains the only surgical option for patients who have failed to obtain satisfactory quality of life with non-operative measures.

Of the population greater than 50 years of age in the United States, 4.5% have had a total knee arthroplasty (TKA) and 2.3% have had a total hip arthroplasty (THA) [6]. Each year in the, over one million TKA and THA procedures are performed in the United States and this rate is expected to increase to nearly two million annually by 2030 [7]. Of patients undergoing TKA and THA, over half are obese and this proportion is increasing [8]. Unfortunately, obese patients undergoing TKA and THA are at significantly increased risks of complications including infection and need for revision [9, 10]. This has spurred consideration and even implementation at some centers of BMI cut-offs [11, 12] and interest in weight loss programs including consideration of bariatric surgery to potentially reduce these risks [13, 14].

A. S. McLawhorn (✉) · D. C. Landy
Hospital for Special Surgery, New York, NY, USA
e-mail: mclawhorna@hss.edu

© Springer Nature Switzerland AG 2021
J. Alverdy, Y. Vigneswaran (eds.), *Difficult Decisions in Bariatric Surgery*,
Difficult Decisions in Surgery: An Evidence-Based Approach,
https://doi.org/10.1007/978-3-030-55329-6_12

Table 12.1 Articles reporting association between bariatric surgery and total knee arthroplasty Outcomes

Article	Data Source	Comparison	Outcome
National or State Database Analyses (NHS, Medicare, and New York State)			
Werner et al. (2015) [15]	Medicare	Morbidly obese patients not having undergone bariatric surgery without additional adjustment	Bariatric surgery prior to TKA was associated with a significantly lower 90-day rate of major medical complications
Nickel et al. (2016) [16]	Medicare	Morbidly obese patients not having undergone bariatric surgery without additional adjustment	Bariatric surgery prior to TKA was associated with a significantly higher rate of 30-day medical complications and significantly higher rates of orthopedic complications
Lee et al. (2018) [17]	Medicare	Patients not having undergone bariatric surgery and adjusted for demographic and clinical characteristics using regression	Bariatric surgery prior to TKA was associated with a significantly lower periprosthetic infection rate but a significantly higher revision rate
McLawhorn et al. (2018) [18]	New York	Morbidly obese patients not having undergone bariatric surgery and matched on demographic and clinical factors using propensity scoring	Bariatric surgery prior to TKA was associated with reduced in-hospital and 90-day post-operative complications but not associated with revision
Individual Institution Analyses			
Severson et al. (2012) [19]	Mayo Clinic	Obese patients undergoing TKA before bariatric surgery with no additional adjustment	Bariatric surgery prior to TKA was not associated with 90-day complications or revision
Martin et al. (2015) [20]	Mayo Clinic	Patients not having undergone bariatric surgery were matched by age, sex, date of surgery, and BMI (a comparison group for both pre- and post-bariatric surgery BMI)	Bariatric surgery prior to TKA was associated with a higher re-operation rate compared to both groups and a higher revision rate and peri-prosthetic infection rate compared to the post-bariatric surgery BMI group

In this chapter, we review the available literature surrounding patient optimization prior to TKA and THA as an indication for bariatric surgery (Tables 12.1, 12.2, 12.3).

12.2   Search Strategy

When PubMed was searched using medical subject headings (MeSH) terms for hip osteoarthritis or knee osteoarthritis combined with bariatric surgery, only 26 results were returned. When the search was broadened by replacing the specific terms for

Table 12.2 Articles reporting association between bariatric surgery and total hip arthroplasty outcomes

Article	Data Source	Comparison	Outcome
National or State Database Analyses (NHS, Medicare, and New York State)			
Lee et al. (2018) [17]	Medicare	Patients not having undergone bariatric surgery and adjusted for demographic and clinical characteristics using regression	Bariatric surgery prior to THA was significantly associated with higher periprosthetic infection rates and non-statistically significantly with higher revision rates
Nickel et al. (2018) [21]	Medicare	Morbidly obese patients not having undergone bariatric surgery without additional adjustment	Bariatric surgery prior to THA was not associated with 90-day post-operative medical complications or infection but was associated with higher revision and dislocation rates at 90 days.
McLawhorn et al. (2018) [18]	New York	Morbidly obese patients not having undergone bariatric surgery and matched on demographic and clinical factors using propensity scoring	Bariatric surgery prior to THA was associated with lower in-hospital complications but not 90-day post-operative complications or revision rates.
Individual Institution Analyses			
Watts et al. (2016) [22]	Mayo Clinic	Patients not having undergone bariatric surgery were matched by age, sex, date of surgery, and pre-bariatric surgery BMI)	Bariatric surgery prior to THA was associated with a significantly lower revision rate and non-significantly lower periprosthetic infection rate

hip and knee osteoarthritis with the MeSH term for generic arthritis, 98 results were returned which entirely subsumed the prior 26 results. These 98 unique articles as well as their references were reviewed.

12.3   Results

12.3.1 Analyses of National and State Databases

Kulkarni et al. used the Hospital Episode Statistics database to identify all patients who were obese and underwent both bariatric surgery and either TKA or THA between 2005 and 2009 in the NHS [23]. Patients who underwent both procedures within 6 months were excluded and patients undergoing THA and TKA were combined. The 90 patients who underwent their bariatric surgery prior to total joint arthroplasty (TJA) were compared to 53 patients who underwent TJA prior to their bariatric surgery without further adjustment. While the differences between groups did reach statistical significance, patients who had bariatric surgery first appeared to

Table 12.3 Articles reporting association between bariatric surgery and combined total knee and hip arthroplasty outcomes

Article	Data Source	Comparison	Outcome
National or State Database Analyses (NHS, Medicare, and New York State)			
Kulkarni et al. (2011) [23]	NHS	Obese patients undergoing TKA or THA before bariatric surgery were combined with no stratification or additional adjustment	Bariatric surgery prior to TJA was associated with a non-statistically significant lower rate of 30-day joint infection and 30-day readmission
Individual Institution Analyses			
Inacio et al. (2014) [24]	Kaiser Permanente	Patients not having undergone bariatric surgery but who could have due to a BMI over 40 or a BMI over 35 and another comorbidity with no additional adjustment or formal statistical comparisons	Bariatric surgery prior to TJA was not obviously associated with 90-day readmission or revision rates
Nearing et al. (2017) [25]	La Crosse, WI	Obese patients undergoing TKA or THA before bariatric surgery with no additional adjustment	Bariatric surgery prior to TJA was not associated with 30-day complication rates though there was a non-statistically significant association with increased manipulation rates and decreased revision rates

be at a lower risk of 30-day joint infection, 1.1% compared to 3.7%, and 30-day readmission, 1.1% compared to 7.5%.

Werner et al. used the PearlDiver platform to identify all patients undergoing TKA from 2005 to 2011 within the Medicare data [15]. These patients were grouped by the presence of morbid obesity based on ICD-9 diagnoses codes, and the morbidly obese patients were further subdivided by having had bariatric surgery, including laparoscopic banding or gastric bypass, using CPT codes. In total, 219 patients were identified as having undergone bariatric surgery prior to TKA and these patients were compared to 11,294 morbidly obese patients who were not known to have undergone bariatric surgery. The demographics of these patients were significantly different with 64% of the bariatric surgery group under 65 years of age compared to only 19% of patients without a known bariatric surgery history. The prevalence of coded medical comorbidities also significantly varied between groups such as with 62% of the bariatric surgery group having sleep apnea compared to only 37% of patients without a known bariatric surgery history. Though analyses did not adjust for these differences between groups, patients having undergone bariatric surgery were significantly less likely to have had major medical complications in the 90-days following their TKA compared to patients without a known bariatric surgery history, 10% versus 19%.

Interestingly, a separate study by Nickel et al. also using the PearlDiver platform to identify patients within the Medicare data who had a TKA for osteoarthritis from 2005 to 2010 reported different results [16]. They compared 5,918 patients who had a history of bariatric surgery prior to TKA to 26,616 patients who had a BMI over 40 but had not undergone bariatric surgery. Again, the demographics and comorbidity profiles of the patient groups were significantly different. Though analyses did not adjust for these differences, patients having undergone bariatric surgery were significantly more likely to have had medical complications in the 30-days following their TKA compared to patients without a history of bariatric surgery including specifically for venous thromboembolism, pneumonia, and myocardial infarction. This study also reported that the patients having undergone bariatric surgery were significantly more likely to have had an orthopedic complication with their TKA at 2-years follow-up compared to patients without a history of bariatric surgery including infection, extensor mechanism rupture, and osteolysis. The authors of this second study attributed their disparate findings to methodological differences introduced in patient identification within the underlying database.

Lee et al. also used Medicare data but limited their analysis to only patients 65 years of age or over who underwent either TKA or THA from 1999 to 2012 [17]. They then identified patients who had bariatric surgery in the past 2 years and compared them to other patients using a regression model to adjust for medical comorbidities and other patient characteristics such as age, sex, and socioeconomic status. Patients having undergone bariatric surgery were significantly less likely to have a periprosthetic infection following TKA but were significantly more likely to have revision. The authors did not discuss how these findings related to TKA were disparate from those of Nickel et al. though such differences may again reflect alternate approaches to coding or be due to the use of regression to adjust for other patient factors. Patients having undergone bariatric surgery were significantly more likely to have a periprosthetic infection following THA and also were more likely to have revision though this association did reach statistical significance.

A separate study by Nickel et al. using the PearlDiver platform to identify patients within the Medicare data who had a THA for osteoarthritis from 2005 to 2012 reported somewhat disparate results from the prior Lee et al. study [21]. They compared 1545 patients who had a history of bariatric surgery prior to THA to 6918 patients who had a BMI over 40 but had not undergone bariatric surgery. While demographics and comorbidity profiles of the patient groups were significantly different and not adjusted for, patients having undergone bariatric surgery were similarly likely to have an infection following THA compared to patients without a history of bariatric surgery but were more likely to have a revision or dislocation at both 90 days, 1% compared to 0.4% for dislocation, and at 2 years, 2.5% compared to 0.9% for dislocation. Additionally, the authors looked at medical complications within the first 30 days following THA. Unlike the findings reported by Nickel et al. using similar methods to study patients undergoing TKA, a history of bariatric surgery was not associated with increased medical complications following THA when compared to obese patients without a history of bariatric surgery.

McLawhorn et al. used data from the New York Statewide Planning and Research Cooperative to identify all morbidly obese patients residing in New York State and having a single TKA or THA at a non-federal hospital in New York State between 1997 and 2011 [18]. Propensity scoring was used to match morbidly obese patients receiving bariatric surgery prior to the TKA or THA to those not receiving surgery based on demographic and clinical factors. The 2636 patients having bariatric surgery prior to TKA had a reduced risk of both in hospital complications and 90-day post-operative complications though there was no clinically or statistically significant difference in revision rates with a hazard ratio of 0.90. The 792 patients having bariatric surgery prior to THA had a reduced risk of in hospital complications but not 90-day post-operative complications. For the THA patients, there was also no clinically or statistically significant difference in revision rates with a hazard ratio of 0.91. For both TKA and THA, the most common in-hospital complication was other and the most common 90-day post-operative complication was infection. For TKA but not THA, the bariatric surgery group had a lower 90-day infection rate, 2.4% compared to 1.3%.

12.3.2 Analyses of Individual Institution Data

Severson et al. used data from the Mayo Clinic registry to identify all patients who underwent both bariatric surgery and TKA at May clinic from 1996 to 2008 [19]. They compared the 39 patients who had TKA prior to bariatric surgery to 61 patients who had TKA more than 2 years after bariatric surgery. Limited information was provided regarding the comorbidity profiles of the groups and no statistical adjustments were made to comparisons though at least for age, there were significant differences. While the sample sizes were limited, there were no statistically or obvious clinically significant differences between patients having TKA prior to bariatric surgery compared to patients having TKA 2-years after bariatric surgery with regard to either 90-day complication rates, 21% compared to 16%, or revision, 5% compared to 8%.

In a separate study using data from the Mayo Clinic registry, Martin et al. identified all 91 patients undergoing TKA after bariatric surgery from 1998 to 2012 [20]. These patients were then matched to 91 patients undergoing TKA by the pre-bariatric surgery BMI and to 182 patients undergoing TKA by the post-bariatric surgery BMI. Patients were additionally matched for age, sex, and date of surgery. The rate of re-operation in the bariatric surgery group was higher compared to patients matched on the pre-bariatric surgery BMI, hazard ratio of 2.55, and compared to patients matched on the post-bariatric surgery BMI, hazard ratio of 2.4. The most common reason for re-operation was a manipulation under anesthesia for stiffness. There were no statistically significant differences in revision or periprosthetic infection between patients having bariatric surgery and those matched on pre-bariatric surgery BMI. There were statistically significant increased rates of revision and periprosthetic infection for patients having bariatric surgery compared to those matched on post-bariatric surgery BMI with a hazard ratio for revision of 2.2 and for infection of 2.6.

Watts et al. used data from the Mayo Clinic registry to identify all 42 patients who underwent 47 THAs following bariatric surgery and matched these cases to 94 THAs by pre-bariatric surgery BMI, gender, age, and date of surgery [22]. Revision rates were significantly higher in the patients who had not undergone bariatric surgery with a hazard ratio of 5.4. There was also a non-statistically significant difference in periprosthetic infection rates with a 5-year infection-free survival rate of 96% in the bariatric surgery group compared to 90% in the matched control group.

Inacio et al. used data from Kaiser Permanente to identify all patients who underwent a first, unilateral TKA or THA between 2005 and 2011 for osteoarthritis [24]. They then created three study groups including a group of 69 patients who underwent TJA greater than 2 years after bariatric surgery, a group of 102 patients who underwent TJA within 2 years of bariatric surgery, and a group of 11,032 patients who had not undergone bariatric surgery but could have due to either a BMI over 40 or a BMI over 35 and an additional comorbidity such as diabetes. There were significant differences between the groups with respect to age and comorbidities. Though analyses did not adjust for differences between the groups and no formal statistical comparisons were made, the 90-day readmission rates were 7.2% for patients who had TJA greater than 2 years after bariatric surgery, 2.5% for patients who had TJA within 2 years of bariatric surgery, and 5.9% for the control group who did not undergo bariatric surgery. Similarly, the revision rates were 2.9% for patients who had TJA greater than 2 years after bariatric surgery, 4.9% for patients who had TJA within 2 years of bariatric surgery, and 2.8% for the control group who did not undergo bariatric surgery.

Nearing et al. used data from their hospital system in La Crosse, WI to identify all patients who underwent bariatric surgery and TKA or THA between 2001 and 2014 and then compared the 66 patients who underwent bariatric surgery prior to TJA to the 36 patients who underwent bariatric surgery after TJA [25]. The two groups had relatively similar age, sex, and comorbidity distributions and no adjustments were made to comparisons. There were no significant differences in 30-day complication rates based on the timing of bariatric surgery in relation to TJA. And while these differences did not reach statistical significance, bariatric surgery prior to TJA was associated with increased manipulation rates, 9% compared to 0%, and decreased revision rates, 11% compared to 2%.

12.3.3 Analyses of Secondary Data

McLawhorn et al. evaluated the use of bariatric surgery prior to TKA compared to performing TKA without bariatric surgery using decision analysis methods [26]. They made assumptions regarding the probability of transitioning to one several variable health states for following either bariatric surgery or TKA. Of note, their analysis assumed that bariatric surgery prior to TKA would result in a 66% chance of losing enough weight to assume the risk profile of a nonobese patient and that nonobese patients were 77% less likely to require revision TKA, repeat revision TKA, or chronic failed revision TKA compared to obese patients. The authors also assigned values to the various health states as well estimated costs associated with the various required interventions. In total and based on these assumptions, their data simulation study suggested that bariatric surgery prior to TKA may be cost-effective. In a similar study looking at bariatric surgery prior to THA, Prekumar et al. found bariatric surgery prior to arthroplasty to be cost effective though under similar assumptions [27].

Li et al. performed a meta-analysis including results from many of the studies referenced above to empirically assess the association between bariatric surgery prior to TJA and outcomes [28]. Their search strategy did not include some of the above results, their analyses did not always exclude studies which used a shared data-source such as Medicare data, and some outcomes were not measured consistently across studies. With those limitations in mind, the authors reported that bariatric surgery prior to TJA was associated with lower short-term medical complication rates following both TKA and THA but was not associated with long-term periprosthetic infection rates, dislocation rates, or revision rates.

12.4 Personal View of the Data

The available evidence does not support the use of bariatric surgery for the sole purpose of reducing the risks of complications after TJA. While prior evidence is conflicting regarding whether bariatric surgery significantly modifies the increased risks associated with obesity following TJA, it should be appreciated that patients are not expected to lose significant weight after TJA either [29, 30]. Additionally, some patients may have significant improvement of their arthritic symptoms after bariatric surgery and not require TKA [31, 32]. There is currently an ongoing multicenter observational trial which will provide the first prospective data regarding the association of bariatric surgery prior to planned TKA and outcomes [33]. In the absence of this data, we would encourage both orthopedic surgeons and bariatric surgeons not to be overly optimistic in assuming that bariatric surgery and associated weight loss will translate directly to improved outcomes following TJA. Decision making must be done at the level of the individual patient and should consider the other risks and benefits.

12.5 Recommendations Based on the Data

- We recommend that patients with morbid obesity should not undergo bariatric surgery for the sole purpose of reducing the risk of complications following TJA.
- Especially given the relatively older age of many patients considering TJA, we recommend orthopedic surgeons and bariatric surgeons consider together with patients the scope of potential benefits and risks of bariatric surgery prior to TJA.

References

1. Nguyen US, Zhang Y, Zhu Y, Niu J, Zhang B, Felson DT. Increasing prevalence of knee pain and symptomatic knee osteoarthritis: survey and cohort data. Ann Intern Med. 2011;155:725–32.
2. Zheng H, Chen C. Body mass index and risk of knee osteoarthritis: systematic review and meta-analysis of prospective studies. BMJ Open. 2015;5(12):e007568.

3. Hoogeboom TJ, den Broeder AA, de Bie RA, van den Ende CH. Longitudinal impact of joint pain comorbidity on quality of life and activity levels in knee osteoarthritis: data from the Osteoarthritis Initiative. Rheumatology. 2013;52:543–6.
4. Jeong H, Baek SY, Kim SW, Eun YH, Kim IY, Lee J, Jeon CH, Koh EM, Cha HS. Comorbidities and health-related quality of life in Koreans with knee osteoarthritis: data from the Korean National Health and Nutrition Examination Survey (KNHANES). PLoS One. 2017 Oct;12:e0186141.
5. Scott CEH, MacDonald DJ, Howie CR. 'Worse than death' and waiting for a joint arthroplasty. Bone Joint J. 2019;101-B:941–50.
6. Maradit Kremers H, Larson DR, Crowson CS, Kremers WK, Washington RE, Steiner CA, Jiranek WA, Berry DJ. Prevalence of total hip and knee replacement in the United States. J Bone Joint Surg Am. 2015;97:1386–97.
7. Sloan M, Premkumar A, Sheth NP. Projected volume of primary total joint arthroplasty in the U.S., 2014 to 2030. J Bone Joint Surg Am. 2018;100:1455–60.
8. George J, Klika AK, Navale SM, Newman JM, Barsoum WK, Higuera CA. Obesity epidemic: is its impact on total joint arthroplasty underestimated? An analysis of national trends. Clin Orthop Relat Res. 2017;475:1798–806.
9. Alvi HM, Mednick RE, Krishnan V, Kwasny MJ, Beal MD, Manning DW. The effect of BMI on 30 day outcomes following total joint arthroplasty. J Arthroplast. 2015;30:1113–7.
10. D'Apuzzo MR, Novicoff WM, Browne JA. The John Insall Award: morbid obesity independently impacts complications, mortality, and resource use after TKA. Clin Orthop Relat Res. 2015;473:57–63.
11. Workgroup of the American Association of Hip and Knee Surgeons Evidence Based Committee. Obesity and total joint arthroplasty: a literature based review. J Arthroplast. 2013;28:714–21.
12. Leopold SS. Editorial: The shortcomings and harms of using hard cutoffs for BMI, hemoglobin A1C, and smoking cessation as conditions for elective orthopaedic surgery. Clin Orthop Relat Res. 2019;477:2391–4.
13. Bronson WH, Fewer M, Godlewski K, Slover JD, Caplan A, Iorio R, Bosco J. The ethics of patient risk modification prior to elective joint replacement surgery. J Bone Joint Surg Am. 2014;96:e113.
14. Chen MJ, Bhowmick S, Beseler L, Schneider KL, Kahan SI, Morton JM, Goodman SB, Amanatullah DF. Strategies for weight reduction prior to total joint arthroplasty. J Bone Joint Surg Am. 2018;100:1888–96.
15. Werner BC, Kurkis GM, Gwathmey FW, Browne JA. Bariatric surgery prior to total knee arthroplasty is associated with fewer postoperative complications. J Arthroplast. 2015;30:81–5.
16. Nickel BT, Klement MR, Penrose CT, Green CL, Seyler TM, Bolognesi MP. Lingering risk: bariatric surgery before total knee arthroplasty. J Arthroplast. 2016;31:207–11.
17. Lee GC, Ong K, Baykal D, Lau E, Malkani AL. Does prior bariatric surgery affect implant survivorship and complications following primary total hip arthroplasty/total knee arthroplasty? J Arthroplast. 2018;33:2070–4.
18. McLawhorn AS, Levack AE, Lee YY, Ge Y, Do H, Dodwell ER. Bariatric surgery improves outcomes after lower extremity arthroplasty in the morbidly obese: a propensity score-matched analysis of a New York Statewide Database. J Arthroplast. 2018;33:2062–9.
19. Severson EP, Singh JA, Browne JA, Trousdale RT, Sarr MG, Lewallen DG. Total knee arthroplasty in morbidly obese patients treated with bariatric surgery: a comparative study. J Arthroplast. 2012;27:1696–700.
20. Martin JR, Watts CD, Taunton MJ. Bariatric surgery does not improve outcomes in patients undergoing primary total knee arthroplasty. Bone Joint J. 2015;97-B:1501–5.
21. Nickel BT, Klement MR, Penrose C, Green CL, Bolognesi MP, Seyler TM. Dislocation rate increases with bariatric surgery before total hip arthroplasty. Hip Int. 2018;28:559–65.
22. Watts CD, Martin JR, Houdek MT, Abdel MP, Lewallen DG, Taunton MJ. Prior bariatric surgery may decrease the rate of re-operation and revision following total hip arthroplasty. Bone Joint J. 2016;98-B:1180–4.
23. Kulkarni A, Jameson SS, James P, Woodcock S, Muller S, Reed MR. Does bariatric surgery prior to lower limb joint replacement reduce complications? Surgeon. 2011;9:18–21.

24. Inacio MC, Paxton EW, Fisher D, Li RA, Barber TC, Singh JA. Bariatric surgery prior to total joint arthroplasty may not provide dramatic improvements in post-arthroplasty surgical outcomes. J Arthroplast. 2014;29:1359–64.
25. Nearing EE, Santos TM, Topolski MS, Borgert AJ, Kallies KJ, Kothari SN. Benefits of bariatric surgery before elective total joint arthroplasty: is there a role for weight loss optimization? Surg Obes Relat Dis. 2017;13:457–62.
26. McLawhorn AS, Southren D, Wang YC, Marx RG, Dodwell ER. Cost-effectiveness of bariatric surgery prior to total knee arthroplasty in the morbidly obese: a computer model-based evaluation. J Bone Joint Surg Am. 2016;98:e6.
27. Premkumar A, Lebrun DG, Sidharthan S, et al. Bariatric surgery prior to total hip arthroplasty is cost-effective in morbidly obese patients. J Arthroplast. 2020;35:1766–75.
28. Li S, Luo X, Sun H, Wang K, Zhang K, Sun X. Does prior bariatric surgery improve outcomes following total joint arthroplasty in the morbidly obese? A meta-analysis. J Arthroplast. 2019;34:577–85.
29. Inacio MC, Silverstein DK, Raman R, Macera CA, Nichols JF, Shaffer RA, Fithian D. Weight patterns before and after total joint arthroplasty and characteristics associated with weight change. Perm J. 2014;18:25–31.
30. Ast MP, Abdel MP, Lee YY, Lyman S, Ruel AV, Westrich GH. Weight changes after total hip or knee arthroplasty: prevalence, predictors, and effects on outcomes. J Bone Joint Surg Am. 2015;97:911–9.
31. Richette P, Poitou C, Garnero P, Vicaut E, Bouillot JL, Lacorte JM, Basdevant A, Clément K, Bardin T, Chevalier X. Benefits of massive weight loss on symptoms, systemic inflammation and cartilage turnover in obese patients with knee osteoarthritis. Ann Rheum Dis. 2011;70:139–44.
32. Chen SX, Bomfim FA, Youn HA, Ren-Fielding C, Samuels J. Predictors of the effect of bariatric surgery on knee osteoarthritis pain. Semin Arthritis Rheum. 2018;48:162–7.
33. Benotti PN, Still CD, Craig Wood G, Seiler JL, Seiler CJ, Thomas SP, Petrick AT, Suk M, Irving BA, Trial Investigators SWIFT. Surgical weight-loss to improve functional status trajectories following total knee arthroplasty: SWIFT trial: Rationale, design, and methods. Contemp Clin Trials. 2018;69:1–9.

Part III

Preoperative Preparation

The Ideal Preoperative Bariatric Surgery Diet

13

Megan Miller, Deborah Hutcheon, and Shanu N. Kothari

13.1 Introduction

Multiple schools of thought exist among medical and allied health professionals for the ideal approach to prepare patients for metabolic and bariatric surgery (MBS) [1, 2]. One school of thought focuses on prescribing a calorie-controlled preoperative diet for days to weeks immediately before surgery [1] in order to achieve multiple positive patient outcomes including formation of healthy diet and lifestyle habits; a reduction in body weight, liver size, fat mass, and body mass index (BMI) [3–5]; improvement in cardiometabolic biomarkers [4]; and provision of optimal nutrition [6]. Such outcomes are believed to facilitate improved laparoscopic access to the abdominal cavity [5, 7–9], reduce risk of perioperative complications [6, 9], support post-operative recovery and healing [6, 10], and increase patient potential to maintain life-long weight management directives following surgery [11–13].

A consensus remains to be set on national standards for preoperative diet preparation [1, 2]. Instead, existing recommendations place the onus on surgeons in collaboration with their allied healthcare team to determine when to prescribe a preoperative diet and which evidence-based intervention to use depending on desired outcomes [1, 2]. To support clinical decision making, this chapter explores existing literature to define preoperative dietary approaches, including composition, calorie prescription, and duration, that have been studied to promote preoperative weight loss and other perioperative outcomes in adult patients seeking MBS. Primary outcomes of interest include change in total body weight (TBW), liver size/volume,

M. Miller (✉) · D. Hutcheon
Minimal Access and Weight Management Institute, Prisma Health, Greenville, SC, USA
e-mail: Meg.Miller2@prismahealth.org; Deborah.Hutcheon@prismahealth.org

S. N. Kothari
Department of Surgery, Prisma Health, Greenville, SC, USA
e-mail: Shanu.Kothari@prismahealth.org

© Springer Nature Switzerland AG 2021
J. Alverdy, Y. Vigneswaran (eds.), *Difficult Decisions in Bariatric Surgery*,
Difficult Decisions in Surgery: An Evidence-Based Approach,
https://doi.org/10.1007/978-3-030-55329-6_13

Table 13.1 Patients, intervention, comparator, outcomes (PICO) literature search terms

P (Patients)	I (Intervention)	C (Comparator)	O (Outcomes)
Adult patients with bariatric surgery (adjustable gastric banding, gastric bypass, gastric sleeve)	Preoperative diet	Not applicable	Total body weight loss, liver size/volume reduction, blood pressure, blood glucose, blood lipids, surgical access, conversion rate, operation time, hospital length of stay, major complication rate

and cardiometabolic biomarkers (e.g., blood pressure, blood glucose, blood lipids) from baseline to endpoint while patients followed the preoperative diet. Secondary outcomes of interest include intraoperative (e.g., ease of surgical access, procedure conversion rate, and operation time) and post-operative outcomes (e.g., post-operative hospital length of stay [LOS] and major complications). This chapter aims to answer the following clinical question: In adult (age $\geq$ 18 years) patients who are candidates for MBS (adjustable gastric banding [AGB], sleeve gastrectomy [SG], or Roux-en-Y gastric bypass [RYGB]), what effect does following a calorie-controlled diet during the immediate preoperative period (up to twelve weeks prior to surgery) have on TBW, liver size/volume, and cardiometabolic biomarkers prior to surgery as well as intraoperative and post-operative outcomes?

13.2 Search Strategy

An electronic search of PubMed, Cochrane, Elsevier, Oxford Academic, ScienceDirect, and Embase databases was completed to obtain relevant primary literature including randomized controlled trials (RCTs), prospective and retrospective cohort studies, non-RCTs, and non-controlled trials investigating perioperative outcomes of preoperative dietary interventions prescribed for $\leq$12 weeks to adult candidates for MBS. The search was limited to human studies involving adults (age $\geq$ 18) undergoing AGB, SG, or RYGB published in full text and in the English language from 2000 to 2020. Search terms included key words and/or medical subject headings of bariatric surgery, weight loss, preoperative/preoperative period, and preoperative diet/diet (Table 13.1). Studies were excluded if the diet protocol (i.e., composition) was not defined, protocols were not administered under free-living conditions (i.e., administration during hospitalization), or at least one primary or secondary outcome of interest was not clearly reported. Four RCTs, four non-RCTs, seven non-controlled trials, three prospective cohort studies, and three retrospective cohort studies were included in the analysis. Data were classified using the GRADE system.

13.3 Results

According to results presented in Table 13.2, very low calorie diets (VLCDs) and low calorie diets (LCDs) are the most common preoperative diet interventions prescribed and studied in adult candidates for MBS. Diet administration varied from 2

Table 13.2 Change in total body weight and liver size/volume among metabolic and bariatric surgery patients while following a preoperative diet

Author (Year)	Location	N[a]	Age (years)[b]	Sex	Baseline BMI (kg/m²)[b]	Surgery type	Diet duration	Diet intervention	Total body weight loss[b]	Liver size/volume reduction[b]	Study type (quality of evidence)
Fris (2004)	New Zealand	40	41 (median)	90% female	47.0 (median)	LAGB	2 weeks	OPTIFAST® VLCD™ 456 kcal/day	4.1%	5.1%	Non-controlled trial (low)
Colles et al. (2006)	Australia	32	48	59% male	47.3	LAGB	12 weeks	OPTIFAST® VLCD™ + low calorie foods 800 kcal/day	10.6%	18.7%	Prospective cohort study (low)
Lewis et al. (2006)	Australia	18	50 (median)	94% female	44.0 (median)	LAGB	6 weeks	OPTIFAST® VLCD™ + low calorie foods 800 kcal/day	7.6% (median, estimate)	12.1% (median, estimate)	Non-controlled trial (low)
Benjaminov et al. (2007)	Israel	14	34 (median)	64% female	45.9	LAGB	4 weeks	Low carbohydrate diet 54 ± 22 g or 14 ± 4% kcal carbohydrate/day (mean) 1520 ± 285 total kcal/day (mean)	3.7% (estimate)	8.1%	Non-controlled trial (low)
Wahlroos et al. (2007)	Australia	14	17 to 64 (range)	100% female	45.0	LAGB	6 weeks	OPTIFAST® VLCD™ + low calorie foods 800 kcal/day	7.6%	NR	Non-RCT (low)

(continued)

Table 13.2 (continued)

Author (Year)	Location	N[a]	Age (years)[b]	Sex	Baseline BMI (kg/m²)[b]	Surgery type	Diet duration	Diet intervention	Total body weight loss[b]	Liver size/volume reduction[b]	Study type (quality of evidence)
Carbajo et al. (2010)	Spain	60 vs 60	38 (both groups)	62% female vs 72% female	45.1 vs 43.6	LRYGB	3 weeks	Vegestart Complet® + liquids 800 kcal/day vs. high protein, no carbohydrate solid diet + liquids undefined calorie prescription	7.5% (estimate) vs. 4.1% (estimate)	NR	RCT (moderate)
Edholm et al. (2011)	Sweden	15	34	100% female	42.9	LRYGB	4 weeks	Modifast® 800 to 1100 kcal/day	6.2% (estimate)	12%	Non-RCT (low)
Van Nieuwenhove et al. (2011)	Europe (Sweden, Lithuania, Spain, Belgium, Netherlands)	137 vs 136	40 (both groups)	70% female vs 68% female	43.4 vs 43.3	LRYGB	2 weeks	OPTIFAST® 800-800 kcal/day vs. no pre-op diet restriction	3.8% vs 0.3% (estimate)	NR	Multicenter RCT (moderate)
Collins et al. (2011)	United States	30	53	90% male	56.0	LRYGB	9 weeks (mean)	OPTIFAST® 800® 800 kcal/day	12.1%	18.0%	Retrospective cohort study (low)

						Laparoscopic bariatric Surgery[c]					
Brody et al. (2011)	United States	21	48	86% female	44.5		4 weeks	Solid food LCD + Nuvista® 1200 to 1500 kcal/day	3.1% (estimate)	43.4%	Non-controlled trial (low)
Gonzalez-Perez et al. (2013)	Mexico	20	35	85% female	46.0 (median)	LRYGB	6 weeks	Solid food VLCD 800 kcal/day	NR	20.3% (median)	Non-controlled trial (low)
Biro et al. (2013)	United States	51	NR	63% female	NR	LAGB LSG LRYGB	2 weeks	Liquid LCD 1100 to 1300 kcal/day	NR	NR	Retrospective cohort study (low)
Faria et al. (2015)	Brazil	57 vs 47	37 vs 36	79% female vs 85% female	42.4 vs 39.7	LRYGB	2 weeks	Liquid food VLCD 760 ± 26 kcal/day vs. solid food VLCD 754 ± 23 kcal/day	3.5% vs 2.5%	NR	RCT (moderate)
Ruiz-Tovar et al. (2015)	Spain	20 vs 20 vs 20	43 (all groups)	80% female vs 75% female vs 70% female	47.5 vs 47.8 vs 48.1	LSG	2 weeks	Solid food LCD 900 kcal/day vs. Supressi® 900 kcal/day vs. Atempero® 900 kcal/day	NR	NR	RCT (moderate)
Edholm et al. (2015)	Sweden	10	43	100% female	42.0	LRYGB	4 weeks	Modifast® 800 to 1100 kcal/day	6.5% (estimate)	18%	Prospective cohort study (low)

(continued)

Table 13.2 (continued)

Author (Year)	Location	Nᵃ	Age (years)[b]	Sex	Baseline BMI (kg/m²)[b]	Surgery type	Diet duration	Diet intervention	Total body weight loss[b]	Liver size/volume reduction[b]	Study type (quality of evidence)
Leonetti et al. (2015)	Italy	50 vs 30	48 vs 43	62% female vs 60% female	53.5 vs 54.8	VSG	4 weeks	Formula VLCKD → solid + liquid VLCD→ solid + liquid LCD 560 to 595 kcal/day → 810 kcal/day→1100 kcal/day vs. solid food LCD 1200 kcal/day	8.5%[d] (estimate) vs. 4.6% (estimate)	NR	Non-RCT (low)
Schiavo et al. (2015)	Italy	37	46	100% male	45.2	LSG	8 weeks	Mediterranean protein-enriched solid food LCD 1200 kcal/day	16.7%	29.1%	Non-controlled trial (low)
Nielsen et al. (2016)	Denmark	30	39	73% female	46.0	RYGB	8 weeks	Cambridge Weight Plan® liquid + solid food LCD 1030 kcal/day	10%	NR	Non-controlled trial (low)
Bennasar-Remolara et al. (2016)	Spain	42	44	69% female	NR	RYGB	4 weeks	Optifast® VLCD 600 kcal/day	8.6%	NR	Retrospective cohort study (low)

Albanese et al. (2019)	Italy	106 vs 72	44 vs 43	75% female vs 83% female	43.1 vs 46.3	LSG	3 weeks	Solid food VLCD 800 kcal/day vs. liquid + solid food VLCKD 700 kcal/day	4.0% (estimate) vs 4.6% (estimate)	NR	Non-RCT (low)
Sivakumar et al. (2020)	Australia	44	44	75% female	43.4	Bariatric Surgery[c]	2 weeks	Optifast® VLCD + very low starch vegetables with olive oil 600 to 700 kcal/day	3.6%	NR	Prospective cohort study (low)

BMI body mass index, *LAGB* laparoscopic adjustable gastric band, *LCD* low calorie diet, *LRYGB* laparoscopic Roux-en-Y gastric bypass, *LSG* laparoscopic sleeve gastrectomy, *NR* none reported, *RCT* randomized controlled trial, *VLCD* very low calorie diet, *VLCKD* very low calorie ketogenic diet

[a]Represents number of subjects who followed the defined diet intervention

[b]Data expressed as means unless otherwise indicated

[c]Surgery type not specified

[d]Analysis based on per protocol $n = 48$

weeks to 12 weeks with the most frequent duration of administration being 2 weeks (6 studies) [3, 6, 9, 14–16] or 4 weeks (6 studies) [7, 8, 10, 17–19]. Key outcomes reported included TBW loss (18 studies) [3–5, 7, 8, 10, 15–25], reduction in liver size/volume (10 studies) [3–5, 7, 8, 17, 18, 22, 23, 26], reduction in systolic and diastolic blood pressure (6 studies) [4, 15, 18, 19, 21, 24], improvement in blood glucose (7 studies) [4, 7, 18, 20, 21, 23, 24], improvement in lipid profile (8 studies) [4, 7, 15, 18–20, 23, 24], easier laparoscopic surgical access (4 studies) [5, 7–9], and attenuated inflammatory response post-surgery (2 studies) [6, 10].

Before analyzing the results, it is important to understand differences between a VLCD and a LCD, particularly related to diet composition and weight loss potential. A VLCD provides ≤800 kcal per day [27] with approximately 40% calories from carbohydrate, 15% calories from fat, and 45% calories from protein [28]. Adequate protein estimated at 0.8 g to 1.5 g per kilogram ideal body weight per day is encouraged to preserve lean body mass and induce loss of fat mass [28]. The calorie prescription and macronutrient composition of the VLCD creates a significant calorie deficit leading to rapid weight loss of on average 3.3 to 5.5 lb. per week [28].

A LCD is defined as a diet that provides 800 to 1500 kcal per day comprised of 10% to 65% calories from carbohydrate, 10% to 40% calories from fat, and 12% to 30% calories from protein [27]. This calorie prescription creates a calorie deficit of at least 500 kcal per day leading to gradual, steady weight loss of 0.5 to 2 lb. per week [27].

Of the 21 studies identified, twelve used a VLCD providing on average 456 to 800 kcal per day [3–5, 9, 10, 15, 16, 20–22, 25, 26]. The majority of these studies ($n = 8$) used Optifast® VLCD [3–5, 10, 16, 20] or Optifast® 800 [9, 22] medically supervised meal replacement products either alone [3, 9, 10, 22] or in combination with a limited amount of low-calorie foods [4, 5, 16, 20] to provide a total daily intake of 456 to 800 kcal per day. The remaining nine studies prescribed a LCD providing on average 800 to 1500 kcal per day [6–8, 14, 17–19, 23, 24]. Diet approaches varied significantly among the LCD studies with the most similar interventions being a medically supervised meal replacement diet ($n = 2$, both using Modifast® providing 800 to 1100 kcal per day [8, 18] or a combination meal replacement product and primarily solid food based diet ($n = 2$) providing 1030 kcal per day [24] or 1200 to 1500 kcal per day [17]. Two studies used conventional solid food-based LCD approaches—one a low carbohydrate diet providing approximately 1500 kcal per day [7] and the second a protein-rich Mediterranean diet providing 1200 kcal per day [23].

Typically, the longer patients are on a preoperative diet and the lower the daily calorie prescription, the greater the TBW loss and reduction in liver size/volume achieved. For example, studies of 2 weeks duration providing 456 to 800 kcal per day resulted in an average 2.5% to 4.1% TBW loss [3, 9, 15, 16] and 5.1% liver size/volume reduction [3]; studies of 4 weeks duration providing 800 to 1100 kcal per day resulted in an average 6.2% to 8.5% TBW loss [8, 18, 19] and 12% to 43.4% liver size/volume reduction [8, 17, 18] (compared to studies of 4 weeks providing 1200 to 1500 kcal per day resulting in 3.1% to 4.6% TBW loss [7, 17, 19] and 8.1% liver size/volume reduction [7]); studies of 6 weeks duration providing 800 kcal per day resulted in an average 7.6% TBW loss [5, 20] and 12% to 20.3% liver size/volume reduction [5, 26]; studies of 8 weeks duration providing 1030 to 1200 kcal

Table 13.3 Change in preoperative cardiometabolic biomarkers among metabolic and bariatric surgery patients while following a preoperative diet

Author (Year)	Surgery type	Diet duration	Diet intervention	SBP	DBP	FG	Fasting insulin	Total cholesterol	TG	LDL-C	HDL-C	CRP	AST	ALT	Other
Colles et al. (2006)	LAGB	12 weeks	OPTIFAST® VLCD™ + low calorie foods 800 kcal/day	↓[a]	↓[a]	↓[a]	↓[a]	↓[a]	↓[a]	↓[a]	NC	↓	↓	↓	↓[a] HbA1c
Benjaminov et al. (2007)	LAGB	4 weeks	Low carbohydrate diet 54 ± 22 g or 14 ± 4% kcal carbohydrate/day (mean) 1520 ± 285 total kcal/day (mean)	NR	NR	↓	NR	↓	↑	↓	↓[a]	NR	↑	↑	NR
Wahlroos et al. (2007)	LAGB	6 weeks	OPTIFAST® VLCD™ + low calorie foods 800 kcal/day	NR	NR	↓	↓	↓[a]	↓	↓	↓[a]	NR	NR	NR	NR
Carbajo et al. (2010)	LRYGB	3 weeks	Vegestart Complet® + liquids 800 kcal/day vs. high protein, no carbohydrate solid diet + liquids undefined calorie prescription	↓[a]	↓[a]	↓[a]	NR	NR	NR	NR	NR	NR	NR	NR	NR
Collins et al. (2011)	LRYGB	9 weeks (mean)	OPTIFAST® 800® 800 kcal/day	NR	NR	NR	NR	NR	NR	NR	NR	NR	NR	NR	Significant percentage (≥40%) of patients with improvement or resolution of poorly controlled DM, HTN or DJD during diet.
Biro et al. (2013)	LAGB LSG LRYGB	2 weeks	Liquid LCD 1100 to 1300 kcal/day	NR	NR	NR	NR	NR	NR	NR	NR	NR	NR	NR	Rapid responders to LCD experienced >50% reduction in insulin dosage during LCD.

(continued)

Table 13.3 (continued)

Author (Year)	Surgery type	Diet duration	Diet intervention	SBP	DBP	FG	Fasting insulin	Total cholesterol	TG	LDL-C	HDL-C	CRP	AST	ALT	Other
Faria et al. (2015)	LRYGB	2 weeks	Liquid food VLCD 760 ± 26 kcal/day vs. solid food VLCD 754 ± 23 kcal/day	↓	NR	NR	↓	↓	↓	NR	↓	↓	NR	NR	NR
Edholm et al. (2015)	LRYGB	4 weeks	Modifast® 800 to 1100 kcal/day	↓ᵃ	↓	↓	↓ᵃ	↓ᵃ	↓ᵃ	↓ᵃ	↓ᵃ	NR	↑ᵃ	↑	NR
Leonetti et al. (2015)	VSG	4 weeks	Formula VLCKD → solid + liquid VLCD → solid + liquid LCD 560 to 595 kcal/day → 810 kcal/day → 1100 kcal/day vs. Solid food LCD 1200 kcal/day	↓	↓	NR	NR	↓	↓	↓	↓	NR	↓	↓	Improved fasting glucose levels for patients with T2DM on formula diet allowing for a reduction in T2DM medications (oral hypoglycemic agents and insulin dosage) prior to surgery.
Schiavo et al. (2015)	LSG	8 weeks	Mediterranean protein-enriched solid food LCD 1200 kcal/day	NR	NR	↓ᵃ	↓ᵃ	↓ᵃ	↓ᵃ	↓ᵃ	↑	NR	↓ᵃ	↓ᵃ	NR
Nielsen et al. (2016)	RYGB	8 weeks	Cambridge Weight Plan® + Solid Food LCD 1030 kcal/day	↓ᵃ	↓ᵃ	↓ᵃ	↓ᵃ	↓ᵃ	↓ᵃ	↓ᵃ	↓ᵃ	↓ᵃ	NR	NR	Improved blood pressure for patients with HTN allowing for reduction in HTN medications prior to surgery.

ALT alanine aminotransferase, *AST* aspartate aminotransferase, *CRP* c-reactive protein, *DBP* diastolic blood pressure, *DJD* degenerative joint disease, *DM* diabetes mellitus, *FG* fasting glucose, *HbA1c* hemoglobin A1c, *HDL-C* high density lipoprotein cholesterol, *HTN* hypertension, *LAGB* laparoscopic adjustable gastric band, *LCD* low calorie diet, *LDL-C* low density lipoprotein cholesterol, *LRYGB* laparoscopic Roux-en-Y gastric bypass, *LSG* laparoscopic sleeve gastrectomy, *NC* no change, *NR* none reported, *SBP* systolic blood pressure, *T2DM* type 2 diabetes mellitus, *TG* triglycerides, *VLCD* very low calorie diet

ᵃDenotes change is statistically significant change from baseline

Table 13.4 Change in operative outcomes among metabolic and bariatric surgery patients who followed a preoperative diet

Author (Year)	Surgery type	Diet duration	Diet intervention	Procedure complexity	Procedure conversion	Operation duration	Hospital LOS	Major complications	Other
Colles et al. (2006)	LAGB	12 weeks	OPTIFAST® VLCD™ + low calorie foods 800 kcal/day	NR	None	NR	No extended LOS	None	NR
Lewis et al. (2006)	LAGB	6 weeks	OPTIFAST® VLCD™ + low calorie foods 800 kcal/day	Surgeon subjective perception that laparoscopic access and liver retraction was easy.	NR	NR	NR	NR	NR
Benjaminov et al. (2007)	LAGB	4 weeks	Low carbohydrate diet 54 ± 22 g or 14 ± 4% kcal carbohydrate/day (mean) 1520 ± 285 total kcal/day (mean)	Surgeon subjective perception that laparoscopic access and liver retraction was easy.	NR	NR	NR	NR	NR
Edholm et al. (2011)	LRYGB	4 weeks	Modifast® 800 to 1100 kcal/day	Surgeon objective assessment of low surgical complexity.	None	Decrease in operation time compared to control group but not statistically different.	Increase in hospital LOS compared to control group but not statistically different.	None	NR

(continued)

Table 13.4 (continued)

Author (Year)	Surgery type	Diet duration	Diet intervention	Procedure complexity	Procedure conversion	Operation duration	Hospital LOS	Major complications	Other
Van Nieuwenhove et al. (2011)	LRYGB	2 weeks	OPTIFAST® 800 800 kcal/day vs. no diet restriction	Surgeon objective assessment of low surgical difficulty.	None	No difference in operation time between diet groups.	NR	Statistically significant lower 30 day complication rate compared to control group.	NR
Collins et al. (2011)	LRYGB	9 weeks (mean)	OPTIFAST® 800 800 kcal/day	NR	NR	Mean 156.1 minutes	Mean 3.5 days	None	NR
Biro et al. (2013)	LAGB LSG LRYGB	2 weeks	Liquid LCD 1100 to 1300 kcal/day	NR	NR	NR	NR	NR	Rapid response to LCD is indicative of higher potential for early remission of T2DM and greater post-op weight loss.
Faria et al. (2015)	LRYGB	2 weeks	Liquid food VLCD 760 ± 26 kcal/day vs. solid food VLCD 754 ± 23 kcal/day	NR	NR	Decrease in operation time with more visceral fat loss using liquid diet compared to food diet.	NR	NR	NR

Author (Year)	Surgery type	Diet duration	Diet intervention	Procedure complexity	Procedure conversion	Operation duration	Hospital LOS	Major complications	Other
Ruiz-Tovar et al. (2015)	LSG	2 weeks	Solid food LCD 900 kcal/day vs. Supressi® 900 kcal/day vs. Atempero® 900 kcal/day	NR	NR	No significant difference in operation time between diet groups.	No significant difference in hospital LOS between groups.	No significant difference in major complications between groups.	High protein and immunonutrition diets resulted in statistically significant reduction in CRP, AST, ALT, and pain rating 24 hours post-surgery.
Nielsen et al. (2016)	RYGB	8 weeks	Cambridge Weight Plan® + solid food LCD 1030 kcal/day	NR	NR	NR	NR	NR	Preoperative weight loss was not associated with postoperative weight loss at 18 months post-operation.
Albanese et al. (2019)	VSG	3 weeks	Solid food VLCD 800 kcal/day vs. liquid + solid food VLCKD 700 kcal/day	NR	NR	Decrease in operation time for VLCKD compared to VLCD but not significantly different.	Decrease in hospital LOS for VLCKD compared to VLCD but not significantly different.	NR	NR

ALT alanine aminotransferase, *AST* aspartate aminotransferase, *CRP* c-reactive protein, *LAGB* laparoscopic adjustable gastric band, *LCD* low calorie diet, *LOS* length of stay, *LRYGB* laparoscopic Roux-en-Y gastric bypass, *LSG* laparoscopic sleeve gastrectomy, *NR* none reported, *T2DM* type 2 diabetes mellitus, *VLCD* very low calorie diet, *VLCKD* very low calorie ketogenic diet per day resulted in an average 10% to 16.7% TBW loss [23, 24] and 29.1% liver size/volume reduction [23]; and one study of 12 weeks duration providing 800 kcal per day resulted in 10.6% TBW loss and 18.7% liver size/volume reduction [4].

It appears that medically supervised meal replacement diets that include liquid products (i.e., shakes or soups) either alone or in combination with some solid food and solely liquid diets using conventional food and beverage products result in the greatest weight loss when also considering calorie prescription and diet duration. For example, when provided for 2 weeks, Optifast® VLCD plus low calorie foods, Optifast® 800, and a fully liquid VLCD, all providing 600 to 800 kcal per day, achieved similar average losses in TBW (3.5% to 3.8%) [9, 15, 16]. These findings are in comparison to a fully solid-food based VLCD (approximately 750 kcal per day) resulting in average losses of 2.5% TBW [15].

Regardless of diet duration, calorie prescription or diet composition, preoperative VLCDs and LCDs providing 800 kcal to 1500 kcal per day for 2 weeks to 12 weeks result in significant reductions in systolic blood pressure (SBP) [4, 18, 21, 24] and diastolic blood pressure (DBP) [4, 21, 24], fasting glucose (FG) [4, 21, 23, 24], hemoglobin A1c [4], fasting insulin [4, 18, 23, 24], total cholesterol [4, 18, 20, 23, 24], triglycerides [4, 18, 23, 24], and low density lipoprotein cholesterol [4, 18, 24] between baseline and diet completion (Table 13.3). The only consistent negative cardiometabolic outcome demonstrated by preoperative VLCDs and LCDs is a significant reduction in high density lipoprotein cholesterol [7, 18, 20, 24].

For blood pressure, provision of 800 to 1100 kcals per day using medically supervised meal replacement products either alone or in combination with low calorie foods and beverages for 3 to 12 weeks resulted in a 5.6% to 11% reduction in SBP [4, 18, 21, 24] and 8.4% to 11% reduction in DBP [4, 21, 24]. Additionally, Nielsen et al. found that patients with hypertension (HTN) following their 1030 kcal per day diet for 8 weeks experienced significant improvement in blood pressure to the point that they were able to reduce their HTN medication use prior to surgery [24].

For FG, average reductions varied by calorie prescription, diet composition, and duration. Nielsen et al. saw an average 9 mg/dL reduction in FG (mean baseline 106.2 mg/dL vs mean endpoint 97.2 mg/dL, $p < 0.01$) among candidates for RYGB who followed a 1030 kcal per day diet for 8 weeks. Carbajo et al. saw an average 17 mg/dL reduction in FG (mean baseline 118.4 mg/dL vs 101.9 mg/dL, $p < 0.0001$) in as little as 3 weeks among candidates for RYGB who followed an 800 kcal per day diet. Using a protein-enriched Mediterranean diet providing 1200 kcal per day for 8 weeks in candidates for SG, Schiavo et al. demonstrated an average 26.5 mg/dL reduction in FG (mean baseline 118.6 mg/dL vs. mean endpoint 92.1 mg/dL, $p < 0.01$). Similarly, using an 800 kcal diet (Optifast® VLCD plus low calorie foods) for 12 weeks in candidates for AGB, Coles et al. demonstrated an average 27 mg/dL reduction in FG (mean baseline 136.8 mg/dL vs mean endpoint 109.8 mg/dL, $p = 0.011$).

Regardless of a reduction in FG, preoperative VLCDs and LCDs appear to have other positive benefits for blood glucose management, particularly in MBS candidates with type 2 diabetes mellitus (T2DM). Leonetti et al. found that in candidates for SG who followed a combination medical meal replacement formula and conventional solid and liquid food-based diet that progressed from being very low calorie to low calorie (ending in 1100 kcal per day) for 4 weeks, blood glucose improved in patients with T2DM to the point that the majority of these patients were able to reduce their oral hypoglycemic and insulin medication dosages prior to surgery. A similar response was seen by Biro et al. [14] when candidates for AGB, SG, and RYGB followed a liquid LCD providing 1100 to 1300 kcal per day for 2 weeks. In their study, patients with T2DM who were deemed rapid responders, meaning they lost weight quickly on the diet, experienced an over 50% reduction in their insulin dosage prior to surgery. These patients also had a greater potential for early remission of T2DM following surgery [14]. Furthermore, Collins et al. saw at least 40% of their patients who followed the Optifast® 800 diet (800 kcal per day) for an average of 9 weeks experience either improvement or resolution of their T2DM, HTN, and degenerative joint disease while on the diet [22].

Pertaining to intraoperative and postoperative outcomes (Table 13.4), 11 studies reviewed reported at least one relevant outcome [4–9, 14, 15, 22, 24, 25]; however only five studies utilized a control or comparison group to determine whether a preoperative diet results in superior outcomes [6, 8, 9, 15, 25]. Edholm et al. [8] in their non-RCT found that patients in their LCD group (Modifast® 800 to 1100 kcal per day) demonstrated lower surgical complexity and a decrease in operation time (mean 169 ± 34.5 minutes) compared to patient in their control group (mean 172 ± 32.9 minutes), but the difference in operation time was not statistically significant between groups. Hospital LOS was slightly longer among patients in the LCD group (mean 4.9 ± 2.1 days versus 4.3 ± 1.0 days), but this difference was also not statistically significant [8]. Van Nieuwenhove et al. in their multicenter RCT also found that patients in their VLCD group who followed the Optifast® 800 diet for 2 weeks demonstrated lower surgical difficulty and a statistically significant lower 30 day complication rate compared to the control group (8 complications VLCD vs 18 complications control, $p = 0.04$), but there was no significant difference in operation time between diet groups (mean 80 ± 23 minutes VLCD vs. 81 ± 21 minutes control) [9]. Albanese et al. in their non-RCT found that patients following a very low calorie ketogenic diet (700 kcal per day) for 3 weeks experienced a shorter operation time (mean 59.8 ± 18.7 minutes vs 69 ± 31.7 minutes) and hospital LOS (mean 3.0 ± 0.2 days vs 3.2 ± 2.4 days) compared to patients following a solid food VLCD (800 kcal per day), but the difference between groups for both outcomes was not statistically significant [25].

In contrast, Ruiz-Tovar et al. in their RCT found no significant difference in operation time (mean 92.2 ± 14.7 minutes), hospital LOS (mean 3 days) or major complications among their three diet groups, each providing 900 kcal per day either through solid food, a high protein meal replacement product, or an immunonutrition meal replacement product [6]. Faira et al. also found in their RCT that there was no difference in operation time between their two VLCD groups, one a liquid VLCD and the other a solid food VLCD, both providing nearly 800 kcal per day and followed for 2 weeks; however they did find an inverse relationship between operation time (decrease) and the amount of visceral adipose tissue patients in the liquid diet group lost (increase) while following the diet [15].

Although VLCDs and LCDs are considered safe and effective, patients may experience side effects. The most common side effects reported by patients in the studies reviewed include hunger [4, 15, 23, 24, 26], diarrhea [19, 21, 24, 26], constipation [4, 19, 24], nausea/vomiting [19, 21, 26], headache [21, 23, 24], dizziness/lightheadedness [4, 24], and fatigue [24]. The majority of these side effects were reported upon initiation of the prescribed diet and subsided over time. Additional side effects patients experienced included cold intolerance [4, 24], abdominal pain [24], other gastrointestinal problems [23], irritability [24], dry skin [4], flatulence [24], and bad breath [24]. For constipation, which was the most common side effect in the study by Colles et al. [4], treatment should address increasing fluid and vegetable intake. A fiber supplement and mild laxative may also be prescribed [4].

Additional considerations with use of VLCDs and LCDs, particularly those using medically supervised or commercially available meal replacement products, include taste, hunger/satiety, and overall acceptability. Colles et al. found that taste acceptance and satiety of their Optifast® VLCD plus low calorie food diet (800 kcal per day) was greatest during the first 4 weeks of the diet and declined thereafter [4]. Carbajo et al. found patients provided higher taste satisfaction ratings for their solid food diet compared to their liquid diet, but patients reported no difference in satiety between the diets, both followed for 3 weeks [21]. In contrast, Faria et al. found patients reported more hunger with their liquid VLCD than with their solid food VLCD, both when followed for 2 weeks [15]. And, Edholm et al. found that patients following the Modifast® diet (liquid) for 4 weeks reported a desire for solid foods [18].

13.4   Recommendations Based on the Data

The available clinical evidence supports weight reduction, cardiometabolic, intra-operative and postoperative benefits of preoperative diet initiation in patients pursuing MBS. A preoperative VLCD or LCD providing 800 to 1100 kcal per day using medically supervised meal replacement products, either alone or in combination with low calorie food, for two to four weeks is recommended to initiate small to moderate TBW loss and liver size/volume reduction, clinically meaningful improvement in cardiometabolic outcomes, and improved laparoscopic surgical access (evidence quality moderate, strong recommendation). No evidence exists to support use of a preoperative diet less than two weeks in duration. Longer duration preoperative diets providing up to 1500 kcal per day for 6 to 12 weeks may benefit patients needing a greater reduction of TBW and liver size/volume while continuing to support improvement in cardiometabolic outcomes (evidence quality low, conditional recommendation). There is insufficient evidence to support the use of preoperative VLCDs or LCDs for the sole purpose of a reduction of operative time, hospital LOS, and post-operative complication rates (evidence quality low, strong recommendation).

Meal replacement product and liquid-based VLCDs and LCDs appear to achieve clinically meaningful improvements in weight, liver size/volume, cardiometabolic biomarkers, and surgical access in a shorter time frame (2 to 4 weeks) when compared to solid food-based VLCDs and LCDs; therefore a solid food-based VLCD or LCD should be conducted over a longer period of time (4 to 6 weeks) to achieve similar results (evidence quality low, conditional recommendation). High protein immunonutrition meal replacement products as part of a preoperative LCD used for at least two weeks prior to surgery may significantly attenuate inflammatory and pain response following surgery (evidence quality moderate, conditional recommendation). Finally, diets administered for up to 4 weeks and combining both liquid and solid conventional food and beverages may be better accepted and followed by patients based on taste and satiety (evidence quality low, conditional recommendation).

13.5   Summary of Recommendation Options

- Healthcare providers should recommend that adult patients undergoing MBS complete a medically prescribed VLCD (800 kcal per day) or a LCD (800 to 1100 kcal per day) using medically supervised meal replacement products, either alone or in combination with low calorie food, for 2 to 4 weeks immediately before surgery to achieve at least 3% TBW loss, at least 5% reduction in liver size/volume, improvement in cardiometabolic biomarkers (e.g., blood pressure, blood glucose, and blood lipids), and improvement in surgical access (evidence quality low to moderate, strong recommendation).
- Patients should not be prescribed a preoperative VLCD or LCD for the sole purpose of reduction in operation time, hospital LOS, and major complications (evidence quality low, strong recommendation).
- Medically supervised meal replacement products or immunonutrition oral nutrition supplements used either alone or in combination with low calorie foods as part of a VLCD or LCD supports maintenance of adequate nutrition both prior to and immediately following surgery (evidence quality low, weak recommendation).
- Patient monitoring by a qualified health professional is recommended to individualize the diet prescription and maximize compliance and beneficial effects of the preoperative VLCD or LCD (evidence quality very low; weak recommendation).

13.6   Personal View of the Data and Recommendations

Preoperative VLCDs and LCDs demonstrate a clinically significant positive impact on weight loss, liver size/volume reduction, key cardiometabolic and nutrition-related biochemical markers, and surgical access. Unfortunately, there is not a significant amount of moderate to strong evidence to support the development of a consensus on the best preoperative diet for patients undergoing MBS. For most patients prescribed a VLCD or LCD by their surgical healthcare team, there is an initial period (days to weeks) of adjustment, which should be taken into consideration when determining the optimal diet composition and duration. The number of related and complicating co-morbidities that patients have should also be taken into consideration to determine which preoperative diet outcomes may be priority for patients to achieve (i.e., weight loss vs liver size/volume reduction vs cardiometabolic biomarker improvement). Based on comorbidities, a VLCD or LCD may not be medically appropriate for all patients (i.e., chronic kidney disease). Additionally, the financial implications of using medically supervised meal replacement products versus a food-based diet should be considered [29]. These factors increase the value of clinical judgement and individualized patient assessment by a licensed and experienced clinical professional to establish a feasible, patient-centered approach. A minimum of a three-week preoperative diet would provide patients with time to demonstrate their ability to follow a prescribed diet and adopt healthy lifestyle habits prior to surgery, decrease patient burden related to duration and cost of the diet, and improve patient monitoring and counseling opportunities by the clinical team. Unknowns remain including the role of exercise to influence TBW loss, liver size/volume reduction, and changes in biochemical markers while patients follow a preoperative VLCD or LCD.

References

1. Brethauer S. ASMBS position statement on preoperative supervised weight loss requirements. Surg Obes Relat Dis. 2011;7(3):257–60.
2. Kim JJ, Rogers AM, Ballem N, Schirmer B, American Society for Metabolic and Bariatric Surgery Clinical Issues Committee. ASMBS updated position statement on insurance mandated preoperative weight loss requirements. Surg Obes Relat Dis. 2016;12(5):955–9.
3. Fris RJ. Preoperative low energy diet diminishes liver size. Obes Surg. 2004;14(9):1165–70.
4. Colles SL, Dixon JB, Marks P, Strauss BJ, O'Brien PE. Preoperative weight loss with a very-low-energy diet: quantitation of changes in liver and abdominal fat by serial imaging. Am J Clin Nutr. 2006;84(2):304–11.
5. Lewis MC, Phillips ML, Slavotinek JP, Kow L, Thompson CH, Toouli J. Change in liver size and fat content after treatment with Optifast very low calorie diet. Obes Surg. 2006;16(6):697–701.
6. Ruiz-Tovar J, Zubiaga L, Diez M, et al. Preoperative regular diet of 900 kcal/day vs balanced energy high-protein formula vs immunonutrition formula: effect on preoperative weight loss and postoperative pain, complications and analytical acute phase reactants after laparoscopic sleeve gastrectomy. Obes Surg. 2016;26(6):1221–7.
7. Benjaminov O, Beglaibter N, Gindy L, et al. The effect of a low-carbohydrate diet on the nonalcoholic fatty liver in morbidly obese patients before bariatric surgery. Surg Endosc. 2007;21(8):1423–7.
8. Edholm D, Kullberg J, Haenni A, et al. Preoperative 4-week low-calorie diet reduces liver volume and intrahepatic fat, and facilitates laparoscopic gastric bypass in morbidly obese. Obes Surg. 2011;21(3):345–50.
9. Van Nieuwenhove Y, Dambrauskas Z, Campillo-Soto A, et al. Preoperative very low-calorie diet and operative outcome after laparoscopic gastric bypass: a randomized multicenter study. Arch Surg. 2011;146(11):1300–5.

10. Bennasar Remolar MA, Martinez Ramos D, Ortega Serrano J, Salvador Sanchis JL. Nutritional alterations after very low-calorie diet before bariatric surgery. Cir Esp. 2016;94(3):159–64.
11. Livhits M, Mercado C, Yermilov I, et al. Does weight loss immediately before bariatric surgery improve outcomes: a systematic review. Surg Obes Relat Dis. 2009;5(6):713–21.
12. Sarwer DB, Wadden TA, Moore RH, et al. Preoperative eating behavior, postoperative dietary adherence, and weight loss after gastric bypass surgery. Surg Obes Relat Dis. 2008;4(5):640–6.
13. Patel P, Hartland A, Hollis A, et al. Tier 3 multidisciplinary medical weight management improves outcome of Roux-en-Y gastric bypass surgery. Ann R Coll Surg Engl. 2015;97(3):235–7.
14. Biro SM, Olson DL, Garren MJ, Gould JC. Diabetes remission and glycemic response to pre-bariatric surgery diet. J Surg Res. 2013;185(1):1–5.
15. Faria SL, Faria OP, de Almeida CM, Ito MK. Effects of a very low calorie diet in the preoperative stage of bariatric surgery: a randomized trial. Surg Obes Relat Dis. 2015;11(1):230–7.
16. Sivakumar J, Chong L, Ward S, Sutherland TR, Read M, Hii MW. Body composition changes following a very-low-calorie pre-operative diet in patients undergoing bariatric surgery. Obes Surg. 2020;30(1):119–26.
17. Brody F, Vaziri K, Garey C, et al. Preoperative liver reduction utilizing a novel nutritional supplement. J Laparoendosc Adv Surg Tech A. 2011;21(6):491–5.
18. Edholm D, Kullberg J, Karlsson FA, Haenni A, Ahlstrom H, Sundbom M. Changes in liver volume and body composition during 4 weeks of low calorie diet before laparoscopic gastric bypass. Surg Obes Relat Dis. 2015;11(3):602–6.
19. Leonetti F, Campanile FC, Coccia F, et al. Very low-carbohydrate ketogenic diet before bariatric surgery: prospective evaluation of a sequential diet. Obes Surg. 2015;25(1):64–71.
20. Wahlroos S, Phillips ML, Lewis MC, et al. Rapid significant weight loss and regional lipid deposition: implications for insulin sensitivity. Obes Res Clin Pract. 2007;1(1):1–78.
21. Carbajo MA, Castro MJ, Kleinfinger S, et al. Effects of a balanced energy and high protein formula diet (Vegestart complet(R)) vs. low-calorie regular diet in morbid obese patients prior to bariatric surgery (laparoscopic single anastomosis gastric bypass): a prospective, double-blind randomized study. Nutr Hosp. 2010;25(6):939–48.
22. Collins J, McCloskey C, Titchner R, et al. Preoperative weight loss in high-risk super-obese bariatric patients: a computed tomography-based analysis. Surg Obes Relat Dis. 2011;7(4):480–485.25.
23. Schiavo L, Scalera G, Sergio R, De Sena G, Pilone V, Barbarisi A. Clinical impact of Mediterranean-enriched-protein diet on liver size, visceral fat, fat mass, and fat-free mass in patients undergoing sleeve gastrectomy. Surg Obes Relat Dis. 2016;11(5):1164–70.
24. Nielsen LV, Nielsen MS, Schmidt JB, Pedersen SD, Sjodin A. Efficacy of a liquid low-energy formula diet in achieving preoperative target weight loss before bariatric surgery. J Nutr Sci. 2016;5:e22.
25. Albanese A, Prevedello L, Markovich M, Busetto L, Vettor R, Foletto M. Pre-operative very low calorie ketogenic diet (VLCKD) vs. very low calorie diet (VLCD): surgical impact. Obes Surg. 2019;29(1):292–6.
26. Gonzalez-Perez J, Sanchez-Leenheer S, Delgado AR, et al. Clinical impact of a 6-week preoperative very low calorie diet on body weight and liver size in morbidly obese patients. Obes Surg. 2013;23(10):1624–31.
27. Jensen MD, Ryan DH, Apovian CM, et al. 2013 AHA/ACC/TOS guideline for the management of overweight and obesity in adults: a report of the American College of Cardiology/American Heart Association Task Force on Practice Guidelines and the Obesity Society. Circulation. 2014;129(25 Suppl 2):S102–38.
28. Tsai AG, Wadden TA. The evolution of very-low-calorie diets: an update and meta-analysis. Obesity. 2006;14(8):1283–93.
29. Hutcheon D, Hale A, Ewing J, Miller M, Couto F, Bour E, Cobb W, Scott J. Short-term preoperative weight loss and postoperative outcomes in bariatric surgery. J Am Coll Surg. 2018;226(4):514–24.

Is Routine Upper Endoscopy and *H. pylori* Testing Indicated in Advance of Bariatric Surgery?

14

Matthew August Odenwald and Robert T. Kavitt

14.1 Introduction

Bariatric surgery continues to be the only durable approach to long-term weight loss for the obese population and improves multiple weight-related comorbidities. Although safe with low complication rates, the most common procedures roux-en-y gastric bypass (RYGB) and sleeve gastrectomy (LSG) can still be associated with risks and adverse events.

Due to the construct of the gastrojejunostomy, RYGB is associated with the risk of marginal ulcers, estimated to occur between 0.6 and 16% [1, 2]. However, the true incidence may be much higher as these reports only include ulcers that are diagnosed on upper endoscopy, and many marginal ulcers are likely treated without endoscopic documentation. Multiple modifiable risk factors are associated with marginal ulcer development, including smoking, alcohol use, diabetes, NSAID use, surgical technique, and possibly *H. pylori* infection [3–5]. If left untreated, marginal ulcers can cause bleeding, strictures, and eventually obstruction. Additionally, because RYGB excludes of part of the stomach, a rare but potentially fatal adverse event is undetected abnormalities of this excluded stomach, such as ulcers or cancer, that are not easily accessed endoscopically after RYGB.

LSG, although thought of as a simpler bariatric operation, can also be associated with certain morbidity postoperatively. The most common being gastroesophageal

M. A. Odenwald
Department of Medicine, Section of Gastroenterology, Hepatology, and Nutrition,
The University of Chicago, Chicago, IL, USA
e-mail: Matthew.Odenwald@uchospitals.edu

R. T. Kavitt (✉)
Center for Esophageal Diseases, Department of Medicine, Section of Gastroenterology,
Hepatology, and Nutrition, The University of Chicago, Chicago, IL, USA
e-mail: rkavitt@bsd.uchicago.edu

© Springer Nature Switzerland AG 2021
J. Alverdy, Y. Vigneswaran (eds.), *Difficult Decisions in Bariatric Surgery*,
Difficult Decisions in Surgery: An Evidence-Based Approach,
https://doi.org/10.1007/978-3-030-55329-6_14

reflux disease and associated Barrett's esophagus. In patients undergoing LSG, 84.1% who had GERD symptoms previously, continued to have GERD symptoms postoperatively, and 8.6% developed new-onset GERD symptoms postoperatively [6]. This is in contrast to 62.8% resolution of GERD symptoms in patients undergoing RYGB [6]. Given the inability to resolve gastric reflux and the high incidence of new-onset reflux after LSG, both erosive esophagitis and Barrett's esophagus are generally considered contraindications to sleeve gastrectomy and thus important to identify preoperatively.

14.1.1 Preoperative Screening Guidelines

Given the potentially modifiable risk profile of these adverse events, preoperative screening is important to minimize postoperative complications. However, the recommended preoperative evaluation prior to bariatric surgery is controversial, and there is a wide range of surgical practices. This is highlighted by differing statements from multiple international societies. The European Association for Endoscopic Surgery (EAES) recommends either a barium swallow or EGD prior to bariatric surgery [7]. Conversely, the most recent guidelines co-published by the American Society for Gastrointestinal Endoscopy (ASGE), the Society of American Gastrointestinal and Endoscopic Surgeons (SAGES), and the American Society for Metabolic and Bariatric Surgery (ASMBS) in 2015 suggest an individualized approach to both upper endoscopy and *H. pylori* testing and eradication prior to bariatric surgery [8]. These conflicting guidelines raise the question of whether EGD and *H. pylori* testing should be routinely performed before bariatric surgery.

14.2 Search Strategy

We searched PubMed with the terms "bariatric surgery" AND "preoperative endoscopy." We also searched PubMed with the terms "bariatric surgery" AND "preoperative *Helicobacter pylori* testing." Evaluated articles were limited to those published in English and focused on outcomes after either Roux-en-Y gastric bypass or sleeve gastrectomy procedures. Studies from 1990 through 2020 were assessed; the majority of studies cited in this chapter were published within the past 10 years. No randomized controlled trials were available. When available, large cohort studies were given preference. The data was classified using the GRADE system. The most recent American and European guidelines were also reviewed and included.

P (Patients)	I (Intervention)	C (Comparator)	O (Outcomes)
Patients undergoing Roux-en-Y gastric bypass or sleeve gastrectomy	Preoperative endoscopy	Patients not undergoing preoperative endoscopy	Adverse postoperative events: leak, marginal ulcer, gastric cancer, reflux
Patients undergoing Roux-en-Y gastric bypass or sleeve gastrectomy	Preoperative *H. pylori* testing and eradication	Patients not tested for *H. pylori*	Adverse postoperative events: leak, marginal ulcer, gastric cancer

14.3   Results

14.3.1 Routine Upper Endoscopy Prior to Bariatric Surgery

The goal of preoperative endoscopy with EGD is to identify patients with anatomic abnormalities that would alter surgical management in one of three ways: delay the operation to allow for medical treatment, change the recommended surgical approach or technique, or cancel the operation altogether with the ultimate goal of decreasing postoperative complications. Conditions that may alter the operative plan include hiatal hernias, esophagitis, mucosal ulcers, tumors, and vascular abnormalities. One difficulty in determining which patients should be screened is that the correlation of symptoms and endoscopic findings is poor [9, 10], which has led some to advocate for universal preoperative endoscopy. However, the impact of specific endoscopic findings depends on the procedure planned, and the utility of implementing routine preoperative EGD depends on prevalence of abnormalities and the frequency with which abnormal findings will change management.

While no randomized controlled trials exist to guide practice, multiple retrospective case series from bariatric surgery centers have been published in an attempt to help determine the diagnostic yield of routine preoperative EGDs [9, 11–15]. In each of these studies, the most common EGD result was a normal EGD with 21.8–70.7% of all EGDs performed showing no endoscopic abnormality. The prevalence of specific pathologies in these selected studies is the following: Hiatal hernia (9.0–27.5%), benign gastric or duodenal polyps (1.2–6.7%), esophagitis (1.1–16.6%), gastritis (13.7–37.6%), duodenitis (2.2–7.8%), *H. pylori* infection (2.0–44.7%), peptic ulcer disease (0.2–23%), and gastric cancer (0.0–0.8%) (Table 14.1). While abnormal findings were common in each of these studies, the interpretation and subsequent management was not uniform, making it difficult to determine best practice.

These findings can be grouped into categories of findings that either (1) have no impact on medical or surgical management, (2) result in additional medical management, or (3) change surgical management. A meta-analysis by Bennett, et al. analyzed 48 studies and determined that preoperative EGD changed medical management in 27.5% of cases, but only in 2.5% of cases when not counting *H. pylori* eradication [15]. The medical changes were commonly *H. pylori* eradication, which can be reliably done using non-invasive testing, and the addition of a PPI, which is now standard practice for many bariatric surgeons regardless of preoperative endoscopic findings. Similarly, surgical management was affected by 7.8% of preoperative EGDs; however, after removing entities with a variable effect on operative management, such as hiatal hernias and peptic ulcers, EGDs effected surgical management in only 0.4% of cases [15]. However, 7.5% of the changes were major changes in the operative plan such as switching from a LSG to a RYGB or adding a gastrectomy to an RYGB [15]. These findings were supported by a subsequent similar meta-analysis [16]. Findings that typically do not delay surgery include benign gastric or duodenal polyps and hiatal hernia, although hiatal hernias are typically repaired at the time of bariatric surgery. Gastritis, duodenitis, and peptic ulcer disease often change medical management in that their presence results in initiation of

Table 14.1 Summary of studies assessing findings on preoperative endoscopy

Endoscopic finding / Study	Kuper et al. [9]	Loewen et al. [11]	Munoz et al. [12]	Azagury et al. [10]	Peromaa-Haavisto et al. [13]	Schigt et al. [14]	Bennett et al. [15]	Parikh et al. [16]
Normal EGD	21.80%	70.70%	54.00%	54.00%	55.80%	48.90%		
Hiatal hernia	27.50%	9.00%	10.70%	16.93%	25.40%	21.80%	21.10%	19.70%
Gastric polyp	2.90	3.10%	1.30%	1.25%	6.70%	Not reported	Not reported	Not reported
Duodenal polyp		1.30%	Not reported	Not reported	Not reported	Not reported	Not reported	Not reported
H. pylori	8.70%	2.00%	44.70%	39.00%	12.00%	25.80%	20.20%	19.70%
Esophagitis	11.60%	1.10%	16.00%	6.58%	13.20%	16.60%	14.40%	17.00%
Barrett's esophagus	1.40%	Not reported	0.16% (1 patient)	1.25%	0.90%	1.30%	2.10%	0.10%
Esophageal cancer	2.90%	Not reported	Not reported	Not reported	Not reported	Not reported	0.20%	0.08% (combined with gastric)
Gastritis	36.20%	13.6%%	21.00%	26.3%	13.70%	24.30%	37.60%	34.60%
Duodenitis	4.30%	4.30%	7.80%	2.19%	Not reported	4.40%	5.20%	5.00%
Gastric or duodenal erosions		0.70%	Not reported	Not reported	Not reported	Not reported	Not reported	Not reported
Gastric or duodenal ulcers	23.20%	0.20%	5.30%	2.19%	2.90%	1.00%	5.40%	2.30%
Gastric cancer		Not reported	0.16% (1 patient)	Not reported	Not reported	0.80%	0.40%	0.08% (cobined with esophageal)
Vascular lesion	Not reported	0.20%	Not reported	Not reported	Not reported	Not reported	Not reported	Not reported
Type of study	Retrospective case series	Retrospective case series	Retrospective case series	Retrospective case series	Retrospective case series	Retrospective case series	Meta-analysis	Meta-analysis
Quality of evidence	Low	Low	Low	Low	Low	Low	Moderate	Moderate

a proton pump inhibitor (PPI) and testing and eradication of *H. pylori*. However, data supports the practice of routine perioperative PPI use to decrease the risk of marginal ulcer development, and *H. pylori* can be diagnosed with less expensive, non-invasive testing [17–19]. These endoscopic findings are therefore unlikely to change current management. While both reflux esophagitis or Barrett's esophagus are treated with PPI and surveillance upper endoscopy, these endoscopic findings may change treatment with sleeve gastrectomy given that sleeve gastrectomy often results in worsening gastroesophageal reflux and can exacerbate both conditions. In the case of RYGB, however, these findings would not change either medical or operative management, as PPI use is routine in this setting and post-surgical anatomy would not preclude routine surveillance of Barrett's esophagus. Given poor correlation between symptom and endoscopic findings, we advocate for routine upper endoscopy in patients who are planning to undergo sleeve gastrectomy to evaluate for the presence of reflux esophagitis and Barrett's esophagus, and if these pathologies are found, we recommend discussing a change in surgical approach to a RYGB. The prevalence and impact of *H. pylori* infection on bariatric surgery is the topic of the next section.

One of the most feared long-term adverse events of a RYGB is developing pathology such as gastric cancer developing in the relatively inaccessible excluded stomach. Discovering precancerous lesions or gastric cancer on preoperative EGD can either result in offering concurrent gastrectomy or deferring bariatric surgery altogether for oncologic therapy. Gastric cancer in those undergoing bariatric surgery is an exceedingly rare entity, and the above studies reported rates of diagnosing gastric cancer on preoperative endoscopy ranging from 0.0–0.8%. Similarly, studies reporting development of gastric cancer in the excluded stomach after RYGB have been limited to a few case reports [20–23]. Harper et al. report a patient who did not undergo preoperative EGD and was diagnosed with disseminated gastric cancer only 1 year after a RYGB operation [20]. While it is difficult to justify the potential risk and cost of routine endoscopic screening to diagnose such a rare entity, the consequence of missing gastric cancer, however rare, has led some to interpret such cases as reason to do preoperative screening in all patients [12]. However, a normal preoperative endoscopy and eradication of risk factors such as *H. pylori* does not guarantee a cancer-free excluded stomach in the long-term. This is evidenced by Tinoco et al. who reported the development of gastric cancer in the excluded stomach 10 years after a bypass operation in a patient that underwent preoperative *H. pylori* eradication [21]. It is not reported whether this patient had a preoperative EGD. Escalona et al. also report development of gastric cancer in the remnant stomach 8 years postoperatively in a center that routinely performs preoperative endoscopy [24]. Corsini et al. report a patient who had preoperative endoscopy showing intestinal metaplasia and *H. pylori*, which was eradicated preoperatively [22]. The patient unfortunately developed an aggressive gastric carcinoma 4 years after RYGB [14]. Given the presence of metaplasia preoperatively, it can be argued that this previously asymptomatic patient should have either been offered a different operation, such as a sleeve gastrectomy or resection of the remnant stomach at time of bypass, or undergone surveillance endoscopy of his excluded stomach postoperatively.

The utility of routine preoperative EGD for purposes of detecting gastric cancer in the excluded stomach is very low. Similarly, given the low incidence of gastric cancer in the Western world, gastric cancer screening programs have not been implemented for the general population [25, 26]. This is different in high-risk areas such as Japan and South Korea, where the incidence of gastric cancer is high and routine screening is performed [26]. If the patient had no indication for screening other than an upcoming bariatric surgery, we advise against EGD for these purposes.

14.3.2 Routine *H. Pylori* Testing Prior to Bariatric Surgery

H. pylori is the most common chronic human infection with estimates that more than half of the world's population is infected [27], and most patients who are infected are asymptomatic. The prevalence of *H. pylori* infection is strongly influenced by geography with fewer people being infected in developed countries than in developing countries, where *H. pylori* infection is nearly universal [27]. Conflicting reports regarding the prevalence of *H. pylori* infections in the population with obesity have been published, and published rates have ranged from 8.7% to 85.5% in different cohort studies [9, 28]. Discrepancies can be attributed to many factors including study design, method for detecting *H. pylori*, and most importantly, geographic location of the study, making comparing these retrospective studies very difficult. Similarly, some have observed a significant increase in BMI after *H. pylori* eradication, whereas others report an increased prevalence of *H. pylori* infection in patients with obesity. As such, *H. pylori* has been proposed to play both a pathogenic and protective role in the development of obesity [29], potentially through altering circulating ghrelin levels [30]. In those who are infected, obesity is an independent risk factor for treatment failure for *H. pylori* eradication with clarithromycin-based triple therapy [31].

The focus of this chapter, however, is to discuss the utility of routine preoperative *H. pylori* testing and eradication prior to bariatric surgery. Verma, et al. retrospectively analyzed 611 patients with morbid obesity (average BMI of 47.9 kg/m^2) who routinely underwent EGD with biopsies to test for *H. pylori* prior to bariatric surgery [32]. *H. pylori* was found in 23.7% of patients with similar BMI in both infected and uninfected patients. Infected patients had a much higher rate of abnormal preoperative endoscopy with chronic active gastritis being the most common finding. However, the implications of preoperative *H. pylori* infection on postoperative outcomes was not reported [32]. The aim of a universal test and eradicate strategy would be to minimize adverse postoperative events, including viscus perforation, marginal ulcer development, gastrointestinal bleeding, continued foregut symptoms, and cancer development, especially in the relatively inaccessible excluded stomach after RYGB.

14.3.2.1 Perforation

Perforated ulcers are an uncommon but detrimental adverse event after bariatric surgery. To determine the effect of routine *H. pylori* screening on postoperative outcomes in bariatric surgery patients, Hartin, et al. performed a retrospective chart review of 183 patients who underwent bariatric surgery over a 40-month period [33]. Of these patients, 125 were not tested for *H. pylori* preoperatively, and 58 were tested and treated if positive (seven patients [12%] were positive). In this single-center cohort there was a statistical difference in the rate of perforated ulcers with six patients suffering perforation in the untested group and 0 having perforation in the group who was tested and treated [33]. While this lends support to the idea of universal preoperative testing and eradication, this does not prove a pathogenic role of *H. pylori* in perforated ulcers, and this data should be interpreted with caution as it was a single center, single surgeon study. Moreover, the practice of routine *H. pylori* testing was started later in this surgeon's practice, and many factors, including increased surgeon experience may have contributed to the improved outcomes in later years.

14.3.2.2 Marginal Ulcer Development

Marginal ulceration refers to mucosal erosion at the gastrojejunal anastomosis, most commonly on the jejunal side. Development is multifactorial and has been associated with multiple modifiable risk factors including corticosteroid use, smoking status, and NSAID use [4]. The role of *H. pylori* infection on anastomotic ulcer development is controversial, and many cite the typical anatomical location of marginal ulcers on the jejunal side of the anastomosis as empiric evidence discounting the effect of *H. pylori* on marginal ulcer development. Nevertheless, some case series have reported an association between marginal ulcers and *H. pylori.* Schirmer et al. analyzed a consecutive case series of 560 patients undergoing RYGB, and midway through the case series the center changed preoperative practice to routinely test for *H. pylori* with biopsies and eradicate the infection if found [34]. They found that marginal ulcers developed significantly less often in patients who underwent routine *H. pylori* screening (2.4% vs. 6.8%) [34], suggesting that routine *H. pylori* eradication prior to bariatric surgery may prevent marginal ulcers. However, this report does not control for changes in operative technique or increased operative experience that naturally occurs over time and can affect rates of postoperative ulcers. Rasmussen et al. published a retrospective review of 260 patients undergoing RYGB with an overall marginal ulcer rate of 7% [3]. *H. pylori* was routinely screened for with a serum assay and treated with 14 day triple therapy if present. Patients with marginal ulcers were much more likely to have been *H. pylori* positive when compared to patients who did not develop marginal ulcers (32% vs 12%) [3].

Multiple similar studies have been published showing no association between *H. pylori* infection and marginal ulcer formation. For example, in their retrospective analysis of 448 patient undergoing bariatric surgery, Loewen et al. reported a postoperative ulcer rate of 13% that was statistically associated with preoperative gastritis and duodenitis but not *H. pylori* status [11]. Similarly, Papasavas et al. retrospectively compared rates of ulceration in patients who underwent *H. pylori* serum testing and eradication (259 patients) and those who were not tested (153 patients) [35]. They found that both groups had similar rates of indication for postoperative EGDs (5% in tested group vs. 3.7% in untested group), and in the group of patients that was tested, there were similar rates of positive EGD findings in those testing positive and undergoing eradication (3.6%) and those testing negative (5.6%) [35]. This led to their conclusion that *H. pylori* testing and treatment does not lower rate of marginal ulceration or pouch gastritis. Rawlins et al. retrospectively reviewed 228 patients who underwent RYGB to determine the utility of preoperative serum *H. pylori* screening [36]. Sixty-eight of the 228 patients were serum positive, and 24 were persistently positive on follow-up endoscopy despite 14 day triple therapy, highlighting a high rate of treatment failure in this population [36]. Postoperative outcomes of marginal ulceration were very rare (5 total) with 4 occurring in the group that was negative preoperatively and only 1 occurring in the group that was positive and treated for *H. pylori* preoperatively [36]. However, the rate of marginal ulceration was too low to determine if there was a true difference.

Two studies have actually shown a negative association between anastomotic ulcers and *H. pylori* infection. Yang et al. retrospectively reviewed 636 patients who were screened for *H. pylori* with serum IgG prior to either RYGB or laparoscopic adjustable gastric banding [37]. They found that 39% of patients were seropositive regardless of symptoms and that patients who developed postoperative ulcers actually tended to be positive for *H. pylori* less often (27.3% vs 43.3%), although this was not statistically significant [37]. Finally, Kelly et al. reported that 7.6% of *H. pylori* positive patients compared to 17.1% of *H. pylori* negative patients had marginal ulcers, which was statistically significant [38]. Mechanistically, this negative association may be explained by chronic gastropathy and subsequent decreased acidity preventing ulceration; however, this is not proven. From these multiple studies it is clear that more work needs to be done to elucidate the true risk of *H. pylori* infection on marginal ulcer development, especially in the current age where PPIs are commonly used perioperatively to prevent marginal ulceration. Given the lack of strong evidence to the contrary, it is still reasonable to routinely screen and treat for *H. pylori* in the preoperative period, and PPIs should be routinely prescribed in the postoperative period to decrease the incidence of marginal ulceration.

14.3.2.3 Cancer in the Excluded Stomach

As discussed above, reports of cancer in the excluded stomach are rare and limited to case reports. However, from very limited data, *H. pylori* eradication does not seem to prevent this rare entity as preoperative testing and eradication was performed in many of these cases [21, 22]. This may be due to either *H. pylori* reinfection or alternative risk factors of developing gastric cancer such as age, family history, smoking status, and diet. However, the rarity of gastric cancer in the excluded stomach after RYGB limits our ability to study the effect of *H. pylori* eradication on development of cancer in the excluded stomach. It is reasonable to test for and eradicate *H. pylori* even if it does not have impact on immediate surgical outcomes as *H. pylori* is a carcinogen, and eradication can decrease the incidence of gastric cancer in patients without premalignant lesions [39–41]. This is especially true with RYGB when the excluded stomach is much more difficult to access.

14.4   Recommendations Based on the Data

Given the poor correlation between symptoms and endoscopic findings, we strongly recommend routine upper endoscopy in patients who are planning to undergo sleeve gastrectomy for the purposes of evaluating for reflux esophagitis and Barrett's esophagus. If these pathologies are found, we strongly recommend changing the planned surgical approach to a RYGB. In the case of planning for a RYGB, the utility of routine preoperative EGD for purposes of detecting gastric cancer in the excluded stomach is very low, and if the patient had no indication for screening other than an upcoming bariatric surgery, we weakly advise against EGD for these purposes. We weakly recommend routinely testing for and treating *H. pylori* in the preoperative period as a means of potentially decreasing marginal ulcer development and diminishing risk of gastric cancer.

14.5   A Personal View of the Data

Given the rapidly increasing incidence of obesity and the increasing prevalence of bariatric surgery, it will be extremely important to better define the ideal preoperative evaluation, including whether routine EGD and *H. pylori* testing are warranted. The above discussion highlights the lack of randomized controlled trials in the field, as the majority of data is from retrospective reviews of all cases performed at single centers. The best way to define the utility of preoperative EGD and *H. pylori* testing will be through a large, multicenter randomized controlled trial that directly addresses both the prevalence of abnormal EGD findings and *H. pylori* infection and the effect on surgical planning and surgical outcomes. Until such a definitive study is performed, we recommend the following: (1) perform preoperative EGD in all patients planning to undergo LSG in order to assess for reflux esophagitis and Barrett's esophagus; (2) do not perform routine EGD in patients planning to undergo RYGB unless there is another reason to perform EGD; and (3) it is reasonable to test for and eradicate *H. pylori* in all patients prior to bariatric surgery given the conflicting results of prevalence and effect on postoperative outcomes and known carcinogenic effect of *H. pylori*.

14.6   Recommendations

- For patients planning to undergo sleeve gastrectomy, we recommend routine preoperative endoscopy to assess for reflux esophagitis and Barrett's esophagus (Evidence quality moderate; strong recommendation).

- For patients undergoing roux-en-Y gastric bypass, we recommend against routine preoperative endoscopy unless there is another indication to perform EGD (Evidence quality low; weak recommendation).
- We recommend routine preoperative testing and eradication of *H. pylori* (Evidence quality low; weak recommendation).

References

1. Sanyal AJ, Sugerman HJ, Kellum JM, Engle KM, Wolfe L. Stomal complications of gastric bypass: incidence and outcome of therapy. Am J Gastroenterol. 1992;87(9):1165.
2. Sapala JA, Wood MH, Sapala MA, Flake TM Jr. Marginal ulcer after gastric bypass: a prospective 3-year study of 173 patients. Obes Surg. 1998;8(5):505–16.
3. Rasmussen JJ, Fuller W, Ali MR. Marginal ulceration after laparoscopic gastric bypass: an analysis of predisposing factors in 260 patients. Surg Endosc. 2007;21(7):1090–4.
4. Coblijn UK, Lagarde SM, de Castro SM, Kuiken SD, van Wagensveld BA. Symptomatic marginal ulcer disease after Roux-en-Y gastric bypass: incidence, risk factors and management. Obes Surg. 2015;25(5):805–11.
5. Azagury DE, Abu Dayyeh BK, Greenwalt IT, Thompson CC. Marginal ulceration after Roux-en-Y gastric bypass surgery: characteristics, risk factors, treatment, and outcomes. Endoscopy. 2011;43(11):950–4.
6. DuPree CE, Blair K, Steele SR, Martin MJ. Laparoscopic sleeve gastrectomy in patients with preexisting gastroesophageal reflux disease : a national analysis. JAMA Surg. 2014;149(4):328–34.
7. Sauerland S, Angrisani L, Belachew M, Chevallier JM, Favretti F, Finer N, et al. Obesity surgery: evidence-based guidelines of the European Association for Endoscopic Surgery (EAES). Surg Endosc. 2005;19(2):200–21.
8. American Societyfor Gastrointestinal Endoscopy Standards of Practice Commitee, Evans JA, Muthusamy VR, Acosta RD, Bruining DH, Chandrasekhara V, et al. The role of endoscopy in the bariatric surgery patient. Gastrointest Endosc. 2015;81(5):1063–72.
9. Kuper MA, Kratt T, Kramer KM, Zdichavsky M, Schneider JH, Glatzle J, et al. Effort, safety, and findings of routine preoperative endoscopic evaluation of morbidly obese patients undergoing bariatric surgery. Surg Endosc. 2010;24(8):1996–2001.
10. Azagury D, Dumonceau JM, Morel P, Chassot G, Huber O. Preoperative work-up in asymptomatic patients undergoing Roux-en-Y gastric bypass: is endoscopy mandatory? Obes Surg. 2006;16(10):1304–11.
11. Loewen M, Giovanni J, Barba C. Screening endoscopy before bariatric surgery: a series of 448 patients. Surg Obes Relat Dis. 2008;4(6):709–12.
12. Munoz R, Ibanez L, Salinas J, Escalona A, Perez G, Pimentel F, et al. Importance of routine preoperative upper GI endoscopy: why all patients should be evaluated? Obes Surg. 2009;19(4):427–31.
13. Peromaa-Haavisto P, Victorzon M. Is routine preoperative upper GI endoscopy needed prior to gastric bypass? Obes Surg. 2013;23(6):736–9.
14. Schigt A, Coblijn U, Lagarde S, Kuiken S, Scholten P, van Wagensveld B. Is esophagogastroduodenoscopy before Roux-en-Y gastric bypass or sleeve gastrectomy mandatory? Surg Obes Relat Dis. 2014;10(3):411–7. quiz 565-6
15. Bennett S, Gostimir M, Shorr R, Mallick R, Mamazza J, Neville A. The role of routine preoperative upper endoscopy in bariatric surgery: a systematic review and meta-analysis. Surg Obes Relat Dis. 2016;12(5):1116–25.

16. Parikh M, Liu J, Vieira D, Tzimas D, Horwitz D, Antony A, et al. Preoperative endoscopy prior to bariatric surgery: a systematic review and meta-analysis of the literature. Obes Surg. 2016;26(12):2961–6.
17. Coblijn UK, Lagarde SM, de Castro SM, Kuiken SD, van Tets WF, van Wagensveld BA. The influence of prophylactic proton pump inhibitor treatment on the development of symptomatic marginal ulceration in Roux-en-Y gastric bypass patients: a historic cohort study. Surg Obes Relat Dis. 2016;12(2):246–52.
18. Ying VW, Kim SH, Khan KJ, Farrokhyar F, D'Souza J, Gmora S, et al. Prophylactic PPI help reduce marginal ulcers after gastric bypass surgery: a systematic review and meta-analysis of cohort studies. Surg Endosc. 2015;29(5):1018–23.
19. Gumbs AA, Duffy AJ, Bell RL. Incidence and management of marginal ulceration after laparoscopic Roux-Y gastric bypass. Surg Obes Relat Dis. 2006;2(4):460–3.
20. Harper JL, Beech D, Tichansky DS, Madan AK. Cancer in the bypassed stomach presenting early after gastric bypass. Obes Surg. 2007;17(9):1268–71.
21. Tinoco A, Gottardi LF, Boechat ED. Gastric Cancer in the excluded stomach 10 years after gastric bypass. Case Rep Surg. 2015;2015:468293.
22. Corsini DA, Simoneti CA, Moreira G, Lima SE Jr, Garrido AB. Cancer in the excluded stomach 4 years after gastric bypass. Obes Surg. 2006;16(7):932–4.
23. Tornese S, Aiolfi A, Bonitta G, Rausa E, Guerrazzi G, Bruni PG, et al. Remnant gastric cancer after Roux-en-Y gastric bypass: narrative review of the literature. Obes Surg. 2019;29(8):2609–13.
24. Escalona A, Guzman S, Ibanez L, Meneses L, Huete A, Solar A. Gastric cancer after Roux-en-Y gastric bypass. Obes Surg. 2005;15(3):423–7.
25. Siegel RL, Miller KD, Jemal A. Cancer statistics, 2019. CA Cancer J Clin. 2019;69(1):7–34.
26. Bray F, Ferlay J, Soerjomataram I, Siegel RL, Torre LA, Jemal A. Global cancer statistics 2018: GLOBOCAN estimates of incidence and mortality worldwide for 36 cancers in 185 countries. CA Cancer J Clin. 2018;68(6):394–424.
27. Hooi JKY, Lai WY, Ng WK, Suen MMY, Underwood FE, Tanyingoh D, et al. Global prevalence of *Helicobacter pylori* infection: systematic review and meta-analysis. Gastroenterology. 2017;153(2):420–9.
28. Al-Akwaa AM. Prevalence of *Helicobacter pylori* infection in a group of morbidly obese Saudi patients undergoing bariatric surgery: a preliminary report. Saudi J Gastroenterol. 2010;16(4):264–7.
29. Carabotti M, D'Ercole C, Iossa A, Corazziari E, Silecchia G, Severi C. *Helicobacter pylori* infection in obesity and its clinical outcome after bariatric surgery. World J Gastroenterol. 2014;20(3):647–53.
30. Nweneka CV, Prentice AM. *Helicobacter pylori* infection and circulating ghrelin levels - a systematic review. BMC Gastroenterol. 2011;11:7.
31. Abdullahi M, Annibale B, Capoccia D, Tari R, Lahner E, Osborn J, et al. The eradication of *Helicobacter pylori* is affected by body mass index (BMI). Obes Surg. 2008;18(11):1450–4.
32. Verma S, Sharma D, Kanwar P, Sohn W, Mohanty SR, Tortolani AJ, et al. Prevalence of *Helicobacter pylori* infection in bariatric patients: a histologic assessment. Surg Obes Relat Dis. 2013;9(5):679–85.
33. Hartin CW Jr, ReMine DS, Lucktong TA. Preoperative bariatric screening and treatment of *Helicobacter pylori*. Surg Endosc. 2009;23(11):2531–4.
34. Schirmer B, Erenoglu C, Miller A. Flexible endoscopy in the management of patients undergoing Roux-en-Y gastric bypass. Obes Surg. 2002;12(5):634–8.
35. Papasavas PK, Gagne DJ, Donnelly PE, Salgado J, Urbandt JE, Burton KK, et al. Prevalence of *Helicobacter pylori* infection and value of preoperative testing and treatment in patients undergoing laparoscopic Roux-en-Y gastric bypass. Surg Obes Relat Dis. 2008;4(3):383–8.
36. Rawlins L, Rawlins MP, Brown CC, Schumacher DL. Effect of *Helicobacter pylori* on marginal ulcer and stomal stenosis after Roux-en-Y gastric bypass. Surg Obes Relat Dis. 2013;9(5):760–4.

37. Yang CS, Lee WJ, Wang HH, Huang SP, Lin JT, Wu MS. The influence of *Helicobacter pylori* infection on the development of gastric ulcer in symptomatic patients after bariatric surgery. Obes Surg. 2006;16(6):735–9.
38. Kelly JJ, Perugini RA, Wang QL, Czerniach DR, Flahive J, Cohen PA. The presence of *Helicobacter pylori* is not associated with long-term anastomotic complications in gastric bypass patients. Surg Endosc. 2015;29(10):2885–90.
39. Polk DB, Peek RM Jr. *Helicobacter pylori*: gastric cancer and beyond. Nat Rev Cancer. 2010;10(6):403–14.
40. Parsonnet J, Friedman GD, Vandersteen DP, Chang Y, Vogelman JH, Orentreich N, et al. *Helicobacter pylori* infection and the risk of gastric carcinoma. N Engl J Med. 1991;325(16):1127–31.
41. Wong BC, Lam SK, Wong WM, Chen JS, Zheng TT, Feng RE, et al. *Helicobacter pylori* eradication to prevent gastric cancer in a high-risk region of China: a randomized controlled trial. JAMA. 2004;291(2):187–94.

Manometry is Useful Prior to Bariatric Surgery

15

Anna M. Lipowska

15.1 Introduction

Esophageal dysmotility is common in morbidly obese patients. Multiple studies have suggested that individuals with morbid obesity have a significantly increased prevalence of esophageal motor disorders compared to their non-obese peers, including abnormal lower esophageal sphincter (LES) function and altered peristalsis. In addition, current literature suggests that bariatric surgery affects esophageal motility and health, thus increasing the importance of including an evaluation of swallowing disorders in the preoperative stage.

Per current clinical practice guidelines, esophageal manometry is not routinely performed as part of the preoperative work-up of all patients undergoing bariatric surgery [1]. However, there is mounting evidence of the usefulness of manometry prior to bariatric surgery and many institutions are incorporating the performance of manometry into their preoperative protocols. Different bariatric surgical techniques can influence both LES pressures as well as peristalsis, thus the choice of therapy should be carefully and individually considered for each surgical candidate. Understanding physiologic changes that occur as a result of bariatric surgery can help guide what preoperative evaluation should be performed and when to use caution in choosing surgical options. This chapter will address whether esophageal manometry testing should be included as a part of preoperative testing in bariatric surgery and discuss the changes in esophageal mechanics related to bariatric surgery.

A. M. Lipowska (✉)
Division of Gastroenterology and Hepatology, Department of Medicine, University of Illinois Chicago, Chicago, IL, USA
e-mail: lipowska@uic.edu

© Springer Nature Switzerland AG 2021
J. Alverdy, Y. Vigneswaran (eds.), *Difficult Decisions in Bariatric Surgery*,
Difficult Decisions in Surgery: An Evidence-Based Approach,
https://doi.org/10.1007/978-3-030-55329-6_15

15.2 Search Strategy

A literature search of English language publications in the medical database (PubMed) from 1999 to 2019 was used to identify published data on the use of manometry in bariatric surgery. Terms used in the search were "manometry", "motility disorder", "esophageal function", "esophageal motor disorder", "dysmotility", and "preoperative", "weight loss surgery", "bariatric surgery". Due to low numbers of high evidence papers, the majority of the studies were prospective or retrospective cohort studies, with no randomized controlled trials available. The data was classified using the GRADE system.

15.3 Results

15.3.1 Prevalence of Esophageal Disorders in Morbidly Obese Patients

When completing the bariatric preoperative evaluation, it is important to understand that individuals with morbid obesity have a significantly increased prevalence of esophageal motor disorders compared to individuals without obesity. Morbid obesity has been found to be associated with increased dysmotility of both the LES and the esophageal body. The mechanism responsible for alterations in motility in this population remains to be clearly defined. One proposed mechanism suggests that intake of food high in fat content leads to lower LES pressure through the secretion of hormones such as secretin and cholecystokinin [2]. The reported prevalence of both any abnormal manometric findings and of specific diagnosed esophageal disorders significantly varies between studies. (Table 15.1) This may be in part due to the dynamic landscape of manometry interpretation and continuously evolving understanding of esophageal mechanics.

Reported general abnormal esophageal motility in morbid obesity ranged from 17% on the conservative side to up to 61% [3, 8]. In comparison to healthy controls, Iovino et al. demonstrated significantly lower LES pressure in the morbidly obese [10]. Other authors have also found a hypotensive LES as the most common pathology on manometry in this population [7, 9]. The prevalence of a hypotensive LES was reported to range from 6.8% to 25% [3, 5]. Jaffin and colleagues studied 111 morbidly obese patients seeking bariatric surgery, finding that 61% had abnormal manometric findings [3]. This included 25% of patients with a hypotensive LES and 21% with a hypertensive disorder of the esophageal body. Interestingly, 59% of patients with abnormal manometry were asymptomatic, raising concern for abnormal visceral sensation in the morbidly obese population. A more recent evaluation of 221 patients who underwent preoperative manometric testing revealed disturbed manometry in 33.4%, of which 64% had a hypotensive LES [7]. This subset of patients was more likely to have erosive esophagitis and pathologic pH reflux monitoring; however, reflux symptoms did not appear to significantly differ between

Table 15.1 Prevalence of esophageal disorders in morbidly obese patients prior to bariatric surgery[a]

Author	N	Surgery type	Study type (quality of evidence)	Abnormal manometry (%)	Lower esophageal sphincter (LES) pathology	Peristaltic pathology
Jaffin et al. (1999) [3]	111	All	Prospective cohort (low)	61.0	25.0% hypotensive LES	14.4% Nutcracker esophagus, 21.0% hypertensive peristalsis
Hong et al. (2004) [4]	61	All	Retrospective cohort (low)	54.0	16.0% hypotensive LES, 18.0% hypertensive LES	5.0% Nutcracker esophagus, 3.0% diffuse esophageal spasm
Kristo et al. (2019) [5]	147	All	Prospective cohort (low)	34.0	6.8% hypotensive LES, 14.3% hypertensive LES	7.5% Jackhammer esophagus, 4.1% distal esophageal spasm
Merrouche et al. (2007) [6]	100	LAGB, RYGB	Prospective cohort (low)	N/A	11.0% incompetent LES	41.0% decreased amplitude of contractions
Mora et al. (2016) [7]	221	All	Prospective cohort (low)	33.4	21.2% hypotensive LES, 0.4% hypertensive LES	9.5% Nutcracker esophagus, 1.3% diffuse esophageal spasm
Schneider et al. (2018) [8]	610	SG, RYGB	Retrospective cohort (low)	17.0	13.0% abnormal LES	2.8% abnormal peristalsis
Suter et al. (2004) [9]	345	All	Prospective cohort (low)	25.6	17.7% hypotensive LES, 1.2% hypertensive LES	4.8% Nutcracker esophagus

[a]Bariatric surgery includes Laparoscopic adjustable gastric band (LAGB), Sleeve gastrectomy (SG), Roux-en-Y gastric bypass (RYGB)

subjects with normotensive and hypotensive LES, suggesting that reflux symptoms alone may not be a reliable measure of underlying pathology.

Kristo et al. published a prospective analysis of 147 individuals with morbid obesity who underwent esophageal function testing, aimed to investigate the prevalence and to characterize the pathology in this population [5]. They found that 34%

of patients had a motility disorder per the Chicago Classification, 14.3% had a hypertensive LES and 6.8% a hypotensive LES. Interestingly, the hypercontractility disorder Jackhammer esophagus was discovered in 7.5% of subjects. Older studies have also described an increased prevalence of elevated contraction amplitudes on manometry in the morbidly obese, although many noted hypertensive peristalsis called Nutcracker esophagus, which has since been omitted from the most recent Chicago Classification due to its unclear clinical significance [3, 4]. Comparison of these studies is difficult given that manometry interpretation guidelines have significantly changed over the course of time, but it raises the suspicion of undiagnosed hypertensive esophageal body disorders in this population. As newer longitudinal studies suggest that a quarter of Jackhammer esophagus patients progress to achalasia, this even further highlights the importance of a careful preoperative evaluation of esophageal health prior to bariatric surgery [11].

15.3.2 Preoperative Evaluation

Multiple components of the preoperative evaluation may raise suspicion of an underlying esophageal motor disorder and help guide the decision to pursue esophageal manometric testing, including an assessment of symptomatology, results of other preoperative testing and the choice of surgical technique. A detailed history can elucidate symptoms concerning for esophageal dysmotility such as dysphagia or regurgitation. Presence of these symptoms can accentuate concern for an underlying disorder, but may also shed light into potential postoperative outcomes. Symptoms to consider include reflux, as was studied by Kavanaugh and colleagues who developed a protocol at their center requiring foregut testing for all bariatric surgical candidates with symptoms of reflux who were being evaluated for SG [12].

Notably, patients with morbid obesity and underlying esophageal disorders may not present with typical gastrointestinal symptoms. In fact, studies have raised concern that dysphagia symptoms are unreliable to identify underlying abnormal esophageal dysmotility in patients with morbidly obesity. Instead, for example, patients may experience respiratory symptoms as a manifestation of their underlying pathology, leading to a possible missed diagnosis preoperatively [13]. Additionally, the perception of esophageal symptoms may itself be altered in the setting of underlying obesity. The autonomic nervous system may be susceptible to obesity-induced perturbations, causing dysregulation of sensory pathways [14].

In rare cases, other preoperative testing such as upper endoscopy and barium esophagram may pick up esophageal motor changes that need to be confirmed on manometry, such as achalasia [8]. A meta-analysis of preoperative esophagogastroduodenoscopy before bariatric surgery did not recommend manometry to be performed routinely in asymptomatic average-risk patients, and did not find that a significant portion of patients had pathologic findings requiring referral for further manometric testing [15]. However, in patients for whom this testing is indicated, findings on upper endoscopy that could trigger the need for manometry include the presence of liquid stasis in the esophagus and a puckered tight LES. Similarly, although not routinely recommended, barium swallow can be included in preoperative work up. On barium swallow, discovery of a bird's beak appearance, esophageal dilation, or severe peristaltic abnormality can reinforce the importance of diagnostic manometry prior to surgery.

15.3.3 Bariatric Surgery and Esophageal Mechanics

In both patients with and without underlying esophageal dysmotility, bariatric surgery has been found to be associated with changes in esophageal mechanics. A number of prospective and retrospective cohort studies exist evaluating key preoperative esophageal characteristics that influence bariatric surgery outcomes as well as how bariatric surgery can influence esophageal motility. (Table 15.2) Unfortunately, there is a lack of large randomized controlled trials to better define the risks and benefits of each surgery in how it impacts esophageal function and how specific procedure techniques could be improved to lead to better outcomes. In this chapter we will focus on three most studied bariatric surgical procedures, laparoscopic adjustable gastric band (LAGB), sleeve gastrectomy (SG) and roux-en-Y gastric bypass (RYGB) and their associated changes in motility.

15.3.3.1   Laparoscopic Adjustable Gastric Band

The important question of how preoperative manometry influences outcomes in bariatric surgery has been studied mostly in LAGB patients. Lew and colleagues reviewed preoperative manometry data on 77 LAGB patients, finding that 18% of them had an abnormal manometry [29]. While abnormal baseline manometry did not appear to impact weight loss and reflux symptoms, severe postoperative emesis did occur in this patient group, with majority of these patients categorized as having either decreased or ineffective peristalsis. The clinical significance of altered LES pressure was studied by Suter et al., who looked at whether preoperative testing including manometry correlated with outcomes in 134 patients after LAGB surgery [30]. Their group found that patients with higher preoperative LES pressure were more likely to develop long reflux episodes and poor late food tolerance. In a retrospective analysis of 68 patients undergoing LABG, 44.3% were found to have an incompetent LES preoperatively [31]. LES incompetence was associated with a statistically significant increase in reoperation, leading the authors to recommend consideration of preoperative manometry before LAGB and standardization of this into their practice.

Klaus et al. conducted a prospective study of 164 patients with preoperative GERD symptoms undergoing LAGB, finding that patients who remained symptomatic after surgery (31.7%) were more likely to have poorer preoperative esophageal body motility and deterioration of LES relaxation after surgery [32]. Importantly, one third of postoperatively symptomatic patients developed esophageal dilatation following LAGB. Other groups have also demonstrated evidence of concerning esophageal dilatation after LAGB [11, 21]. A retrospective review of 121 patients one year post surgery revealed that 14% had esophageal dilatation on barium

Table 15.2 Effect of bariatric surgery on esophageal motility

Author	N	Surgery type	Study type (quality of evidence)	Significant effect on LES	Significant effect on peristalsis
Tolone et al. (2019) [16]	12	LAGB	Prospective cohort (low)	Increased LES pressure	No significant change
Iovino et al. (2002) [10]	43	LAGB	Prospective cohort (low)	Increased LES pressure	No significant change
Merrouche et al. (2007) [6]	60	LAGB	Prospective cohort (low)	Increased LES pressure	No comment
de Jong et al. (2010) [17]	N/A	LAGB	Systematic Review (moderate)	Increased LES pressure	Increased disturbed peristalsis
Korenkov et al. (2002) [18]	20	LAGB	Prospective cohort (low)	No significant change	No significant change
Suter et al. (2005) [19]	43	LAGB	Prospective cohort (low)	No significant change	Weakened contractions
Weiss et al. (2002) [20]	52	LAGB	Prospective cohort (low)	Decreased LES relaxation	Esophageal stasis, esophageal dilation
Milone et al. (2008) [21]	121	LAGB	Retrospective cohort (low)	No comment	Esophageal dilatation
Petersen et al. (2012) [22]	37	SG	Prospective cohort (low)	Increased LES pressure	No comment
Tolone et al. (2019) [16]	26	SG	Prospective cohort (low)	No significant change	Increased ineffective peristalsis
Del Genio et al. (2014) [23]	25	SG	Prospective cohort (low)	No significant change	Increased ineffective peristalsis
Valezi et al. (2017) [24]	73	SG	Prospective cohort (low)	Decreased LES pressure	Decreased normal peristalsis
Braghetto et al. (2010) [25]	20	SG	Prospective cohort (low)	Decreased LES pressure	No comment
Tolone et al. (2019) [16]	18	RYGB	Prospective cohort (low)	No significant change	No significant change
Korenkov et al. (2002) [18]	30	RYGB	Prospective cohort (low)	No significant change	No significant change
Ortega et al. (2004) [26]	40	RYGB	Prospective cohort (low)	No significant change	No significant change
Merrouche et al. (2007) [6]	36	RYGB	Prospective cohort (low)	No significant change	No comment
Valezi et al. (2012) [27]	81	RYGB	Prospective cohort (low)	No significant change	Increased abnormal peristalsis
Mejia-Rivas et al. (2008) [28]	20	RYGB	Prospective cohort (low)	No significant change	Decreased amplitude of contractions

LAGB laparoscopic adjustable gastric band, *SG* sleeve gastrectomy, *RYGB* roux-en-Y gastric bypass swallow [21]. This anatomic change was associated with increased emesis and reflux symptoms.

In the postoperative period, impairment of LES relaxation as well as weakened esophageal peristalsis have been found on multiple studies after LAGB [10, 17, 19, 20]. Tolone et al. performed high resolution manometry and pH testing pre- and post-operatively in 112 patients undergoing one of seven bariatric surgeries [16]. There was no difference in LES pressures before and after therapy for all bariatric procedures except for LAGB who experienced an increase in pressure. Furthermore, several LAGB patients developed pseudoachalasia syndrome postoperatively. A systematic review by de Jong and colleagues demonstrated that all but one patient experienced increase in LES pressure after surgery and most patients had decreased LES relaxation [17]. Furthermore, evidence of disturbed peristalsis was found in four out of six studies that had adequate data on manometry. In a prospective study of 43 LAGB patients esophageal body contractions weakened and there was a trend towards postoperative motility disorders, however the LES appeared unaffected by surgery [19]. This led the authors to recommend that manometry be performed routinely prior to LAGB. On the contrary, a small prospective study of LAGB and RYGB patients showed no effect of gastric reduction surgery on postoperative esophageal function, with 20 LAGB patients undergoing pre- and post-operative manometry [18]. This study was noted to have a smaller sample size compared to others, and notably of the LAGB patients only one had preoperative dysmotility and 18% had weak LES pressure, which likely influenced the result. Overall, the majority of studies suggest that preoperative dysmotility in LAGB patients is associated with increased adverse outcomes such as vomiting, reflux, and potential need for reoperation. Furthermore, LAGB placement in general appears to increase LES pressure, impair LES relaxation, and potentially disturbs peristalsis which can lead to esophageal stasis in patients with poor underlying motility and rarely to pseudoachalasia.

15.3.3.2 Sleeve Gastrectomy

Research to date is limited on the effects of sleeve gastrectomy on esophageal function. Studies demonstrate a trend towards delayed esophageal emptying and are inconsistent on changes to the lower esophageal sphincter [22, 23, 25, 33]. It is thought that the large variance may be due to the number of different surgical techniques available during sleeve creation.

A study of 73 patients undergoing SG described a significant decrease in LES pressures postoperatively, with the number of patients with LES hypotonia progressing from 8% to 32% after surgery [24]. The authors also found a significant decrease in the number of patients with normal peristalsis after surgery. Tolone et al. demonstrated that the frequency of ineffective peristalsis significantly increased in patients after sleeve gastrectomy, while not being significantly altered following other bariatric operations [16]. Patients after SG also had greater intragastric pressure and gastroesophageal pressure gradients compared to prior, leading to a large increase in esophageal acid exposure.

Braghetto and colleagues sought to describe changes in the LES after SG, studying 20 patients prospectively until 6 months after surgery [25]. They discovered that resting LES pressures reduced significantly postoperatively, with 85% of patients having an incompetent LES. A longer prospective study 13 months postoperatively showed no change in LES function, however there was a significant increase in ineffective peristalsis and incomplete bolus transit [23]. On the other hand, a small prospective study of 37 patients demonstrated a significant increase in LES pressure postoperatively, which the authors credited to their utilized surgical strategy [22]. Chiu and colleagues attempted to consolidate the available data on the effect of SG on GERD into consensus unsuccessfully, and while a similar effort has not been performed to date for esophageal function, it is clear that great variability in results exists between studies [34]. In summary, SG appears to alter esophageal function with a greater number of studies suggesting decreasing LES pressure and weakened peristalsis postoperatively; however, more objective data is needed to improve our understanding.

15.3.3.3   Roux-en-Y Gastric Bypass

Compared to other bariatric surgeries, RYGB has been found to lead to the least functional impairment of the LES and esophageal body. In a prospective study of multiple bariatric surgeries, the frequency of ineffective peristalsis and LES pressure was found to be unchanged before and after RYGB [16]. Three other small prospective studies demonstrated no LES dysfunction or change in motility pre- and post-operatively after RYGB [6, 18, 26]. Comparatively, a study of RYGB patients without GERD symptoms showed postoperatively no significant difference in all manometric variables except for peristalsis [27]. A different group looked at 20 patients after RYGB, describing that the percentage of patients with altered esophageal function diminished from 35% to 25% [28]. In this cohort, there was no observed change in basal LES pressure, but the amplitude of esophageal contractions decreased after RYGB. Overall, RYGB is found to have the least impact on LES function compared to LAGB and SG, and the majority of studies did not find a significant change in motility postoperatively.

15.4   Conclusions

Bariatric surgery has been found to impact esophageal function and may lead to esophageal motor impairment. The increased prevalence of esophageal motility disorders in patients with morbid obesity augments the importance of a thorough preoperative evaluation. There is currently inadequate evidence for routine preoperative manometry testing in all patients undergoing bariatric surgery. However, for patients with concerning symptoms of an underlying esophageal motor disorder, manometry is a useful tool in the preoperative setting. In patients undergoing LAGB, the presence of preoperative abnormal peristalsis may increase adverse outcomes postoperatively. There is increasing evidence that preoperative esophageal manometry should be considered in patients undergoing SG given its effect on LES function and peristalsis, although larger and higher quality studies are needed in the future to define its benefit. RYGB appears to have the least amount of effect on esophageal motility and should be considered in patients with known esophageal motor disorders. However, bariatric surgery should always be performed with caution in patients with motility disorders.

15.5 A Personal View of the Data

Understanding the increased prevalence of esophageal dysmotility in morbid obesity, we perform a detailed review of any symptomatology that could reveal an underlying esophageal motor disorder and trigger the need for esophageal manometry testing in all patients undergoing a preoperative bariatric surgery evaluation. Symptoms are interpreted with caution as patients with morbid obesity may not present with typical symptoms and symptom perception itself may be altered in the setting of obesity. If manometry reveals a significantly hypotensive LES, RYGB may be considered over SG given that it is the least likely to lead to worsening reflux. LAGB is a rarely recommended treatment for morbid obesity, in part due to the significant rate of esophageal dysmotility and esophageal dilatation after LAGB. Future high quality studies are needed to improve our understanding of how underlying esophageal disorders can affect postoperative outcomes and of the effect of bariatric surgery on esophageal function.

15.6 Recommendations

1. Use of esophageal manometry testing is not part of current clinical practice guidelines and is not routinely recommended as part of the pre-operative work-up for asymptomatic patients undergoing bariatric surgery (Evidence quality moderate; strong recommendation)
2. If there is concern for preexisting esophageal dysmotility based on history, symptoms, upper endoscopy, or barium swallow, preoperative manometry testing should be strongly considered as it may influence the chosen surgical approach (Evidence quality moderate; moderate recommendation)
3. Gastric bypass is favored over other surgical approaches in the setting of underlying esophageal dysmotility, as it appears to have the least amount of effect on esophageal motility (Evidence quality low, weak recommendation)

References

1. Mechanick JI, Apovian C, Brethauer S, Garvey WT, Joffe AM, Kim J, et al. Clinical practice guidelines for the perioperative nutrition, metabolic, and nonsurgical support of patients undergoing bariatric procedures – 2019 update: cosponsored by American Association of Clinical

Endocrinologists/American College of Endocrinology, The Obesity Society, American Society for Metabolic & Bariatric Surgery, Obesity Medicine Association, and American Society of Anesthesiologists. Surg Obes Relat Dis. 2019;25(12):1346–59.

2. Nebel O, Castell DO. Inhibition of the lower oesophageal sphincter by fat: a mechanism for fatty food intolerance. Gut. 1973;14(4):270–4.

3. Jaffin B, Knoepflmacher P, Greenstein R. High prevalence of asymptomatic esophageal motility disorders among morbidly obese patients. Obes Surg. 1999;9(4):390–5.

4. Hong D, Khajanchee Y, Pereira N, Lockhart B, Patterson E, Swanstrom L. Manometric abnormalities and gastroesophageal reflux disease in the morbidly obese. Obes Surg. 2004;14(6):744–9.

5. Kristo I, Paireder M, Jomrich G, Felsenreich DM, Nikolic M, Langer FB, et al. Modern esophageal function testing and aastroesophageal reflux disease in morbidly obese patients. Obes Surg. 2019;29(11):3536–41.

6. Merrouche M, Sabate J, Jouet P, Harnois F, Scaringi S, Coffin B, et al. Gastro-esophageal reflux and esophageal motility disorders in morbidly obese patients before and after bariatric surgery. Obes Surg. 2007;17(7):894–900.

7. Mora F, Cassinello N, Mora M, Bosca M, Minguez M, Ortega J. Esophageal abnormalities in morbidly obese adult patients. Surg Obes Relat Dis. 2016;12(3):622–8.

8. Schneider R, Lazaridis I, Kraljevic M, Beglinger C, Wolnerhanssen B, Peterli R. The impact of preoperative investigations on the management of bariatric patients; results of a cohort of more than 1200 cases. Surg Obes Relat Dis. 2018;14(5):693–9.

9. Suter M, Dorta G, Giusti V, Calmes J. Gastroesophageal reflux and esophageal motility disorders in morbidly obese patients. Obes Surg. 2004;14(7):959–66.

10. Iovino P, Angrisani L, Tremolaterra F, Nirchio E, Ciannella M, Borrelli V, et al. Abnormal esophageal acid exposure is common in morbidly obese patients and improves after a successful lap-band system implantation. Surg Endosc. 2002;16(11):1631–5.

11. Huang L, Pimentel M, Rezaie A. Do Jackhammer contractions lead to achalasia? A longitudinal study. Neurogastroenterol Motil. 2017;29(3):e12953.

12. Kavanagh R, Smith J, Bashir U, Jones D, Avgenakis E, Nau P. Optimizing bariatric surgery outcomes: a novel preoperative protocol in a bariatric population with gastroesophageal reflux disease. Surg Endosc. 2019;34(4):1812–8.

13. Almogy G, Anthone G, Crookes P. Achalasia in the context of morbid obesity: a rare but important association. Obes Surg. 2003;13(6):896–900.

14. O'Brien PD, Hinder LM, Callaghan BC, Feldman EL. Neurological consequences of obesity. Lancet Neurol. 2017;16(6):465–77.

15. Bennett S, Gostimir M, Shorr R, Mallick R, Mamazza J, Neville A. The role of routine preoperative upper endoscopy in bariatric surgery: a systematic review and meta-analysis. Surg Obes Relat Dis. 2016;12(5):1116–25.

16. Tolone S, Savarino E, de Bortoli N, Frazzoni M, Frazzoni L, Savarino V, et al. Esophageal high-resolution manometry can unravel the mechanisms by which different bariatric techniques produce different reflux exposures. J Gastrointest Surg. 2019;24(1):1–7.

17. de Jong JR, Besselink MG, van Ramshorst B, Gooszen HG, Smout AJ. Effects of adjustable gastric banding on gastroesophageal reflux and esophageal motility: a systematic review. Obes Rev. 2010;11(4):297–305.

18. Korenkov M, Kohler L, Yucel N, Grass G, Sauerland S, Lempa M, et al. Esophageal motility and reflux symptoms before and after bariatric surgery. Obes Surg. 2002;12(1):72–6.

19. Suter M, Dorta G, Giusti V, Calmes J. Gastric banding interferes with esophageal motility and gastroesophageal reflux. Arch Surg. 2005;140(7):639–43.

20. Weiss H, Nehoda H, Labeck B, Peer-Kuehberger R, Oberwalder M, Aigner F, et al. Adjustable gastric and esophagogastric banding: a randomized clinical trial. Obes Surg. 2002;12(4):573–8.

21. Milone L, Daud A, Durak E, Olivero-Rivera L, Schrope B, Inabnet WB, et al. Esophageal dilation after laparoscopic adjustable gastric banding. Surg Endosc. 2008;22(6):1482–6.

22. Petersen WV, Meile T, Kuper MA, Zdichavsky M, Konigsrainer A, Schneider JH. Functional importance of laparoscopic sleeve gastrectomy for the lower esophageal sphincter in patients with morbid obesity. Obes Surg. 2012;22(3):360–6.
23. Del Genio G, Tolone S, Limongelli P, Brusciano L, D'Alessandro A, Docimo G, et al. Sleeve gastrectomy and development of "de novo" gastroesophageal reflux. Obes Surg. 2014;24(1):71–7.
24. Valezi AC, Herbella FA, Mali-Junior J, Menezes MA, Liberatti M, Sato RO. Preoperative manometry for the selection of obese people candidate to sleeve gastrectomy. Arq Bras Cir Dig. 2017;30(3):222–4.
25. Braghetto I, Lanzarini E, Korn O, Valladares H, Molina JC, Henriquez A. Manometric changes of the lower esophageal sphincter after sleeve gastrectomy in obese patients. Obes Surg. 2010;20(3):357–62.
26. Ortega J, Escudero MD, Mora F, Sala C, Flor B, Martinez-Valls J, et al. Outcome of esophageal function and 24-hour esophageal pH monitoring after vertical banded gastroplasty and roux-en-Y gastric bypass. Obes Surg. 2004;14(8):1086–94.
27. Valezi AC, Herbella FA, Junior JM, de Almeida Menezes M. Esophageal motility after laparoscopic roux-en-Y gastric bypass: the manometry should be preoperative examination Routine? Obes Surg. 2012;22(7):1050–4.
28. Mejia-Rivas MA, Herrera-Lopez A, Hernandez-Calleros J, Herrera MF, Valdovinos MA. Gastroesophageal reflux disease in morbid obesity: the effect of Roux-en-Y gastric bypass. Obes Surg. 2008;18(10):1217–24.
29. Lew JI, Daud A, DiGorgi MF, Olivero-Rivera L, Davis DG, Bessler M. Preoperative esophageal manometry and outcome of laparoscopic adjustable silicone gastric banding. Surg Endosc. 2006;20(8):1242–7.
30. Suter M, Giusti V, Calmes J, Paroz A. Preoperative upper gastrointestinal testing can help predicting long-term outcome after gastric banding for morbid obesity. Obes Surg. 2008;18(5):578–82.
31. Bueter M, Thalheimer A, le Roux CW, Wierlemann A, Seyfried F, Fein M. Upper gastrointestinal investigations before gastric banding. Surg Endosc. 2010;24(5):1025–30.
32. Klaus A, Gruber I, Wetscher G, Nehoda H, Aigner F, Peer R, et al. Prevalent esophageal body motility disorders underlie aggravation of GERD symptoms in morbidly obese patients following adjustable gastric banding. Arch Surg. 2006;141(3):247–51.
33. Tolone S, Savarino E, Yates RB. The impact of bariatric surgery on esophageal function. Ann N Y Acad Sci. 2016;1381(1):98–103.
34. Chiu S, Birch DW, Shi X, Sharma AM, Karmali S. Effect of sleeve gastrectomy on gastroesophageal reflux disease: a systematic review. Surg Obes Relat Dis. 2011;7(4):510–5.

Smoking Cessation Is Essential Prior to Bariatric Surgery

16

Shushmita M. Ahmed and Victoria Lyo

16.1 Introduction

With the rise in obesity throughout the United States, the prevalence of bariatric operations is increasing. In 2018, 252,000 procedures were performed, an increase of 24,000 from the year before, and double the number of procedures performed a decade ago [1, 2]. Bariatric surgery remains a safe treatment for morbidly obese patients, with 30-day mortality rates as low as 0.08% [3]. Serious complications are also rare (<5%); however, overall complication rates range from 13 to 25% [4]. Given the number of operations performed each year, even rare complications translate to hundreds of patients at risk. It is therefore imperative to address modifiable risk factors prior to surgery to optimize patient outcomes.

Smoking is one such modifiable risk factor. Currently, 16.5% of Americans 18 years and older use combustible tobacco (cigarettes, cigars, pipes) and a rising proportion of individuals use vaping devices (electronic-cigarettes and electronic nicotine delivery systems) [5–7]. Among patients undergoing bariatric surgery, a significant proportion have a history of smoking: upwards of 33% of patients were former smokers and 7–27% were current smokers [8–10]. Furthermore, little is known about the prevalence of marijuana smoking in bariatric patients and its effect on bariatric outcomes. The detriments of smoking on postsurgical outcomes after abdominal and orthopedic operations are well documented [11]. In 2002, Moller et al. conducted a randomized controlled trial in which preoperative smokers were assigned to intervention (weekly tobacco cessation counseling, nicotine substitution, and encouragement to quit) vs control (no counseling or information on tobacco risk) arms 6–8 weeks prior to surgery. Wound complications were reduced by 83% and overall complications were reduced by 65% in the intervention group

S. M. Ahmed · V. Lyo (✉)
Department of Surgery, University of California Davis, Sacramento, CA, USA
e-mail: vlyo@ucdavis.edu

© Springer Nature Switzerland AG 2021
J. Alverdy, Y. Vigneswaran (eds.), *Difficult Decisions in Bariatric Surgery*,
Difficult Decisions in Surgery: An Evidence-Based Approach,
https://doi.org/10.1007/978-3-030-55329-6_16

[12]. Lindstrom et al.'s randomized trial in 2008 showed that smoking cessation interventions initiated as late as 4 weeks prior to surgery reduced 30-day postoperative complications by half [13]. Thus, the risks of smoking may be mitigated with timely cessation.

Currently, the American Society for Metabolic and Bariatric Surgery recommends smoking cessation prior to bariatric surgery [14]. The aim of this chapter is to review the data on the effects of smoking on bariatric outcomes to support these recommendations.

16.2   Search Strategy

A PUBMED literature search of all English language publications from 2000 to 2020 was used to identify studies documenting the effect of smoking on perioperative outcomes following bariatric surgery. The following search terms were used: "'smoking' OR 'tobacco' OR 'vaping' OR 'e-cigarette' OR 'marijuana' AND 'outcomes' AND 'bariatric surgery'" and "'risk factors' OR 'predictors' AND 'complications' AND 'bariatric surgery.'" As roux-en-y gastric bypass (RYGB) and sleeve gastrectomy (SG) are the most commonly performed bariatric operations, search terms "gastric bypass" and "sleeve gastrectomy" were added to the above terms. Finally, as wound complications, respiratory failure, ulcers and venous thromboembolism (VTE) have been previously associated with smoking after abdominal surgery, the following terms were used to identify the effects of smoking in the bariatric population: "'respiratory failure' AND 'bariatric surgery' AND 'risk factors,'" "'wound complications' AND 'risk factors' AND 'bariatric surgery,'" "'marginal ulcer' AND 'risk factors' AND 'bariatric surgery,'" and "'venous thromboembolism' AND 'risk factors' AND 'bariatric surgery.'"

16.3   Results

Our search yielded 27 English language studies exploring the effect of smoking on bariatric outcomes. Four of those studies specifically focused on smoking while the rest included smoking within a multivariate analysis of several preoperative risk factors. No randomized controlled trials for smoking cessation have been done in the bariatric population. Study summaries and classification of the data using the GRADE system are found in Table 16.1.

16.3.1 Thirty-Day Complications

Several studies explore the impact of smoking on 30-day complications. Dayer-Jankechova et al. found that among patients with complications following RYGB, smokers had increased risk of major complications compared to nonsmokers (p = 0.016) [16]. Similar findings were shown in analyses of large databases. In

Table 16.1 Summary of data exploring the effects of smoking on bariatric outcomes

Author (year)	Smoking is focused risk factor	N	Study type	Study outcome	Quality of evidence
Blair et al. (2015) [15]	No	66,838	Prospective cohort	Smoking significantly increased risk of postoperative sepsis (OR 1.63, CI: 1.23–2.14; p = 0.0006); 1% additional increase in developing sepsis with each additional pack year	Low
Dayer-Jankechova et al. (2016) [16]	No	1573	Prospective cohort	Among RYGB patients with complications, smoking was associated with increased risk of major complication (p = 0.016)	Very low
El Chaar et al. (2019) [17]	No	101,599	Retrospective cohort	Multivariate analysis showed increase risk of both major complications (OR 1.12, CI: 1.01–1.24, p = 0.04) and readmissions (OR 1.14, CI: 1.03–1.27, p = 0.01)	Low
Finks et al. (2011) [18]	No	25,469	Prospective cohort	Smoking significantly increased risk of serious comorbidity (OR 1.20, CI: 1.02–1.40; p = 0.03)	Low
Gambhir et al. (2019) [19]	No	369,032	Retrospective cohort	Smoking did not increase risk of 30-day DVT (OR 1.0, CI 0.70–1.26; p = 0.72) or PE (OR 0.7, CI: 0.42–1.04; p = 0.10)	Low
Gonzalez et al. (2003) [20]	No	158	Retrospective cohort	Multivariate regression did not show increased risk of ICU admission among smokers (OR 2.04, CI: 0.59–7.06)	Low
Gonzalez et al. (2005) [21]	No	660	Prospective cohort	Smokers were more likely to develop venous thromboembolisms compared to non-smokers (22 vs. 7%, p < 0.01); OR 6.7, CI: 1.90–23.57	Low
Haskins et al. (2014) [22]	Yes	41,445	Prospective cohort	Smoking increases risk of prolonged intubation (OR 2.59), pneumonia (OR 5.92). Reintubation (OR 2.19), sepsis (OR 1.49), shock (OR 1.78) and organ space infection (OR 2.71). All p < 0.05. No increased risk of 30-day mortality	Moderate
Haskins et al. (2017) [23]	Yes	33,714	Prospective cohort	SG patients who smoked within 1 year of operation had increased rate of composite morbidity (4.3 vs. 3.7%, p = 0.04), serious morbidity (0.9 vs. 0.6%, p = 0.003), 30-day mortality (0.2 vs. 0.1%, p = 0.004), and had increased risk of unplanned intubation (OR 1.88, CI: 1.01–3.50)	Low

(continued)

Table 16.1 (continued)

Author (year)	Smoking is focused risk factor	N	Study type	Study outcome	Quality of evidence
Hussain et al. (2018) [24]	No	772	Retrospective cohort	Smoking significantly increased major complication on univariate analysis, but not on multivariate analysis (OR 5.24, CI: 0.60–45.60; p = 0.133)	Low
Inadomi et al. (2017) [25]	Yes	49,772	Prospective cohort	Among RYGB patients, recent smokers with increased risk of serious complication than non-smokers (OR 1.34, CI: 1.01–1.77, p = 0.04); no difference in outcomes for smokers vs non-smokers among SG patients	Low
Livingston et al. (2006) [26]	No	575	Prospective cohort	Veterans' Affairs patients with over 20 pack year history who smoked within 1 year of surgery were more likely to remain intubated 48 h after surgery compared to those with over 20 pack year history who did not smoke within 1 year of surgery, and those with under 20 pack year history and did not smoke within 1 year of surgery (11.1 vs. 5.8 vs. 1.8%, p < 0.05)	Low
Major et al. (2017) [27]	No	408	Retrospective cohort	Smoking did not increase risk of overall complication (OR 0.34, CI: 0.02–5.37; p = 0.442)	Low
Marchini et al. (2012) [28]	No	229	Retrospective cohort	Compared to non-smokers, LOS was increased by 4 days among current smokers and 1 day among those who quit within 1 year prior to surgery (p < 0.01)	Low
Morgan et al. (2015) [29]	No	12,062	Retrospective cohort	Patients with unplanned ICU admission were more likely to be smokers than patients with planned ICU admission (19 vs. 12%, p = 0.05)	Low
Masoomi et al. (2011) [30]	No	304,515	Retrospective cohort	Multivariate analysis showed no increase of VTE among smokers during index hospitalization (OR 0.6, CI: 0.4–0.9)	Very low
Masoomi et al. (2013) [31]	No	304,515	Retrospective cohort	On multivariate regression analysis smoking trended towards increased risk for acute respiratory failure (OR 1.1, CI: 1.0–1.2; p = 0.05)	Low

Study		Sample size	Study type	Findings	Quality
Stenberg et al. (2014) [32]	No	26,173	Prospective cohort	Patients with history of smoking trended towards increased risk of any complication (OR 1.13, CI: 1.00–1.28; p = 0.055) but not serious complication (OR 1.15, CI: 0.95–1.39, p = 0.142)	Low
Young et al. (2015) [33]	No	24,117	Prospective cohort	On multivariate analysis smoking significantly increased risk of serious morbidity (p < 0.05)	Low
Zhang et al. (2005) [34]	No	18,972	Prospective cohort	Smoking significantly increased the risk of long-term mortality (HR 2.05, CI: 1.67–2.52; p < 0.0001)	Low
Azagury et al. (2011) [35]	No	103	Retrospective cohort	Smoking increased risk of marginal ulcer on univariate analysis (OR 2.5, CI 1.5–5; p = 0.02) but not on multivariate analysis (OR 2.4, CI 0.9–7; p = 0.4)	Low
Coblijn et al. (2015) [36]	No	350	Retrospective cohort	Multivariate regression showed increased risk of marginal ulcer with smoking (OR 2.85, CI: 1.03–7.84; p = 0.04)	Low
El Hayak et al. (2012) [37]	No	328	Retrospective cohort	Univariate analysis showed increased risk of marginal ulcer with smoking (OR 1.6, CI:1.01–2.6; p = 0.04); multivariate analysis did not show this (OR 1.5, CI:0.9–2.5; p = 0.07); among those with ulcer, smoking increased risk of non-healing ulcers (OR 14.1, CI:2.5–80.4; p = 0.003)	Low
Spaniolas et al. (2018) [38]	Yes	35,075	Retrospective cohort	Tobacco use significantly increased risk of marginal ulcer (HR 1.56, CI: 1.41–1.73; p < 0.001) long term	Low
Wilson et al. (2006) [39]	No	1001	Retrospective cohort	Smoking at the time of ulcer presentation significantly increased risk of marginal ulcer (OR 30.6, CI 6.4–146; p < 0.001)	Low
Bauer et al. (2018) [40]	Yes (Marijuana)	434	Retrospective cohort	No difference is surgical site infections (p = 0.55), readmissions (p = 0.69), and postoperative emergency department visits (p = 0.57) between marijuana users and nonusers	Low
Shocker et al. (2020) [41]	Yes (Marijuana)	1176	Prospective cohort	No difference in readmission (p = 0.311), reoperation (p = 1.00), VTE (p = 0.316), bleeding (p = 0.154) or infection (p = 0.316) between marijuana users and nonusers	Low

Abbreviations: *RYGB* roux-en-y gastric bypass, *SG* sleeve gastrectomy, *OR* odds ratio, *HR* hazard ratio, *CI* confidence interval, *DVT* deep venous thrombosis, *PE* pulmonary embolism, *ICU* intensive care unit

2014, analysis of the American College of Surgeons National Surgery Quality Improvement Program (NSQIP) database showed that smokers undergoing bariatric surgery had an increase in major complications such as reintubation (OR 2.19), organ space infection (OR 2.71), sepsis (OR 1.49) and shock (OR 1.78) [22]. Among patients undergoing laparoscopic RYGB, smoking also increased the risk of 30-day reoperation by 50% (OR 1.52, CI: 1.02–2.27). Blair et al.'s 2015 NSQIP analysis of patients undergoing laparoscopic RYGB complemented these findings [15]. The authors not only showed an increased risk of sepsis with smoking (OR 1.63), but also that the risk increased by 1% with each additional pack-year. Multivariate analysis of the Metabolic and Bariatric Surgery Accreditation and Quality Improvement Program (MBSAQIP) database showed that among patients undergoing RYGB and SG, smokers had increased risk of major complications (OR 1.14, CI: 1.01–1.24) [17]. Young and colleagues found similar results using the NSQIP database—on multivariate analysis, they too found an increased risk of major complications among smokers compared to nonsmokers in patients undergoing RYGB [33]. The 2011 Michigan Bariatric Surgery Collaborative (MBSC) analysis also found an increased risk of major complications among smokers (OR 1.20, CI: 1.02–1.40) [18]. This study included all bariatric procedures. In 2017, Inadomi et al. analyzed the MBSC as well, but focused on patients undergoing RYGB and SG. A 30% increased risk of major complication was found in smokers among the RYGB group, but no increase was seen amongst those undergoing SG [25]. This is in contrast to Haskins et al.'s 2017 NSQIP analysis which showed an increase in both major complications and overall complications among smokers undergoing SG [23].

Some refute the association between smoking and 30-day complications. Husain et al. studied 772 consecutive patients undergoing RYGB and SG [24]. Smoking was a risk factor for major complications on univariate analysis (OR 3.52, CI: 1.21–10.24; p = 0.031), but not on multivariate regression analysis (OR 5.24, CI: 0.60–45.60; p = 0.133). Analysis of the Scandinavian Obesity Surgery Registry showed mixed results [32]. Smokers were not at increased risk of major complications (OR 1.15, CI: 0.95–1.39), but did trend towards increased risk of overall complications (OR 1.13, CI: 1.00–1.28). When complications were broken down, there was a significant increased risk of pulmonary complications (OR 1.53), wound infections (OR 1.47) and urinary tract infections (OR 1.92). Finally, in a retrospective review of RYGB and SG from a single Polish institution, there was no increase in complications among smokers [27]. Despite some varied data, evidence from large databases (NSQIP, MBSC and MBSAQIP) do support an association between smoking and major complications and warrant the call for smoking cessation.

16.3.2 Pulmonary Complications

Smoking significantly increases the risk of pulmonary complications following abdominal surgery. Haskins et al. demonstrated this association in the bariatric population [22]. Among patients undergoing open procedures, smoking increased the risk of pneumonia (OR 3.06) and prolonged intubation (OR 2.14, CI: 1.21–3.80).

Among those undergoing laparoscopic procedures, smokers again had increased risk of prolonged intubation (OR 1.63, CI: 1.01–2.64) as well increased risk of reintubation (OR 1.61, CI: 1.02–2.54). Among laparoscopic RYGB patients in particular, the risk of pneumonia was increased by 90% (OR 1.90, CI: 1.42–2.54). In 2017, Haskins et al. further demonstrated increased reintubation risk amongst smokers undergoing SG (OR 1.88, CI: 1.01–3.50) [23]. Multivariate analysis of the Nationwide Inpatient Sample database demonstrated increased risk of acute respiratory failure among smokers undergoing any bariatric operation (OR 1.1, CI: 1.0–1.2) [31]. Of note, this database only encompasses hospitalizations during the index bariatric operation and does not account for respiratory failure following discharge (e.g. following readmission for pneumonia). Livingston et al. reported risk factors for bariatric complications within the Veterans' Affairs (VA) population [26]. In this study, patients who smoked within 1 year prior to surgery and those with heavy smoking history were both at risk of prolonged intubation. Thus, these studies support the association between smoking and postoperative pulmonary complications in the bariatric population.

16.3.3 Intensive Care Unit Admission

Studies have shown increased vulnerability of obese patients compared to non-obese patients in the ICU [42]. Therefore, it is important to assess the risk of smoking on ICU admission, especially as the studies above illustrate an association between smoking and prolonged intubation/reintubation. Morgan and colleagues analyzed the Australian Department of Health Data Linkage Unit database [29]. They found that patients with unplanned ICU admissions were more likely to be smokers than patients with planned ICU admissions (19% vs. 12%, p = 0.05). Gonzalez et al. found otherwise [20]. In a retrospective study looking at 158 patients undergoing RYGB, the authors identified 23 patients who required ICU admission greater than 48 h (if ICU admission was planned) or were admitted to the ICU from the floor (unplanned ICU admission). While the prevalence of smoking was significantly greater among these 23 patients (30% vs. 16%, p = 0.04), multivariate regression showed no increased risk of smoking on ICU admission (OR 2.04, CI: 0.59–7.06). The data on this topic is sparse—further studies are required before a conclusive statement can be made regarding the relationship of smoking and ICU admission.

16.3.4 Venous Thromboembolism

Smoking and obesity have both been shown to be independent risk factors for postoperative VTE in the general population. Gonzalez et al. analyzed 660 patients undergoing RYGB, 23 of whom developed postoperative VTE [21]. Multivariate analysis showed increased risk of VTE with smoking (OR 6.7, CI: 1.90–23.57). In contrast, both Gambhir et al. and Masoomi et al. showed no increased risk with smoking [19, 30]. Gambhir and colleagues analyzed the MBSAQIP database and looked at 30-day incidence of VTE among laparoscopic RYGB and SG patients (DVT OR 1.0, CI: 0.70–1.26 and PE OR 0.7, CI: 0.42–1.04). Masoomi and colleagues, on the other hand, looked at NIS data for any bariatric operation. Again, this database only documents VTE occurring during the index hospitalization and fails to capture all VTE presenting after discharge, thereby excluding the majority of post-bariatric VTE [43]. As it stands, further investigation is needed to corroborate 30-day VTE outcomes and no conclusive association between smoking and VTE after bariatric surgery can be made at this time.

16.3.5 Marginal Ulcers

Marginal ulcer is a late occurring complication with variable presentation ranging from mild cases requiring only pharmacotherapy to morbid cases requiring omental patch or anastomotic revisions. Spaniolas and colleagues analyzed New York's Statewide Planning and Research Cooperative System database and identified over 35,000 patients undergoing RYGB [38]. Patients were followed for subsequent diagnoses of marginal ulcers. Marginal ulcer was documented as late as 8 years postoperatively. In this study, smoking at the time of surgery was found to be an independent risk factor for ulcer development (HR 1.56, CI: 1.41–1.73). In addition, preoperative smokers had significantly greater rates of marginal ulcer for each year postoperatively. Coblijn et al. showed similar findings [36]. Studies from Brigham and Women's Hospital (BWH) and Cleveland Clinic had mixed results [35, 37]. In the BWH study, there was a statistically significant increased risk of marginal ulcers with smoking on univariate analysis (OR 2.5, CI: 1.5–5) but not on multivariate analysis (OR 2.4, CI: 0.9–7). Similarly, in the Cleveland Clinic study, smoking risk was significant on univariate analysis (OR 1.6, CI: 1.01–2.6; $p = 0.04$) but only trended in multivariate analysis (OR 1.5, CI: 0.9–2.5; $p = 0.07$). Interestingly, however, among patients with marginal ulcer, preoperative smoking increased the risk of nonhealing ulcer on multivariate analysis (OR 14.1, CI: 2.5–80.4; $p = 0.003$).

One limitation in all of these studies is that the authors did not distinguish patients who continued to smoke after surgery. Smoking recidivism is high, so although patients are required to quit prior to surgery, many patients may resume postoperatively [44, 45]. Thus, the effect of preoperative smoking on long term outcomes may be falsely attributed. Wilson et al.'s study is different from the rest [39]. In this study, the authors classified patients as smokers only if they were smoking at the time of ulcer diagnosis. As a result, they identified current smoking as risk for increased rates of marginal ulcers (OR 30.6, CI: 6.4–146). This still does not show the association between preoperative smoking and marginal ulcers. A study investigating the incidence of marginal ulcers in patients who smoked preoperatively but remained abstinent would better determine the effect of smoking on marginal ulcer development.

16.3.6 Mortality

Mortality is rare following bariatric surgery; thus, few studies have analyzed the effects of smoking in this small population. NSQIP analysis found no increased risk of 30-day mortality among smokers across all procedure types, but did show increased risk among smokers undergoing SG (0.2% in smokers vs. 0.1% in non-smokers, p = 0.004) [22, 23]. Zhang et al. looked at long term mortality [34]. Within the International Bariatric Surgery Registry (IBSR), 19,000 patients underwent bariatric surgery between January 1986 and December 1999 and were followed for an average of 8 years. Preoperative smokers had twice the risk of death compared to nonsmokers. This population underwent surgery over 20 years ago; bariatric surgery has evolved considerably since that time. As it stands, the data is inconclusive to assess the relationship between smoking and mortality. Up to date longitudinal studies are needed to assess both 30-day and long-term mortality outcomes due to smoking.

16.3.7 Length of Stay

In the era of Early Recovery After Surgery, postoperative care is streamlined to allow safe and early discharge. Thus, factors altering this trajectory must be identified and addressed early. Marchini et al. found increased length of stay (LOS) among current and former smokers compared to nonsmokers (p < 0.01) [28]. In Haskins et al.'s study, smokers had increased risk of prolonged stay (LOS > 7 days) with open (OR 1.47; CI: 1.04–2.08; p = 0.03) and laparoscopic operations (OR 1.29, CI: 1.00–1.66; p = 0.05) [22]. Data is limited and while no definitive statement can be made, these studies do suggest an association between longer LOS and smoking.

16.3.8 Marijuana and Vaping Device Use

Only two studies have examined the effect of marijuana on bariatric surgery outcomes. Bauer et al.'s retrospective study of 434 patients undergoing bariatric surgery found no difference in 30-day surgical site infections, readmissions, or postoperative emergency department visits [40]. Similarly, Shockor et al. found no differences in 30-day postoperative complications (including readmission, infection, thromboembolic events, bleeding, or reoperation) in 1176 patients undergoing bariatric surgery [41]. This is in contrast to studies showing increased risk of myocardial infarction and VTE among marijuana users undergoing elective abdominal and orthopedic operations [46, 47]. Thus, while findings from Bauer et al. and Shockor et al.'s studies are consistent, findings documenting the adverse effects of marijuana after major surgery necessitates further data to make a definitive comment on the effects of marijuana on bariatric surgery.

Currently, there are no studies documenting the effects of vaping on bariatric outcomes. With the rise in the prevalence of vaping, this is a necessary next step to identify the risks associated with vaping within the bariatric population.

16.3.9 Other Considerations

Few studies have shown an association between a remote history of smoking and outcomes. Inadomi et al.'s study classified patients into nonsmokers, former smokers (abstinent for >12 months prior to surgery) and recent smokers (abstinent 3–12 months prior to surgery). Former smokers had similar outcomes compared to nonsmokers. Similarly, Livingston et al. grouped patients into a) those with <20 pack year history and >1 year abstinence, b) >20 pack year history and >1 year abstinence, and c) those with >20 pack year history and <1 year abstinence. They found more complications in both recent smokers and patients with heavy smoking history. These studies suggest that longer abstinence is beneficial—however, they do not specify the minimum time required for cessation to offset adverse effects. This is where randomized controlled trials (similar to Moller and Lindstrom's) can have the greatest impact [10, 11].

Another consideration is smoking recidivism. Studies have shown little difference in the rates of pre- and postoperative cigarette use, indicating that despite successful preoperative cessation, patients resume smoking long term [44, 45]. Randomized trials have a role here too—trials testing different cessation strategies can identify methods that allow for the greatest success with preoperative smoking cessation and sustained abstinence.

16.4 Recommendation

Patients undergoing bariatric procedures should quit smoking prior to surgery. The longer the abstinence period, the better. All attempts should be made to encourage continued smoking abstinence postoperatively, including routine screening for smoking at postoperative visits. (Evidence quality low, moderate recommendation).

16.5 Personal View of the Data

In reviewing the literature, we found that the effect of preoperative smoking on postoperative complications is not always clear. While there is strong data to suggest a link between smoking and pulmonary complications, the data linking smoking with VTE, ICU admission, and mortality is mixed. The effect of current smoking on marginal ulceration is strongly supported, but studies designed to evaluate the effect of preoperative smoking on ulcer development should exclude patients who smoke at the time of ulcer detection to determine the true relationship. Nonetheless, we find sufficient evidence to support the recommendation for smoking cessation prior to bariatric surgery. Though randomized controlled trials may be useful to evaluate the direct effect of smoking on outcomes, given the current data, we believe further trials randomizing smokers to bariatric surgery is not ethical. However, randomized trials can aid in identifying the minimum duration of cessation required to mitigate adverse effects as well as methods that best promote preoperative smoking cessation and sustained abstinence.

References

1. English WJ, et al. American Society for Metabolic and Bariatric Surgery 2018 estimate of metabolic and bariatric procedures performed in the United States. Surg Obes Relat Dis. 2020.
2. Nguyen NT, et al. Trends in utilization of bariatric surgery, 2009-2012. Surg Endosc. 2016;30(7):2723–7.
3. Chang SH, et al. The effectiveness and risks of bariatric surgery: an updated systematic review and meta-analysis, 2003-2012. JAMA Surg. 2014;149(3):275–87.
4. Ma IT, Madura JA II. Gastrointestinal complications after bariatric surgery. Gastroenterol Hepatol (N Y). 2015;11(8):526–35.
5. Creamer MR, et al. Tobacco product use and cessation indicators among adults – United States, 2018. MMWR Morb Mortal Wkly Rep. 2019;68(45):1013–9.
6. Hammond D, et al. Prevalence of vaping and smoking among adolescents in Canada, England, and the United States: repeat national cross sectional surveys. BMJ. 2019;365:12219.
7. Miech R, et al. Trends in adolescent vaping, 2017-2019. N Engl J Med. 2019;381(15):1490–1.
8. Mombach KD, et al. Emotional and affective temperaments in smoking candidates for bariatric surgery. PLoS One. 2016;11(3):e0150722.
9. Levine MD, et al. History of smoking and postcessation weight gain among weight loss surgery candidates. Addict Behav. 2007;32(10):2365–71.
10. Healton CG, et al. Smoking, obesity, and their co-occurrence in the United States: cross sectional analysis. BMJ. 2006;333(7557):25–6.
11. Schmid M, et al. Impact of smoking on perioperative outcomes after major surgery. Am J Surg. 2015;210(2):221–9. e6
12. Moller AM, et al. Effect of preoperative smoking intervention on postoperative complications: a randomised clinical trial. Lancet. 2002;359(9301):114–7.
13. Lindstrom D, et al. Effects of a perioperative smoking cessation intervention on postoperative complications: a randomized trial. Ann Surg. 2008;248(5):739–45.
14. Mechanick JI, et al. Clinical practice guidelines for the perioperative nutritional, metabolic, and nonsurgical support of the bariatric surgery patient–2013 update: cosponsored by American Association of Clinical Endocrinologists, the Obesity Society, and American Society for Metabolic & Bariatric Surgery. Surg Obes Relat Dis. 2013;9(2):159–91.
15. Blair LJ, et al. Risk factors for postoperative sepsis in laparoscopic gastric bypass. Surg Endosc. 2016;30(4):1287–93.
16. Dayer-Jankechova A, et al. Complications after laparoscopic Roux-en-Y gastric bypass in 1573 consecutive patients: are there predictors? Obes Surg. 2016;26(1):12–20.
17. El Chaar M, et al. A novel risk prediction model for 30-day severe adverse events and readmissions following bariatric surgery based on the MBSAQIP database. Surg Obes Relat Dis. 2019;15(7):1138–45.
18. Finks JF, et al. Predicting risk for serious complications with bariatric surgery: results from the Michigan Bariatric Surgery Collaborative. Ann Surg. 2011;254(4):633–40.
19. Gambhir S, et al. Venous thromboembolism risk for the contemporary bariatric surgeon. Surg Endosc. 2019.
20. Gonzalez R, et al. Preoperative factors predictive of complicated postoperative management after Roux-en-Y gastric bypass for morbid obesity. Surg Endosc. 2003;17(12):1900–4.
21. Gonzalez R, et al. Predictive factors of thromboembolic events in patients undergoing Roux-en-Y gastric bypass. Surg Obes Relat Dis. 2006;2(1):30–5; discussion 35–6.

22. Haskins IN, Amdur R, Vaziri K. The effect of smoking on bariatric surgical outcomes. Surg Endosc. 2014;28(11):3074–80.
23. Haskins IN, et al. Should recent smoking be a contraindication for sleeve gastrectomy? Surg Obes Relat Dis. 2017;13(7):1130–5.
24. Husain F, et al. Risk factors for early postoperative complications after bariatric surgery. Ann Surg Treat Res. 2018;95(2):100–10.
25. Inadomi M, et al. Effect of patient-reported smoking status on short-term bariatric surgery outcomes. Surg Endosc. 2018;32(2):720–6.
26. Livingston EH, et al. National Surgical Quality Improvement Program analysis of bariatric operations: modifiable risk factors contribute to bariatric surgical adverse outcomes. J Am Coll Surg. 2006;203(5):625–33.
27. Major P, et al. Risk factors for complications of laparoscopic sleeve gastrectomy and laparoscopic Roux-en-Y gastric bypass. Int J Surg. 2017;37:71–8.
28. Marchini JF, et al. Low educational status, smoking, and multidisciplinary team experience predict hospital length of stay after bariatric surgery. Nutr Metab Insights. 2012;5:71–6.
29. Morgan DJ, et al. Incidence and risk factors for intensive care unit admission after bariatric surgery: a multicentre population-based cohort study. Br J Anaesth. 2015;115(6):873–82.
30. Masoomi H, et al. Factors predictive of venous thromboembolism in bariatric surgery. Am J Surg. 2011;77(10):1403–6.
31. Masoomi H, et al. Risk factors for acute respiratory failure in bariatric surgery: data from the Nationwide Inpatient Sample, 2006-2008. Surg Obes Relat Dis. 2013;9(2):277–81.
32. Stenberg E, et al. Early complications after laparoscopic gastric bypass surgery: results from the Scandinavian Obesity Surgery Registry. Ann Surg. 2014;260(6):1040–7.
33. Young MT, et al. Use and outcomes of laparoscopic sleeve gastrectomy vs laparoscopic gastric bypass: analysis of the American College of Surgeons NSQIP. J Am Coll Surg. 2015;220(5):880–5.
34. Zhang W, et al. Factors influencing survival following surgical treatment of obesity. Obes Surg. 2005;15(1):43–50.
35. Azagury DE, et al. Marginal ulceration after Roux-en-Y gastric bypass surgery: characteristics, risk factors, treatment, and outcomes. Endoscopy. 2011;43(11):950–4.
36. Coblijn UK, et al. Symptomatic marginal ulcer disease after Roux-en-Y gastric bypass: incidence, risk factors and management. Obes Surg. 2015;25(5):805–11.
37. El-Hayek K, et al. Marginal ulcer after Roux-en-Y gastric bypass: what have we really learned? Surg Endosc. 2012;26(10):2789–96.
38. Spaniolas K, et al. Association of long-term anastomotic ulceration after Roux-en-Y gastric bypass with tobacco smoking. JAMA Surg. 2018;153(9):862–4.
39. Wilson JA, et al. Predictors of endoscopic findings after Roux-en-Y gastric bypass. Am J Gastroenterol. 2006;101(10):2194–9.
40. Bauer FL, et al. Marijuana's influence on pain scores, initial weight loss, and other bariatric surgical outcomes. Perm J. 2018;22:18–002.
41. Shockcor N, et al. Marijuana use does not affect the outcomes of bariatric surgery. Surg Endosc. 2020.
42. El-Solh A, et al. Morbid obesity in the medical ICU. Chest. 2001;120(6):1989–97.
43. Aminian A, et al. Who should get extended thromboprophylaxis after bariatric surgery? A risk assessment tool to guide indications for post-discharge pharmacoprophylaxis. Ann Surg. 2017;265(1):143–50.
44. Conason A, et al. Substance use following bariatric weight loss surgery. JAMA Surg. 2013;148(2):145–50.
45. Li L, Wu LT. Substance use after bariatric surgery: a review. J Psychiatr Res. 2016;76:16–29.
46. Goel A, et al. Cannabis use disorder and perioperative outcomes in major elective surgeries: a retrospective cohort analysis. Anesthesiology. 2020;132(4):625–35.
47. Vakharia RM, et al. Patients who have cannabis use disorder have higher rates of venous thromboemboli, readmission rates, and costs following primary total knee arthroplasty. J Arthroplasty. 2020;35(4):997–1002.

Part IV

Ethics and Bariatric Surgery

Is the Insurance Requirement for Supervised Weight Loss Prior to Bariatric Surgery an Ethical Strategy to Prevent Non-compliant Patients from Undergoing Surgery?

Colston Edgerton and Scott A. Shikora

17.1 Introduction

Despite decades of fad diets, physician-supervised weight loss programs, commercial programs and medications, bariatric surgery remains the most effective treatment for achieving meaningful and durable weight loss for individuals who suffer from severe obesity [1–4]. However, these procedures are often challenging due to the deranged body habitus, abundant intraabdominal adipose tissue, and enlarged fatty livers encountered in these patients. There is ample published evidence that preoperative or supervised weight loss may be beneficial. Preoperative weight loss has been felt to reduce operative complications by shrinking the intrabdominal fat mass and liver volume, improving the surgeon's visualization and access to the gastrointestinal tract [5, 6]. Preoperative weight loss has also been demonstrated to result in physiologic improvements [7–9], and to improve overall weight loss [10–13]. Adherence to a pre-operative diet and experiencing pre-operative weight loss is believed by some to predict long-term patient compliance, which has been shown to influence outcomes [14, 15]. It is for these reasons that many bariatric programs require patients being evaluated and prepared for bariatric surgery to attempt to lose weight as a requirement for proceeding with surgery. Currently, there is no consensus in the bariatric surgery community as to the application of this process. It varies from mandatory for all patients being considered for surgery, to being reserved only for certain patients such as those with higher body mass indexes (BMI), metabolic syndrome, or large abdominal compartments. Additionally, while it has been demonstrated that a moderate amount of weight loss is physiologically beneficial, the

C. Edgerton · S. A. Shikora (✉)
Center for Metabolic and Bariatric Surgery, Department of Surgery, Brigham and Women's Hospital, Boston, MA, USA
e-mail: cedgerton@bwh.harvard.edu; sshikora@bwh.harvard.edu

© Springer Nature Switzerland AG 2021
J. Alverdy, Y. Vigneswaran (eds.), *Difficult Decisions in Bariatric Surgery*,
Difficult Decisions in Surgery: An Evidence-Based Approach,
https://doi.org/10.1007/978-3-030-55329-6_17

amount of weight loss necessary to result in meaningful perioperative benefits is not known.

In addition to its use by bariatric surgical practices for reducing perioperative complications, preoperative weight loss has been recommended by some medical societies to be part of a comprehensive approach to weight loss. However, it has been used by many health insurance companies as a requirement that patients must satisfy prior to providing coverage for bariatric surgery services. While mandating that patients complete this task, these same companies do not provide or require any specific programs to achieve the necessary weight loss. Additionally, they usually require that all patients participate, leaving the clinician no opportunity to identify patients in whom they believe preoperative weight loss would be beneficial and those they do not. For all patients, the mandate delays surgery and has contributed to patient dropout from bariatric programs [16, 17]. The American Society for Metabolic and Bariatric Surgery (ASMBS), the foremost authority in the specialty of bariatric surgery, performed an extensive literature review and then issued a position statement that called this practice into question, citing that the mandate is based on a paucity of high quality evidence, delays patient care, and lacks individualism for patient care plans [18]. An open letter from the ASMBS to insurance companies in 2015 stated that "policies such as these that delay, impede, or otherwise interfere with life-saving and cost-effective treatment, which has been proved to be true for bariatric surgery to treat morbid obesity, are unacceptable without supporting evidence" [19]. An updated position statement in 2016 echoed this, and again highlighted the lack of high quality evidence to justify its practice [20]. Given that this mandate is determined by the payer rather than the patient, health care provider, or medical societies, the question has arisen: is it ethical?

In order to answer this complex question, one must consider two issues. First, what is the basis for the health insurance carrier to require patients to achieve preoperative weight loss as a condition for coverage, and second, what are the standards by which modern biomedical ethics are defined? This chapter will discuss both topics.

17.2 Search Strategy

To investigate the published literature concerning health insurance carrier mandatory requirement for supervised weight loss, a search was conducted in the English literature using terms "supervised weight loss" AND "bariatric surgery." The databases PubMed, Web of Science, Cochrane Library, JSTOR, and Embase were used. This resulted in 40 references. Of those, 16 were relevant to the primary question and were used for this analysis.

To investigate the ethical considerations of this practice, a search was performed with the following terms "supervised weight loss" AND "bariatric surgery" AND (ethical OR ethics or "biomedical ethics") in PubMed, Web of Science, Cochrane Library, JSTOR, and Embase. This retrieved two references. The first, published in a law journal examines the regulation of medical necessity in the field of bariatric surgery [21]. The second examines outcomes following Roux en Y Gastric Bypass (RYGB) among patients broken down into quartiles of pre-operative weight loss and weight gain. The authors found no significant differences in perioperative and postoperative outcomes, but that patients with the greatest % preoperative excess weight change had the longest intervals from initial visit to operation [22]. Given the limited scope of published studies investigating this specific question, it is more appropriate to identify the terms that have defined modern biomedical ethics, and then examine this practice in the context of each.

17.3 Results

In order to first understand the ethics of the mandated supervised weight loss requirement, one must identify what these policies entail, and their origin. In 1991, the National Institutes of Health (NIH) Consensus Development Conference Panel on Gastrointestinal Surgery for Severe Obesity published its report outlining guidelines and selection criteria for both medical and surgical weight loss [23]. These criteria were based on the published evidence at that time and best practice. The panel concluded "patients seeking therapy for severe obesity for the first time should be considered for treatment in a nonsurgical program with integrated components of a dietary regimen, appropriate exercise, and behavioral modification and support". There was no mention of a weight loss requirement or how it was to be achieved, only that the candidate for surgery should have in the past participated in a nonsurgical weight loss program. Seven years later, the NIH Expert Panel on the Identification, Evaluation, and Treatment of Overweight and Obesity in Adults published their recommendations [24]. In addition to identifying BMI and comorbid criteria, this report recommended that patients could undergo surgery when medical, dietary, and lifestyle methods had not achieved meaningful outcomes. Again, there was no stated requirement for any specific amount of weight loss as mandatory criteria for proceeding with bariatric surgery. While these consensus statements, published in the dawn of the popularity and widespread adoption of bariatric surgery, were meant to promote patient safety, minimize surgical risks, and establish a comprehensive approach to the treatment of morbid obesity, they inadvertently laid the groundwork for the health insurance mandated supervised weight loss requirement.

As the field of bariatric surgery matured, morbidity and mortality declined and patient outcomes improved. The introduction of laparoscopic access further improved results and new less morbid procedures such as the laparoscopic adjustable gastric band were developed. As the criteria for surgery established by the NIH in 1991 were based predominantly on the open gastric bypass procedure, the ASMBS leadership felt that the 13 year old guidelines were outdated and needed to be revised to reflect these practice changes. In 2004 the ASMBS held a Consensus Conference and published updated guidelines that included a statement endorsing attempts at medical weight loss prior surgery, but rejecting that participation in a formal pre-operative program should be a precondition for surgery [25].

The debate on whether health insurance provider mandated supervised medical weight loss should be a prerequisite for paying for bariatric surgery is grounded in the different objectives held by patients, providers and payers. Containing costs is the primary interest for the payer, which is limited to several strategies. Insurers can require clinicians to use resources more efficiently, pay providers less, exclude high risk patients, reduce benefits and services by denying treatment claims, or increase the deductibles and copayments [26]. Often the most immediate and effective way to reduce costs is to limit services [27]. The decision to pay for a surgical procedure is grounded in the balance between cost and quality tradeoffs, which often results in "medical necessity" becoming the least common denominator. When a case of medical necessity is legally contended, it is often fought through external review laws in which an appeal is made to an independent external reviewer [21]. Studies in California and Texas in the past have cited bariatric surgery as the most frequently appealed medical-surgical procedure, and that these denials are more frequently lost than any other appeal [21, 28]. As a result, insurance companies want to avoid the costly monetary and negative publicity of the appeals process. Yet as evidence of its efficacy for weight loss, resolution of comorbidities, and years of life saved has become more proven over time, the case for the medical necessity of bariatric surgery has become harder to debate. Health insurance companies are therefore left with few options on how to curtail the expense incurred by covering bariatric surgery. The NIH recommendations published in the early 1990s provided a justified means by which to delay or even reduce services.

Importantly, the way these mandates and all bariatric services are delivered is not done consistently across states, or even across insurance plans from the same state. The Employee Retirement Income Security Act (ELISA) was passed into law in 1974 for the purpose of protecting employer or union based benefits from state regulation. ELISA was ostensibly designed to protect pensions from being subjected to more restrictive and inconsistent state regulations. ELISA protections were expanded to all employee benefits including health insurance. While the law provided reasonably effective federal protection for pensions against inconsistent state regulations, it did not do this for health insurance benefits [29]. This was thought to be the nidus for further legislation including in obstetrical care where the Newborns' and Mothers' Health Protection Act of 1996 was passed to mandate that health insurance companies had to pay for post-natal obstetrical care for 48 h after vaginal delivery or 96 h following cesarean sections as recommended by the American College of Obstetricians and Gynecologists. Unfortunately, similar protections have not been extended to many other medical treatments. The Affordable Care Act (ACA) sought to change this by dictating that all plans that qualify under this program must cover certain Essential Health Benefits (EHB). While the law laid out 10 categories, it did not itemize services. The Department of Health & Human Services (DHHS) placed the burden on states to define their own EHBs, which was accomplished by selecting packages offered by an existing state plan. As a result, bariatric surgery is listed as an EHB in only 23 states. Furthermore only 12 states cover nutritional counseling, and just 3 states cover weight loss programs. Only one state (Michigan) and the District of Columbia provide comprehensive weight loss services by considering nutritional counseling, medical weight loss programs, and bariatric surgery as EHBs. Therefore, even if certain plans mandate supervised medical weight loss, they may not provide coverage for the very counseling and medical weight loss programs they require. This is in contrast to 45 states that include chiropractor care as an EHB and 31 that include treatment for Temporomandibular Joint disorders [30]. While it is widely recognized that one adverse result of mandatory preoperative participation in a supervised medical weight loss programs is delay in time to surgery, inconsistencies in coverage for the full range of services may explain why some have linked supervised medical weight loss to a higher rate of attrition prior to surgery [16, 17, 31]. In the authors' state of Massachusetts, the state health plan Masshealth has a written policy for the determination of *medical necessity* for bariatric surgery. To meet criteria for necessity, one must provide "Documentation of an attempt of weight loss control through participation in structured program(s) before bariatric surgery monthly for at least four-to-six months in the 2 years before the request for the procedure" [32]. Blue Cross Blue Shield of MA, however, does not include a specified period of time. Their requirements simply state that "Attempts to lose weight led to failure and have been recorded" [33].

One can now consider what is known about these policies in the context of modern biomedical ethics principles. The field of biomedical ethics was reborn in the wake of several notorious experimental research studies that violated the rights of human subjects, such as the Tuskegee Syphilis Study in which human subjects were knowingly subjected to untreated Syphilis [34, 35]. In 1974, the National Commission for the Protection of Human Subjects of Biomedical and Behavioral Research was created and in 1979 The Belmont Report offered a summary of the commission's findings. This document outlined the three pillar foundation of Nonmaleficence, Beneficence, and Justice [36]. Beauchamp and Childress expanded upon these by adding a fourth principle, "Autonomy" in their work *Principles of Biomedical Ethics*, first published in 1979 and now in its fifth edition [37]. These works have defined the cannon of biomedical ethics over the past 40 years and should be the focus of any discussion on ethical considerations in clinical practice. Even so, it is difficult to apply medical ethics that have historically been applied to individual health care providers to health care organizations or insurance companies, where "business ethics" have been the standard. Health care economics create a unique blend of medical and business ethics, two terms that are not synonymous [26]. Some have argued that physician ethics and organizational ethics are distinct, and that a separate standard for health care organizations is necessary [38, 39]. Business ethics are designed to encourage fair practices in a competitive market. These include disseminating truthful and honest information to allow participants in the market to make voluntary choices to buy or sell goods and services. Medical ethics, in contrast, assumes significant inequality in knowledge and skill between physicians and patients, as was highlighted in the unethical Tuskegee Syphilis study. Health care providers therefore have a fiduciary obligation to their patients, whereas businesses have a fiduciary obligation to their shareholders, not their customers. However, because the business of medical organizations and insurance corporations involves the delivery of care on behalf of morally responsible providers, the ethical standards to which they are held should more closely reflect the services rendered [40].

17.3.1 Respect for Patient Autonomy

Autonomy is the idea that people should have the liberty to choose their own actions and course in life, which is predicated on independence from controlling influences. This is the basis for the informed consent process [37]. The issue at hand may not be that patients would not consent to supervised weight loss. Rather, the loss of autonomy could arise when patients are told what type of weight loss program they must participate in, how much weight they are required to lose, and for how long they must attempt to lose weight prior to proceeding with surgery. They may have been attempting this unsuccessfully their entire lives, and the action they are autonomously choosing is to proceed directly with a surgical option.

17.3.2 Beneficence

Beneficence is the obligation to provide benefits and to balance benefits against risks [37]. One way to justify taking away some degree of patient autonomy is often to prove that "it is for the good of the patient". Smoking cessation prior to surgery to minimize wound complications is one example where autonomous patients may prefer to continue smoking, yet the expertise of the medical provider dictates that the benefits of smoking cessation outweigh the risks of permitting its practice. In the case of supervised medical weight loss, the benefit in patient outcomes has not consistently been proven [41]. Even in published series that do show benefit of preoperative weight loss, there is no consensus on the type, duration, and structure of the program to achieve this. Therefore, in order to use this as a justification for limiting the autonomy of the patient and health care team, consistent high-level supportive evidence is needed.

17.3.3 Nonmaleficence

Nonmaleficence is the obligation to "first, do no harm" [37]. Here again we find a balance between risk and benefit. While surgery will always cause some degree of "harm" in the form of pain, bleeding, or other unforeseen risks, the degree of harm must be balanced to a reasonable degree with the likelihood of benefit from the procedure being performed. This has traditionally been viewed in the sense of physical harm but is equally applicable in the context of successful delivery of care. If there is an action that has been shown to delay or limit the number of patients who will eventually receive services that decrease morbidity and mortality, and provide the medical, psychological, and emotional benefit that they seek, this can be considered a form of maleficence [2, 16, 31, 42–48].

17.3.4 Distributive Justice

This principle dictates that the distribution of benefits should be extended in an equitable way to all persons free from bias or prejudice [37]. Aside from the ongoing debate on the effectiveness of supervised weight loss to minimize non-compliance and optimize outcomes, it is perhaps here that the heterogeneity of plans faces the greatest ethical challenge. Why should a patient in Wisconsin not have bariatric surgery, nutrition counseling, or coverage for medical weight loss programs included as an EHB in a health care plan while a patient living across the border in Michigan have all three available? Why should two different plans in the same state require different lengths of supervised weight loss? Herein lies the chasm between biomedical and business ethics. Insurance plans governed by laws in different states, or decisions made by companies to offer different benefits based off premium rates and patient risk is not inherently unethical as defined by fair and balanced business practices in a *competitive* market. But human rights and the delivery of health care is not competitive, it is a medical necessity.

17.4   Recommendations Based on the Data

The issue addressed in this chapter is not focused on whether there is or isn't physiologic and psychologic benefits to weight loss prior to proceeding with a bariatric surgery. While there is ample published evidence to suggest that weight loss prior to bariatric surgery might be beneficial, the data is not conclusive and mostly the interpretation of data extracted from small retrospective reviews of single practice databases. These leave several questions unanswered. Should all patients be required to lose weight or just selected patients? How much weight loss is necessary to be beneficial? Should it be a set amount or individualized? Should there be a time interval for achieving this weight loss and what happens to the patient who is unsuccessful?

The main issue of this chapter is whether it is ethical for the health insurance payer to mandate that patients preoperatively participate for 3–12 months in some form of a weight loss program that will definitely delay their bariatric surgery but may or may not benefit the patient. There are no published studies demonstrating the benefits of such programs. In fact, this approach can be potentially harmful. Jamal et al. compared a group of patients that participated in a mandatory 13 week preoperative dietary counseling (PDC) program prior to proceeding with a gastric bypass to a group of patients who were not obligated to participate in such a program. The researchers found that the presurgery drop out rate was 50% higher in the PDC patients and the weight loss at 1 year was statistically greater in the non-PDC group [31]. Mandating that patients delay their bariatric surgery to complete a weight loss program can also be harmful. Al Harakeh et al. compared the outcomes of 189 patients denied bariatric surgery by their insurance payers with 587 patients that had gastric bypass. The groups were comparable in regard to comorbid conditions. During a 3 year follow up period, the group denied surgery had a statistically greater incidence of new-onset diabetes, hypertension, sleep apnea, GERD, and lipid disorders [48]. Most concerning is the knowledge that without surgery, morbidly obese patients may experience a deterioration in their state of health. The possibility exists that during the participation in a mandatory weight loss program for 3–12 months, some patients may suffer a serious health issue that would render them unfit to withstand a bariatric surgery procedure, or result in a death. Sowenimo et al. observed a 14.3% mortality in patients denied bariatric surgery vs. 2.9 % for those that had surgery [42].

In summary, there is no true evidence of any benefit to subjecting patient to complete a preoperative weight loss program. Mandated participation only succeeds in delaying bariatric surgery which may be harmful for these patients and would not be considered for other medical conditions such as heart disease or diabetes. Therefore, policies that require such participation in fact impede, delay, or interfere with timely (as determined by clinicians) bariatric surgery are unethical. Only clinicians caring for these patients should determine whether preoperative weight loss is deemed necessary and then determine how, how much and how long.

17.5 A Personal View of the Data

Like cancer, diabetes and heart disease, severe obesity is a chronic, progressive disease. It adversely affects nearly every organ system of the body and is associated with several life-threating conditions such as diabetes, heart disease, liver disease and the metabolic syndrome. Bariatric surgery has been proven to achieve meaningful weight loss and dramatic improvement of the comorbid conditions. However, the obesity epidemic has resulted in millions of potential bariatric surgery candidates which would result in a financial crisis for the health insurance companies. In an effort to control costs, many of these payers have imposed mandatory participation in weight loss programs for various lengths (generally 3–12 months). Since these programs are based on time not results, and the insurance companies that require them generally don't create, analyze, or monitor these programs, it is possible that their true goal is cost containment not patient well-being. They delay the process and also result in an increase in attrition.

While this practice may be ethical from a business standpoint, it is the strong belief of these authors that it is medically unethical and harmful for patients.

17.6 Recommendations

- There is no true evidence of any benefit to subjecting patient to complete a preoperative weight loss program.
- Mandated participation only succeeds in delaying bariatric surgery which may be harmful for these patients.

- Policies that require such participation in fact impede, delay, or interfere with timely (as determined by clinicians) bariatric surgery are unethical.
- Only clinicians caring for these patients should determine whether preoperative weight loss is deemed necessary and then determine how, how much and how long.

References

1. Mechanick JI, et al. Clinical practice guidelines for the perioperative nutritional, metabolic, and nonsurgical support of the bariatric surgery patient—2013 update: cosponsored by American Association of Clinical Endocrinologists, the Obesity Society, and American Society for Metabolic & Bariatric Surgery. Obesity. 2013;21(S1):S1–S27.
2. Sjöström L. Review of the key results from the Swedish Obese Subjects (SOS) trial–a prospective controlled intervention study of bariatric surgery. J Intern Med. 2013;273(3):219–34.
3. Adams TD, et al. Health benefits of gastric bypass surgery after 6 years. JAMA. 2012;308(11):1122–31.
4. Courcoulas AP, et al. Weight change and health outcomes at 3 years after bariatric surgery among individuals with severe obesity. JAMA. 2013;310(22):2416–25.
5. Fris RJ. Preoperative low energy diet diminishes liver size. Obes Surg. 2004;14(9):1165–70.
6. Ross R, et al. Influence of diet and exercise on skeletal muscle and visceral adipose tissue in men. J Appl Physiol. 1996;81(6):2445–55.
7. Uusitupa MI, et al. Effects of a very-low-calorie diet on metabolic control and cardiovascular risk factors in the treatment of obese non-insulin-dependent diabetics. Am J Clin Nutr. 1990;51(5):768–73.
8. Loube DI, Loube AA, Mitler MM. Weight loss for obstructive sleep apnea: the optimal therapy for obese patients. J Am Diet Assoc. 1994;94(11):1291–5.
9. Anderson JW, et al. Relationship of weight loss to cardiovascular risk factors in morbidly obese individuals. J Am Coll Nutr. 1994;13(3):256–61.
10. Still CD, et al. Outcomes of preoperative weight loss in high-risk patients undergoing gastric bypass surgery. Arch Surg. 2007;142(10):994–8.
11. Livhits M, et al. Does weight loss immediately before bariatric surgery improve outcomes: a systematic review. Surg Obes Relat Dis. 2009;5(6):713–21.
12. Alami RS, et al. Is there a benefit to preoperative weight loss in gastric bypass patients? A prospective randomized trial. Surg Obes Relat Dis. 2007;3(2):141–5.
13. Riess KP, et al. Effect of preoperative weight loss on laparoscopic gastric bypass outcomes. Surg Obes Relat Dis. 2008;4(6):704–8.
14. Pontiroli AE, et al. Post-surgery adherence to scheduled visits and compliance, more than personality disorders, predict outcome of bariatric restrictive surgery in morbidly obese patients. Obes Surg. 2007;17(11):1492–7.
15. Poole NA, et al. Compliance with surgical after-care following bariatric surgery for morbid obesity: a retrospective study. Obes Surg. 2005;15(2):261–5.
16. Alvarez R, et al. Factors associated with bariatric surgery utilization among eligible candidates: who drops out? Surg Obes Relat Dis. 2018;14(12):1903–10.
17. Eng V, et al. Preoperative weight loss: is waiting longer before bariatric surgery more effective? Surg Obes Relat Dis. 2019.
18. Brethauer S. ASMBS position statement on preoperative supervised weight loss requirements. Surg Obes Relat Dis. 2011;7(3):257–60.
19. Blackstone R, Ponce J, Morton J. Open letter to insurance companies, regarding mandatory pre-bariatric surgery diet regimens. 2015. https://asmbs.org/resources/open-letter-to-insurance-companies-regarding-mandatory-pre-bariatric-surgery-diet-regimens. Accessed 1 Jan 2020.

20. Kim JJ, et al. ASMBS updated position statement on insurance mandated preoperative weight loss requirements. Surg Obes Relat Dis. 2016;12(5):955–9.
21. Hall MA. State regulation of medical necessity: the case of weight-reduction surgery. Duke Law J. 2003;53:653.
22. Blackledge C, et al. Outcomes associated with preoperative weight loss after laparoscopic Roux-en-Y gastric bypass. Surg Endosc. 2016;30(11):5077–83.
23. Hubbard VS, Hall WH. Gastrointestinal surgery for severe obesity. Obes Surg. 1991;1(3):257–65.
24. Heart N, et al. Clinical guidelines on the identification, evaluation, and treatment of overweight and obesity in adults: the evidence report. National Heart, Lung, and Blood Institute; 1998.
25. Buchwald H. Consensus conference statement: bariatric surgery for morbid obesity: health implications for patients, health professionals, and third-party payers. Surg Obes Relat Dis. 2005;1(3):371–81.
26. Mariner WK. Business vs. medical ethics: conflicting standards for managed care. J Law Med Ethics. 1995;23(3):236–46.
27. Schwartz WB, Mendelson DN. Eliminating waste and inefficiency can do little to contain costs. Health Aff. 1994;13(1):224–38.
28. Studdert DM, Gresenz CR. Enrollee appeals of preservice coverage denials at 2 health maintenance organizations. JAMA. 2003;289(7):864–70.
29. Butler PA, Polzer K. Private-sector health coverage: variation in consumer protections under ERISA and state law. 1996. George Washington University, National Health Policy Forum.
30. Weiner J, Colameco C. Essential health benefits: 50-state variations on a theme. 2014.
31. Jamal MK, et al. Insurance-mandated preoperative dietary counseling does not improve outcome and increases dropout rates in patients considering gastric bypass surgery for morbid obesity. Surg Obes Relat Dis. 2006;2(2):122–7.
32. Guidelines for Medical Necessity Determination for Bariatric Surgery. https://www.mass.gov/files/documents/2019/08/15/mg-bariatricsurgery.pdf. Accessed 1 Jan 2020.
33. BCBS Massachusetts – Requirements for weight loss surgery approval. https://www.obesity-coverage.com/bcbs-massachusetts-requirements-for-weight-loss-surgery-approval/. Accessed 1 Jan 2020.
34. Curran WJ. The Tuskegee syphilis study. Mass Medical Soc. 1973.
35. Corbie-Smith G. The continuing legacy of the Tuskegee Syphilis Study: considerations for clinical investigation. Am J Med Sci. 1999;317(1):5–8.
36. Department of Health, E., and Welfare, The National Commission for the Protection of Human Subjects of Biomedical and Behavioral Research. Ethical principles and guidelines for the protection of human subjects of research. The Belmont Report. 1979.
37. Beauchamp TL, Childress JF. Principles of biomedical ethics. USA: Oxford University Press; 2001.
38. Wolf SM. Health care reform and the future of physician ethics. Hastings Cent Rep. 1994;24(2):28–41.
39. Waymack MH. Health care as a business: the ethic of Hippocrates versus the ethic of managed care. Bus Prof Ethics J. 1990:69–78.
40. Sulmasy DP. Physicians, cost control, and ethics. Ann Intern Med. 1992;116(11):920–6.
41. Jantz EJ, et al. Number of weight loss attempts and maximum weight loss before Roux-en-Y laparoscopic gastric bypass surgery are not predictive of postoperative weight loss. Surg Obes Relat Dis. 2009;5(2):208–11.
42. Sowemimo OA, et al. Natural history of morbid obesity without surgical intervention. Surg Obes Relat Dis. 2007;3(1):73–7.
43. Flum DR, Dellinger EP. Impact of gastric bypass operation on survival: a population-based analysis. J Am Coll Surg. 2004;199(4):543–51.
44. MacDonald KG, et al. The gastric bypass operation reduces the progression and mortality of non-insulin-dependent diabetes mellitus. J Gastrointest Surg. 1997;1(3):213–20.
45. Sjöström L, et al. Effects of bariatric surgery on mortality in Swedish obese subjects. N Engl J Med. 2007;357(8):741–52.

46. Adams TD, et al. Long-term mortality after gastric bypass surgery. N Engl J Med. 2007;357(8):753–61.
47. Christou NV, et al. Surgery decreases long-term mortality, morbidity, and health care use in morbidly obese patients. Ann Surg. 2004;240(3):416.
48. Al Harakeh AB, et al. Natural history and metabolic consequences of morbid obesity for patients denied coverage for bariatric surgery. Surg Obes Relat Dis. 2010;6(6):591–6.

Ethical Concerns of Bariatric Surgery in the Pediatric Population

18

Saunders Lin and Manish Tushar Raiji

18.1 Introduction

Approximately 18.5% of youth in the USA meet the criteria for obesity, defined as a body mass index (BMI) $\geq$ 95th percentile for age and sex. 8.5% of those aged 12–19 are categorized as severely obese (BMI $\geq$ 120% of the 95th percentile) [1]. This concerning trend increases the risk of obesity-related morbidity and mortality over time, and children who develop obesity are at higher risk of experiencing complications from their obesity than individuals who develop obesity later in life. Moreover, adolescent obesity predicts adult obesity and its many associated metabolic complications, such as type 2 diabetes (T2D), obstructive sleep apnea, hypertension, nonalcoholic fatty liver disease, and dyslipidemia [2, 3].

Medical intervention programs such as family-based behavioral therapy coupled with caloric reduction and increases in physical activity have varied success rates, with some studies showing it to be only be effective for 50% of patients [4]. In contrast, for carefully screened adolescent candidates, metabolic and bariatric surgery (MBS) has been shown to be more effective for treating severe obesity and related co-morbidities than medical intervention. Despite evidence that bariatric surgery leads to excellent short-term outcomes, the annual number of inpatient bariatric surgery admissions for adolescents (aged $\leq$20 years) remains low [5].

The reason for this is multifactorial, and despite the evidence for short-term success in bariatric surgery, many ethical and moral issues exist in performing bariatric

S. Lin
Department of General Surgery, Oregon Health and Sciences University, Portland, OR, USA
e-mail: lsau@ohsu.edu

M. T. Raiji (✉)
Department of Surgery, Division of Pediatric Surgery, University of Chicago, Chicago, IL, USA
e-mail: mraiji@surgery.bsd.uchicago.edu

© Springer Nature Switzerland AG 2021
J. Alverdy, Y. Vigneswaran (eds.), *Difficult Decisions in Bariatric Surgery*,
Difficult Decisions in Surgery: An Evidence-Based Approach,
https://doi.org/10.1007/978-3-030-55329-6_18

surgery in the pediatric population. This chapter addresses the ethical concerns of bariatric surgery in the pediatric patient through the lens of the four major ethical principles of autonomy, beneficence, nonmaleficence, and justice. These four principles will be used to aid physicians and patients in the bioethical decision making to be considered in the pediatric bariatric surgery patient.

18.2   Search Strategy

A literature search of English language publications from 2000 to 2019 was performed to identify information on ethical principles in the context of pediatric bariatric surgery. Databases searched were PubMed, Embase, Science Citation Index/Social sciences Citation Index, and Cochrane Evidence Based Medicine. Terms used in our search included (Bariatric Surgery OR Metabolic Surgery OR Bariatric Surgical Procedures OR Stomach Stapling) AND (Child OR Adolescent) AND (Ethics OR Moral Policy ORBariatric Surgery/ethics OR ethical OR moral OR autonomy OR benevolence OR non-malfeasance.)

18.2.1   Autonomy

Autonomy in the medical setting refers to the obligation to respect the self-determination of patients who have decision-making capacity. There are a variety of issues that are raised when considering the autonomous decision making for adolescent patients who have not yet reached the age of medical consent.

18.3   Pediatric Patients Are Unable to Provide Their Own Consent

The need for informed decision making or informed consent is paramount in the context of the pediatric bariatric surgical patient. Informed consent involves the permission granted for the performance of a medical or surgical intervention with knowledge of the possible consequences of that treatment. The legal authority to provide informed consent requires the legal ability to form a valid contract and the psychological or developmental ability to make sound decisions [6]. In this context, minors cannot give legal informed consent.

The ethical concerns of informed consent in the pediatric subpopulation is not unique to MBS, and thus the American Academy of Pediatrics (AAP) recommends a two-step approach to informed consent for children: 1) The child must assent to the treatment, and 2) The physician should receive the proxy consent of the parent, also called informed parental permission. Assent, as opposed to consent, refers to the ability of the child to give affirmation to the procedure based on the extent he/she is able to understand the procedure. This understanding stems from an explanation of the procedure itself, the medical condition, a framework of *values* that provides a context for specific value judgments, and the ability for the pediatric patient to reason through all available options and appreciate their effect, including risks and chances of success. This is necessary to demonstrate respect for the patient's emerging autonomy and may help enhance cooperation with medical care [6, 7].

Ethical questions arise concerning when adolescents and children are considered to be old enough to be legally allowed to make their own medical decisions. Minor treatment statutes, known as the mature minor doctrine, allow minors with *adequate decisional capacity and understanding* of their medical condition the right to consent to treatment without parental permission, with examples of this used in both reproductive and mental health. The age for this doctrine varies by state statue, with 16 years being a common cut-off, but with some states using an age as young as 14 years to consent to medical treatment [6].

There is no agreed consensus in the pediatric bariatric surgery literature for the minimum age of operation. In one review article, it was found that physiologic maturity was most often used to calculate minimum age for MBS. Six articles adopted Tanner stage IV and/or 95% of adult height based on bone age, which corresponds to ≥13 years old for girls and ≥15 years old for boys [5]. In contrast, one study by Woolford et al. showed that most physicians thought patients should be at least 18 years old before being considered for surgery [8], while healthcare professionals in a UK study believed 16 years to be an acceptable minimum age [9].

Ethical and moral issues also arise from the parent perspective. Some parents focus on the negative medical and psychosocial impact of obesity in their children or may feel guilt for their child's situation. These parental feeling should have no influence on a child's access to surgery [10], but parental pressures introduce a risk of overt or covert coercion in the child or adolescent's assent. More so, this may lead parents to push for their own wishes to supersede the wishes of their own children. At the same time, parental involvement is relevant in assessing a child's eligibility for surgery, as parental support is important in preadolescent and adolescent post-surgical nutritional management. Balancing the cognitive, emotional, and social development of the child, as well as the familial support available to the child is critical for determining a child's eligibility for MBS, and this balance can be a source of ethical challenges when determining a child's preparedness for MBS [10, 11].

18.4 Primary Care Providers May Not Be Willing to Recommend Bariatric Surgery Despite Their Patient's Wishes

The autonomy of pediatric patients is also impacted by the potential biases that exist within the medical community. Some studies seem to suggest that despite the growing problem of childhood obesity and the potential difficulties encountered with sustaining weight loss using non-operative methods, many of primary care physicians are reluctant to refer adolescents for a bariatric surgical assessment [9]. In one study, 48% participating family physicians and pediatricians indicated that they would not ever refer an obese adolescent for a bariatric operation and 46% indicated that the minimum age at which they would make a referral was 18 years [12]. In another study, although 66.8% of primary care physicians surveyed expected that MBS may be effective in therapy-resistant morbid obesity, only 41.3% would consider referral for surgery [13]. The most important reason for reluctance was the uncertainty about long-term efficacy and safety and the unknown long-term metabolic effects of weight loss surgery in such a young population [13, 14].

Another component affecting providers may be weight discrimination and stigmatization in the medical community. These stereotypes unjustly categorize overweight and obese persons as "lazy, sloppy, unmotivated, noncompliant, and less competent", who are "willful deviants who lack self-discipline" [11]. This biased sentiment may contribute to the unwillingness of primary care providers to refer child or adolescent patients to bariatric surgery centers, despite medical indications and/or the patient's and their parent's desire to pursue surgical intervention.

18.5 The Outcomes of These Procedures Will Be Faced by Patients Well After They Have Attained the Age of Consent

Bariatric surgical procedures including vertical sleeve gastrectomy and Roux-en-Y gastric bypass permanently alter the anatomy and physiology of patients. An ethical concern for the pediatric patient undergoing MBS is that they may assent to the procedure at the time, but regret such an assent later in life. MBS leads to permanent changes in patients' nutritional status, routines, medication regimens, and ability to socialize. These permanent changes may not be fully grasped or may not seem important to children and adolescents at the time of intervention, and may result in procedural regret in the future [10].

Furthermore, long term data in the pediatric population in the context of MBS has yet to be fully vetted [15]. Although there is strong evidence for improved weight reduction and reversal of comorbidities, the potential remains for the development of unforeseen problems much later in life [16]. A thorough and candid discussion about unintended consequences between the pediatric bariatric surgeon, the patient, and his/her family should emphasize what is known and, more importantly, what is unknown about late effects of MBS [17].

18.6 Informed Consent for Bariatric Surgery in the Pediatric Population

The complexity of information necessary for informed consent for MBS can be overwhelming for both adult and pediatric patients. In one study of adult MBS patients, only one-third of patients tested on information about bariatric surgery that

Table 18.1 Principles of informed consent for adolescent bariatric patients

1. Disclosure of the patient's diagnosis, including the degree of morbid obesity and the extent of comorbidities; this should include a discussion in lay language about what is currently understood about the pathophysiology of obesity and its related complications.
2. The nature of the proposed bariatric operation(s); use of visual aids and/or videos may help in describing each procedure.
3. The risks and benefits of the proposed interventions; including explicit discussion of what each complication would mean to the individual patient (i.e., an anastomotic leak is life-threatening and requires urgent reoperation, a slipped AGB must be realigned or replaced).
4. The actions and behaviors the patient will need to continue after the procedure in order for the bariatric operation to be successful in achieving weight loss, reversal of comorbidities, and to remain healthy.
5. An outline of the medical, surgical, and other follow up that will be required in the short- and long-term aspects of postoperative care.
6. Alternatives to the proposed bariatric interventions and their risks and benefits.
7. The risks and benefits of receiving no bariatric intervention or medical treatment.
8. The financial aspects of the proposed bariatric interventions, postoperative care, and costs if complications develop in the short and long term.
9. The outcomes of pediatric bariatric operations by the pediatric surgical team, including how they compare to published outcomes for complications and durable weight loss.
10. If the patient is a candidate for a clinical research trial.

Modified from Caniano [17]

had been provided during preoperative informed consent could correctly answer all questions 1 year post-surgery [18].

Informed consent for a bariatric intervention in a pediatric patient should be a lengthy process that takes place over a several-month period, during which the adolescent and his/her family engage in a medical weight reduction and behavioral modification program. Long term interactions with the pediatric surgeon concurrently during this time reinforces information about specific bariatric options, the risk/benefit profile for each operation, the likelihood of reaching the patient's stated goals, and a frank discussion about the uncertain long-term aspects of treatment [17]. The critical aspects of informed consent for adolescents undergoing bariatric surgery is summarized in Table 18.1.

Patients should not be considered candidates for MBS if they have poorly documented weight loss attempts, inadequate family support, a lack of insight into their problem, impaired decision-making capacity, major unstable psychoses, or suicidal ideation [15].

18.6.1 Beneficence

Beneficence in the context of adolescent obesity refers to the obligation for physicians to seek to reverse the physical and psychological derangements that interfere with well-being of obese pediatric patients [17].

18.7   Medical Weight Loss Has a Very Low Success Rate as Compared to Bariatric Surgery

For the morbidly obese, a twofold increased risk of mortality has been detected as early as the fourth decade of life [15]. Structured diet and exercise programs, which are the first line therapies for obesity, have relatively poor outcomes. Pharmacologic options and meal replacements are being investigated, but data demonstrating the safety and effectiveness of many of these pharmacologic agents is poor and many do not have FDA approval in patients under the age of 18. Protein-sparing modified fasts have been demonstrated as safe and effective methods of weight loss, but only when performed in a supervised inpatient setting, causing long-term recidivism to remain an issue [19].

MBS has been shown to be an effective method to achieve weight loss and reverse obesity related complications. A systematic review and meta-analysis of adolescent MBS demonstrated an average weighted BMI difference from baseline to 1 year of -13.5 kg/m^2 when including all procedures. When analyzed by procedure type, weight loss was greatest for roux-en-y gastric bypass (RYGB) and least for adjustable gastric banding (AGB) [20]. Data from Teen-LABS, a multi-centered longitudinal study, showed that 242 adolescents who underwent MBS at one of five adolescent bariatric centers demonstrated BMI reductions of 15.1 kg/m^2 (28%), 13.1 kg/m^2 (28%), and 3.8 kg/m^2 (8%) among adolescents undergoing RYGB, Vertical Sleeve Gastrectomy (VSG), and ABG procedures, respectively after 3 years [21].

Teen-LABS also demonstrated that by 3 years after surgical intervention, remission of type 2 diabetes occurred in 95% of patients, and remission of abnormal kidney function, pre-diabetes, hypertension, and dyslipidemia occurred in 86%, in 76%, 74%, and 66% of patients, respectively [21]. These data suggest that offering MBS as an option along the spectrum of care for adolescent patients with obesity is in keeping with the principle of beneficence.

18.8   Lack of Guidelines Exist That Define a Reasonable Course of Medical Weight Loss for a Child Prior to Advancing Towards Surgical Intervention

According to Caniano, violation of beneficence in the setting of adolescent morbid obesity include situations in which there was inadequate preoperative evaluation of patient comorbidities and insufficient efforts to achieve weight reduction by medical interventions [17]. Failure of medical therapy for obesity may prompt, under the principle of beneficence, consideration for MBS. Unfortunately, there are no clear guidelines that define a reasonable course of medical weight loss prior to advancing towards surgical intervention. One study interviewing UK physicians and adolescent bariatric surgery care teams showed that 58.4% selected 12 months as an adequate time period. It was also noted that almost 40% of surgeons felt that 6 months was a sufficient period for a weight management program, as opposed to only 17% of the physicians and nurses [9].

18.8.1 Non-maleficence

The principle of non-maleficence refers to the physician's obligation to avoid inflicting harm on a patient. In the context of adolescent obesity, this involves balancing the known long-term risks of obesity with the known short-term risks of obesity surgery and the somewhat nebulous long-term effects of obesity surgery.

18.9 Data Regarding Long-Term Outcomes Is Lacking, Leading to Ethical Constraints When Performing Irreversible Operations

Short term postoperative complications after MBS are well documented and include anastomotic or staple line leak, strictures, postoperative bleeding, bowel obstructions, wound infections, deep venous thrombosis, worsened gastroesophageal reflux, and hospital readmissions [16]. The most significant long-term complications of adolescent MBS are nutritional deficiencies, metabolic complications such as dumping syndrome, and psychological adjustment problems. Furthermore, additional management of excess skin may be required, which would require additional postoperative body contouring surgery [19]. The lack of mature long-term outcomes data for adolescent bariatric surgery patients presents some ethical ambiguity when considering the obligation to avoid causing harm to a patient.

18.10 Our Preoperative Evaluations Center Around Perceived Ability to Maintain a Weight-Loss Diet, But Not on the Resilience of Children Who Face Operative Complications for an Elective Procedure

The potential harms that can occur following bariatric interventions may be difficult for an adolescent patient and her/his family to manage, and complications may have more severe consequences as a result. Adverse events are reported even with very experienced surgeons [10], and a patient may not fully appreciate the impact that complications will have in terms of length of hospitalization, re-operative surgery, and unanticipated long-term problems [17].

Perhaps the best way of addressing this ethical dilemma is to prevent complications as much as possible. This includes procedures performed by only experienced providers in settings that can appropriately care for obese patients, as conditions under which bariatric surgery is performed appears to be highly relevant for the outcome. High quality care includes preoperative evaluation by a multidisciplinary team, an MBS center with competency with children and adolescents, close postoperative care and follow up, and family support [10].

18.11 Mental Disorders Should Be Monitored and Addressed in the Treatment of Severe Obesity to Prevent Any Additional Harm to Adolescent Mental Health

There is a high prevalence of mental health association in the obese pediatric population, with studies demonstrating that up to 30% of adolescents seeking weight-loss surgery self-reported symptoms of clinical depression, had significantly lower health-related quality of life scores, and up to 45% reported binge eating behaviors at some point in their life [22, 23]. Failure of expected results or the development of complications from MBS can exacerbate these psychological stressors. There is an ethical obligation for bariatric surgical centers to care for the potential psychological comorbidities associated with obesity, and this obligation may be amplified when treating adolescents. Ongoing psychosocial evaluation and support with an emphasis on optimizing mental health, social support structure, and adequately assessing whether an adolescent and their guardian fully understand the risk and benefits of MBS are very important to ensure the successful holistic care of obese adolescents [12].

18.11.1 Justice

The ethical principle of justice refers to the mandate that each person receives a fair share of health resources and equitable treatment [17]. Encapsulated within this is an implicit understanding that certain disease processes are unequally distributed amongst different populations based on race, socio-economic status, and other demographic differences. A just medical system of care is capable of addressing the unique needs of different communities.

18.12 Ethnic and Socio-economic Disparities in Terms of Rates of Obesity and Access to Medical and Surgical Care Exist, and Certain Populations May Be Excluded from the More Efficacious Surgical Approach

Pediatric obesity in the US affects one in three socially disadvantaged children, and children raised in low income neighborhoods score worse on most childhood health indicators. In fact, children within the lowest 20th-percentile for socioeconomic status (SES) have a 70% increase in obesity rates when compared to the highest 5th-percentile. Black, Hispanic, and Native American children across all economic strata also have significantly higher rates of obesity. Given these disparities, it is important for surgeons and practitioners to advocate for these patients and note at risk populations may not have ready access to medical weight management and bariatric services [17].

18.13 Conclusions and Recommendations

The treatment of obesity includes a wide range of options, including MBS. The ethical constructs surrounding MBS must be fully developed in order to provide reasonable treatment options for adolescents that appropriately addresses a variety of issues unique to minors. The ethical principles of autonomy, beneficence, nonmaleficence, and justice each raise unique issues that must be carefully considered both from a population perspective, and from the perspective of each individual patient. The ultimate decision as to which pediatric patients are appropriate candidates for MBS must take into consideration a variety of individual, familial, and social factors that impact the physical and mental outcomes associated with the surgical therapy of obesity.

References

1. Skinner AC, Ravanbakht SN, Skelton JA, Perrin EM, Armstrong SC. Prevalence of obesity and severe obesity in US children, 1999–2016. Pediatrics. 2018;141(3).
2. Abdullah A, Wolfe R, Stoelwinder JU, de Courten M, Stevenson C, Walls HL, et al. The number of years lived with obesity and the risk of all-cause and cause-specific mortality. Int J Epidemiol. 2011;40(4):985–96.
3. Kelly AS, Barlow SE, Rao G, Inge TH, Hayman LL, Steinberger J, et al. Severe obesity in children and adolescents: identification, associated health risks, and treatment approaches: a scientific statement from the American Heart Association. Circulation. 2013;128(15):1689–712.
4. Levine MD, Ringham RM, Kalarchian MA, Wisniewski L, Marcus MD. Is family-based behavioral weight control appropriate for severe pediatric obesity? Int J Eat Disord. 2001;30(3):318–28.
5. Childerhose JE, Alsamawi A, Mehta T, Smith JE, Woolford S, Tarini BA. Adolescent bariatric surgery: a systematic review of recommendation documents. Surg Obes Relat Dis. 2017;13(10):1768–79.
6. Unguru Y. Making sense of adolescent decision-making: challenge and reality. Adolesc Med State Art Rev. 2011;22(2):195–206, vii–viii.
7. Katz AL, Webb SA, Committee On B. Informed consent in decision-making in pediatric practice. Pediatrics. 2016;138(2).
8. Woolford SJ, Clark SJ, Gebremariam A, Davis MM, Freed GL. To cut or not to cut: physicians' perspectives on referring adolescents for bariatric surgery. Obes Surg. 2010;20(7):937–42.
9. Penna M, Markar S, Hewes J, Fiennes A, Jones N, Hashemi M. Adolescent bariatric surgery–thoughts and perspectives from the UK. Int J Environ Res Public Health. 2013;11(1):573–82.
10. Hofmann B. Bariatric surgery for obese children and adolescents: a review of the moral challenges. BMC Med Ethics. 2013;14:18.
11. Hunsaker SL, Garland BH, Rofey D, Reiter-Purtill J, Mitchell J, Courcoulas A, et al. A multisite 2-year follow up of psychopathology prevalence, predictors, and correlates among adolescents who did or did not undergo weight loss surgery. J Adolesc Health. 2018;63(2):142–50.
12. van Geelen SM, Bolt IL, van der Baan-Slootweg OH, van Summeren MJ. The controversy over pediatric bariatric surgery: an explorative study on attitudes and normative beliefs of specialists, parents, and adolescents with obesity. J Bioeth Inq. 2013;10(2):227–37.
13. Roebroek YGM, Talib A, Muris JWM, van Dielen FMH, Bouvy ND, van Heurn LWE. Hurdles to take for adequate treatment of morbidly obese children and adolescents: attitudes of general practitioners towards conservative and surgical treatment of paediatric morbid obesity. World J Surg. 2019;43(4):1173–81.

14. Iqbal CW, Kumar S, Iqbal AD, Ishitani MB. Perspectives on pediatric bariatric surgery: identifying barriers to referral. Surg Obes Relat Dis. 2009;5(1):88–93.
15. Inge TH. Bariatric surgery for morbidly obese adolescents: is there a rationale for early intervention? Growth Horm IGF Res. 2006;16 Suppl A:S15-9.
16. Inge TH, Laffel LM, Jenkins TM, Marcus MD, Leibel NI, Brandt ML, et al. Comparison of surgical and medical therapy for type 2 diabetes in severely obese adolescents. JAMA Pediatr. 2018;172(5):452–60.
17. Caniano DA. Ethical issues in pediatric bariatric surgery. Semin Pediatr Surg. 2009;18(3):186–92.
18. Madan AK, Tichansky DS. Patients postoperatively forget aspects of preoperative patient education. Obes Surg. 2005;15(7):1066–9.
19. Thenappan A, Nadler E. Bariatric surgery in children: indications, types, and outcomes. Curr Gastroenterol Rep. 2019;21(6):24.
20. Black JA, White B, Viner RM, Simmons RK. Bariatric surgery for obese children and adolescents: a systematic review and meta-analysis. Obes Rev. 2013;14(8):634–44.
21. Inge TH, Courcoulas AP, Jenkins TM, Michalsky MP, Helmrath MA, Brandt ML, et al. Weight loss and health status 3 years after bariatric surgery in adolescents. N Engl J Med. 2016;374(2):113–23.
22. Zeller MH, Roehrig HR, Modi AC, Daniels SR, Inge TH. Health-related quality of life and depressive symptoms in adolescents with extreme obesity presenting for bariatric surgery. Pediatrics. 2006;117(4):1155–61.
23. Glasofer DR, Tanofsky-Kraff M, Eddy KT, Yanovski SZ, Theim KR, Mirch MC, et al. Binge eating in overweight treatment-seeking adolescents. J Pediatr Psychol. 2007;32(1):95–105.

Adjustable Gastric Banding: Why Did It Fail?

19

Elizaveta Walker and Bruce Wolfe

19.1 Introduction

In the United States, rates of bariatric surgery utilization have steadily grown since its introduction in the 1960s [1]. In the first half of the past decade, Roux-en-Y gastric bypass (RYGB) and adjustable gastric banding (AGB) were utilized for nearly three-fourths of all bariatric procedures performed. At its peak, as many as 25% of bariatric procedures were AGB [2]. However, the declining utilization of AGB in the wake of more contemporary procedures, namely sleeve gastrectomy—accounting for 62% of bariatric procedures in 2018—warrants examination as to the reasons for the procedure's waning use. This chapter will summarize the history and development of AGB, describe the mechanistic features of the once-innovative procedure, discuss the reported outcomes of AGB and conclude with a narrative summary of why AGB has failed.

19.2 History of the Development of Adjustable Gastric Banding

The history of bariatric surgery has been marked with innovation, refinement and evolution. Throughout the development of this field, many procedures have refined prior bariatric techniques to address complications and limitations, though many

E. Walker
OHSU-PSU School of Public Health, Portland, OR, USA
e-mail: walkeliz@ohsu.edu

B. Wolfe (✉)
Oregon Health & Science University, Portland, OR, USA
e-mail: wolfeb@ohsu.edu

© Springer Nature Switzerland AG 2021
J. Alverdy, Y. Vigneswaran (eds.), *Difficult Decisions in Bariatric Surgery*,
Difficult Decisions in Surgery: An Evidence-Based Approach,
https://doi.org/10.1007/978-3-030-55329-6_19

introduced disadvantages of their own. Likewise, AGB was foremost a solution to address complications of previously developed bariatric procedures.

The initial concept underpinning early bariatric procedures was that by creating a short bowel syndrome, malabsorption would occur in otherwise hyperphagic patients resulting in weight loss [3]. Amassing popularity in the 1960s and 1970s, jejunoileal bypass (JIB) was the surgical means by which to mimic outcomes experienced by short bowel patients, namely durable weight loss. The creation of this surgical short gut involved bypass of approximately 90% of the small intestine while the bypassed intestine was retained. While weight loss was successfully achieved in most cases with this approach, complications including liver failure, micronutrient deficiency and related metabolic problems (e.g., kidney stones) were unacceptably common and led to abandonment of this approach.

The emphasis then shifted away from malabsorptive toward "restrictive" procedures, intending to reduce the amount of nutrient intake. Examples of such restrictive procedures included stapling devices and others used to create reduction of stomach size of the opening, or "stoma," into the functional body of the stomach [4, 5]. However, staple line leaks presented a major complication, resulting in prolonged recovery and rare mortality among patients. The introduction of staple line reinforcement was promptly offered as a solution, however this practice has mixed reporting in the literature regarding diminishing leak rates [5].

Subsequently, a variety of versions of gastroplasty were done with variable results [6–8]. Simple partial stapling of the stomach to limit the size of the gastric pouch above the staple line had little success regarding sustained weight loss due to disruption of the staples and dilation of the stoma. Through a variety of modifications, the procedure which emerged as the predominant procedure was the vertical banded gastroplasty (VBG) [9]. In this procedure, a portion of the stomach was separated from the body of the stomach by a staple row. The communication between this small gastric pouch and the body of the stomach was reinforced with prosthetic mesh encircling the outlet or the gastric pouch stoma. The largest reported series of the outcomes following the VBG came from Sweden [10, 11]. A number of important benefits from the weight loss achieved were reported by these investigators and others [12]. Ultimately, a number of limitations and complications were identified with this operative approach, including dilation of the gastric pouch and distal esophagus, erosion of the reinforcing band through the gastric wall, and staple line disruption, all complications which would result in inferior weight loss. Subsequent conversion to a different bariatric procedure such as RYGB was required to achieve satisfactory weight loss.

19.3   Mechanisms of AGB

In order to address these limitations and complications, a gastric band was devised by Kuzmak [13, 14] in which a gastric band encircling the proximal stomach was constructed with an inflatable or adjustable balloon within the lumen of the band, with tubing connecting the subcutaneous port to the balloon inside the band. Thus, the extent of narrowing of the opening between the upper gastric pouch and the body of the stomach could be adjusted according to outcomes. Inadequate weight loss, for example, was managed by tightening of the band whereas persistent vomiting, esophageal or gastric dilatation could be managed by deflation of the band through the subcutaneous port.

19.4 From AGB to LAGB

The development of laparoscopic techniques for bariatric surgery has led to decreased complication rates, decreased peri- and post-operative adverse events, decreased wound complication, and decreased length of stay, among other benefits [15]. The weight loss achieved by the implantation of a LAGB and frequent adjustments, as needed, was originally reported to be favorable by several investigators, including a group from Australia [16–19]. Within randomized control settings, O'Brien and colleagues [19] reported that LAGB was statistically significantly more effective than lifestyle and pharmacologic interventions for weight loss. Further, they reported significant increases in quality-of-life metrics. Other claims by the group included fasting and postprandial prolonged satiety among AGB patients [20, 21].

While the AGB weight loss was inferior to RYGB in other long-term studies, the results reported from Australia consistently reported the weight loss to be nearly as substantial with AGB as following RYGB and equivalent to that achieved with the VBG, advocating for the "broader application of LAGB for the serious and common problem of obesity" ([19], p. 632). The group subsequently went on to report comparable and sustained weight loss in the long-term as compared to other bariatric procedures [18]. Further, these studies reported mean weight loss, thus ignoring the variability of weight loss response among bariatric patients, including subgroups that may experience no weight loss. Reports such as these contributed to the unrealistic expectations regarding AGB weight loss among clinicians, advocates, and patients.

19.5 Widespread Application

The LAGB procedure and device became popular in bariatric surgical programs for several reasons. In addition to the seemingly satisfactory weight loss as described above, the operation itself was intended from the start to be a laparoscopic procedure. The procedure of placing a band or collar about the proximal stomach lent itself well to the laparoscopic approach. There was no division of the stomach or staple line to risk a leak. Thus, the procedure was technically simple, able to be conducted in less time than a RYGB, and perioperative complications were substantially lower than reported for RYGB [2, 22]. These characteristics increased the attractiveness of the LAGB and its uptake among bariatricians.

19.6   Long Term Outcomes

In time, it was increasingly apparent that LAGB weight loss was inferior to that seen with RYGB, by as little as one half as much [23]. In addition to the diminished weight loss, a number of complications occurred including dilation of the gastric pouch, the esophagus, gastroesophageal reflux [22]. Erosion of the band wall or gastric band erosion resulted in loss of the band function and ultimate regain of weight [24]. As a result of these limitations, revisions of the band procedure were commonly done. Most common was a need to replace, or reposition, the subcutaneous port as access of the port would become limited. Over time, removal of the band became a relatively common revisional procedure, often conducted in tandem with a conversion to a RYGB through either a single stage or a two-stage intervention [25]. These conversions led to improved weight loss and reasonable safety [26, 27].

However, one point worth acknowledging when appraising the outcomes of LAGB: the tendency of many LAGB reports to describe weight loss as percent excess weight loss (%EWL), an outdated and largely exaggerated method of reporting, especially in bariatric patients with lower preoperative BMI [28, 29]. While some still argue for its use despite the availability of more robust metrics [30], Mocanu et al. [31] published a systematic review in which they report inconsistencies across bariatric reporting regarding weight loss. The authors warn of the rise in increasing heterogeneity across bariatric terms, outcomes, and reporting criteria, and offer recommendations to address current discrepancies.

19.7   Why Did the LAGB Fail?

Despite the substantial popularity of LAGB in the 1990s and early 2000s, the procedure gradually lost favor, decreased in application and currently is all but expired. The reasons for this failure were numerous.

1. Insufficient or unsatisfactory weight loss. The weight loss required for a successful procedure is a judgment made by patients and their caregivers. Related to this judgment is improvement or remission of obesity-related comorbidities such as Type 2 diabetes, cardiovascular risk, hypertension, asthma, and other complications.
2. As noted above, several complications emerged over time in addition to inadequate weight loss. These complications include malposition of the subcutaneous port precluding adjustment of the tightness of the band, infection, or leak of the port or tubing. Dilation of the gastric pouch, sometimes markedly dilated, as well as distal esophagus limited the effect of the "restriction."
3. Demonstration of the superior weight loss associated with RYGB. The importance and dominance of the variable weight loss following gastric bypass in procedure selection was paramount [32]. Thus, RYGB has continued to increase in numbers whereas the number of bands placed gradually diminished [1].

4. Advent of the sleeve gastrectomy. Sleeve gastrectomy incorporates the positive features associated with RYGB while requiring less operative time than bypass. Further, sleeve gastrectomy complication rates are lower than RYGB or LAGB complication profiles. Further, multiple studies have shown the weight loss following sleeve gastrectomy to be only marginally inferior to that of RYGB but largely superior to LAGB, though long-term studies are still not available due to the procedure's relatively recent introduction in the late 2000s. Although this superiority of RYGB increases over a period of years, the marked short- and medium-term weight loss following sleeve gastrectomy, coupled with its relatively less required technical skill, has led to the high popularity of this procedure. Despite involving a long staple line, sleeve gastrectomy is still a simpler operative procedure as compared with RYGB, with fewer perioperative complications reported in the short-term. Thus, these two procedures have dominated the current landscape of bariatric surgical utilization, resulting in virtual elimination of LAGB as a viable option for today's bariatric candidate.

19.8   Conclusion

In summary, adjustable gastric banding "failed" because of inadequate weight loss, subsequent complications, the frequency by which removals and conversions were conducted, and the advent of more effective procedures. The confluence of these factors has relegated LAGB to be an artifact of this evolving field.

References

1. American Society for Metabolic and Bariatric Surgery (ASMBS). Estimate of Bariatric Surgery Numbers, 2011–2018. Resources. 2018. https://asmbs.org/resources/estimate-of-bariatric-surgery-numbers. Accessed 1 Mar 2020.
2. Flum DR, Belle SH, King WC, Wahed AS, Berk P, Chapman W, Pories W, Courcoulas AP, Mitchell J, Wolfe BM. Longitudinal Assessment of Bariatric Surgery (LABS) Consortium. Perioperative safety in the longitudinal assessment of bariatric surgery. N Engl J Med. 2009;361(5):445–54.
3. Singh D, Laya AS, Clarkston WK, Allen MJ. Jejunoileal bypass: a surgery of the past and a review of its complications. World J Gastroenterol: WJG. 2009;15(18):2277.
4. Champion JK, Williams MD. Prospective randomized comparison of linear staplers during laparoscopic Roux-en-Y gastric bypass. Obes Surg. 2003;13(6):855–9.
5. Giannopoulos GA, Tzanakis NE, Rallis GE, Efstathiou SP, Tsigris C, Nikiteas NI. Staple line reinforcement in laparoscopic bariatric surgery: does it actually make a difference? A systematic review and meta-analysis. Surg Endosc. 2010;24(11):2782–8.
6. Familiari P, Costamagna G, Bléro D, Le Moine O, Perri V, Boskoski I, Coppens E, Barea M, Iaconelli A, Mingrone G, Moreno C. Transoral gastroplasty for morbid obesity: a multicenter trial with a 1-year outcome. Gastrointest Endosc. 2011;74(6):1248–58.
7. Pekkarinen T, Koskela K, Huikuri K, Mustajoki P. Long-term results of gastroplasty for morbid obesity: binge-eating as a predictor of poor outcome. Obes Surg. 1994;4(3):248–55.
8. Terry ML, Vernon A, Hunter JG. Stapled-wedge Collis gastroplasty for the shortened esophagus. Am J Surg. 2004;188(2):195–9.

9. Suter M, Jayet C, Jayet A. Vertical banded gastroplasty: long-term results comparing three different techniques. Obes Surg. 2000;10(1):41–6.

10. Sjöström CD. Surgery as an intervention for obesity. Results from the Swedish obese subjects study. Growth Hormon IGF Res. 2003;13:S22–6.

11. Sjöström L. Review of the key results from the Swedish Obese Subjects (SOS) trial—a prospective controlled intervention study of bariatric surgery. J Intern Med. 2013;273(3):219–34.

12. Torgerson JS, Sjöström L. The Swedish Obese Subjects (SOS) study—rationale and results. Int J Obes. 2001;25(1):S2–4.

13. Kuzmak LI, Coe FL, inventors; Mentor Worldwide LLC, assignee. Gastric banding device. United States Patent US 4,592,339. 1986.

14. Kuzmak LI, inventor; Kuzmak, Lubomyr I., assignee. Laparoscopic adjustable gastric banding device and method for implantation and removal thereof. United States Patent US 5,449,368. 1995.

15. Nguyen N, Brethauer SA, Morton JM, Ponce J, Rosenthal RJ, editors. The ASMBS textbook of bariatric surgery. Cham: Springer International Publishing; 2020.

16. Dixon JB, O'Brien PE. Health outcomes of severely obese type 2 diabetic subjects 1 year after laparoscopic adjustable gastric banding. Diabetes Care. 2002;25(2):358–63.

17. Egberts K, Brown WA, O'Brien PE. Systematic review of erosion after laparoscopic adjustable gastric banding. Obes Surg. 2011;21(8):1272–9.

18. O'Brien PE, Sawyer SM, Laurie C, Brown WA, Skinner S, Veit F, Paul E, Burton PR, McGrice M, Anderson M, Dixon JB. Laparoscopic adjustable gastric banding in severely obese adolescents: a randomized trial. JAMA. 2010;303(6):519–26.

19. O'Brien PE, Dixon JB, Laurie C, Skinner S, Proietto J, McNeil J, Strauss B, Marks S, Schachter L, Chapman L, Anderson M. Treatment of mild to moderate obesity with laparoscopic adjustable gastric banding or an intensive medical program: a randomized trial. Ann Intern Med. 2006;144(9):625–33.

20. Dixon AF, Dixon JB, O'Brien PE. Laparoscopic adjustable gastric banding induces prolonged satiety: a randomized blind crossover study. J Clin Endocrinol Metab. 2005;90(2):813–9.

21. Fielding GA, Duncombe JE. Laparoscopic adjustable gastric banding in severely obese adolescents. Surg Obes Relat Dis. 2005;1(4):399–405.

22. Dorman RB, Miller CJ, Leslie DB, Serrot FJ, Slusarek B, Buchwald H, Connett JE, Ikramuddin S. Risk for hospital readmission following bariatric surgery. PLoS One. 2012;7(3):e32506.

23. Courcoulas AP, King WC, Belle SH, Berk P, Flum DR, Garcia L, Gourash W, Horlick M, Mitchell JE, Pomp A, Pories WJ. Seven-year weight trajectories and health outcomes in the Longitudinal Assessment of Bariatric Surgery (LABS) study. JAMA Surg. 2018;153(5):427–34.

24. Snow JM, Severson PA. Complications of adjustable gastric banding. Surg Clin. 2011;91(6):1249–64.

25. Spaniolas K, Bates AT, Docimo S Jr, Obeid NR, Talamini MA, Pryor AD. Single stage conversion from adjustable gastric banding to sleeve gastrectomy or Roux-en-Y gastric bypass: an analysis of 4875 patients. Surg Obes Relat Dis. 2017;13(11):1880–4.

26. Van Wezenbeek MR, Van Oudheusden TR, de Zoete JP, Smulders JF, Nienhuijs SW. Conversion to gastric bypass after either failed gastric band or failed sleeve gastrectomy. Obesity surgery. 2017;27(1):83–9.

27. Gagner M, Gumbs AA. Gastric banding: conversion to sleeve, bypass, or DS. Surg Endosc. 2007;21(11):1931–5.

28. Pok EH, Lee WJ, Ser KH, Chen JC, Chen SC, Tsou JJ, Chin KF. Laparoscopic sleeve gastrectomy in Asia: long term outcome and revisional surgery. Asian J Surg. 2016;39(1):21–8.

29. van de Laar A. Bariatric Outcomes Longitudinal Database (BOLD) suggests excess weight loss and excess BMI loss to be inappropriate outcome measures, demonstrating better alternatives. Obes Surg. 2012;22(12):1843–7.

30. Park JY, Kim YJ. Reply to the Letter to Editor entitled "The% EBMIL/% EWL double-booby trap. A comment on studies that compare the effect of bariatric surgery between heavier and lighter patients". Obes Surg. 2016;26(3):614–6.

31. Mocanu V, Nasralla A, Dang J, Jacobson M, Switzer N, Madsen K, Birch DW, Karmali S. Ongoing inconsistencies in weight loss reporting following bariatric surgery: a systematic review. Obes Surg. 2019;29(4):1375–87.
32. Varban OA, Cassidy RB, Bonham A, Carlin AM, Ghaferi A, Finks JF. Factors associated with achieving a body mass index of less than 30 after bariatric surgery. JAMA Surg. 2017;152(11):1058–64.

What Is the Role of Bariatric Surgery in the Treatment of Nonalcoholic Steatohepatitis?

Adam C. Sheka and Sayeed Ikramuddin

20.1 Introduction

Nonalcoholic fatty liver disease (NAFLD) is one of the most common liver disorders, affecting about 25% of people worldwide [1]. NAFLD is the hepatic manifestation of metabolic syndrome and is strongly correlated with obesity, dyslipidemia, and type 2 diabetes [2]. Up to 90% of patients undergoing bariatric surgery demonstrate NAFLD at the time of their operation [3]. Nonalcoholic steatohepatitis (NASH) is the inflammatory subtype of NAFLD, occurring in 3–6% of the population [4, 5]. Current guidelines require a histologic diagnosis for NASH, including steatosis as well as evidence of hepatocyte injury (ballooning) and inflammation [2]. NASH may be clinically silent but over time can progress to cirrhosis, and it is a risk factor for hepatocellular carcinoma and need for liver transplant [2]. NASH progresses to cirrhosis in up to 20% of patients, compared to about 4% of all NAFLD patients, and represents the segment of the fatty liver population most in need of targeted therapy [6].

However, there are few specific treatments for NAFLD and NASH. While targeted pharmaceuticals are in phase 3 clinical trials, none are yet approved for NASH therapy. Currently, the primary treatment for NASH is weight loss. At least 7–10% total body weight loss is needed to see histologic improvement [7]. Weight loss of >10% is associated with NASH resolution in 90% of patients and may even improve fibrosis [8]. However, this degree of weight loss is difficult for patients to achieve and maintain, even in monitored clinical trials. Bariatric surgery is the most effective weight-loss therapy but is not currently considered a specific treatment for

A. C. Sheka · S. Ikramuddin (✉)
Department of Surgery, University of Minnesota, Minneapolis, MN, USA
e-mail: ikram001@umn.edu

© Springer Nature Switzerland AG 2021
J. Alverdy, Y. Vigneswaran (eds.), *Difficult Decisions in Bariatric Surgery*,
Difficult Decisions in Surgery: An Evidence-Based Approach,
https://doi.org/10.1007/978-3-030-55329-6_20

NASH by the American Association for the Study of Liver Diseases (AASLD) [2]. This chapter will examine the existing evidence for bariatric surgery as a treatment for NASH and identify knowledge gaps that must be filled by future studies.

20.2 Search Strategy

MEDLINE, EMBASE, CENTRAL, and Google Scholar were searched for published data on the effect of bariatric surgery on nonalcoholic steatohepatitis (Table 20.1). The search included articles written in the English language involving human patients with no limitation by date of publication. Search terms included ("bariatric" OR "sleeve gastrectomy" OR "adjustable gastric band" OR "gastric bypass" OR "Roux-en-Y" OR "duodenal switch" OR "jejunoileal bypass" OR "vertical banded gastroplasty" OR "biliopancreatic diversion") AND ("non alcoholic fatty liver" OR "nonalcoholic fatty liver" OR "NAFL" OR "NAFLD" OR "NASH" OR [nonalcoholic AND steatohepatitis] OR ["non alcoholic" AND steatohepatitis]). The reference lists in retrieved publications, meta-analyses, and clinical reviews were also manually searched for relevant results not included in the initial query.

20.3 Results

After resolving duplicate results, 614 studies were returned by the search strategy. A total of 544 studies were excluded based on a review of titles and abstracts. The full text of the remaining 70 studies was reviewed. Given that current guidelines require a histologic diagnosis for NASH, studies using surrogate markers were excluded, and only the 39 studies that included both pre- or intra-operative as well as post-bariatric surgery biopsies were reviewed for this chapter. Of these 39 studies, 19 (48.7%) contained adequate information about the histologic diagnosis of NASH to draw conclusions from the data; these studies are listed in Table 20.2 [9–27]. Studies using the NAFLD Activity Score (NAS) cutoff as a surrogate for NASH were reviewed but not included in Table 20.2 (n = 9), as this score does not always correlate with a diagnosis of NASH [28–37]. The NAS, which rates the individual components of NASH (steatosis, lobular inflammation, and hepatocellular ballooning) on a numeric scale, is useful for describing changes in NASH and is therefore

Table 20.1 Search and data review strategy

Patients	Intervention	Comparator	Outcomes
Patients with NAFLD or NASH	Bariatric surgery	Other bariatric surgery, lifestyle modification, pharmacologic treatment, or no treatment	Histologic improvement in NASH, development of cirrhosis, development of hepatocellular carcinoma, liver-specific mortality, overall mortality, cost, complications of bariatric surgery

Table 20.2 Studies including paired biopsies evaluating changes in NASH after bariatric surgery

Study	Study type	Procedure type	# of patients with paired biopsies	n (%) of patients with NASH on pre-op biopsy	n (%) of patients with NASH on post-op biopsy	Post-op biopsy interval	Quality	Other findings
Barker et al. 2006 [9]	Retrospective cohort	RYGB	19	19 (100%)	2 (10.5%)	21.4 months	Very low	
de Almeida et al. 2006 [10]	Prospective cohort	RYGB	16	16 (100%)	0 (0%)	23.5 ± 8.4 months	Low	Fibrosis stable or improved in 4 patients with fibrosis on initial biopsy
Dixon et al. 2004 [11]	Prospective cohort	AGB	36	23 (63.9%)	4 (11.1%)	25.6 ± 11 months	Low	Of 4 with persistent NASH, 2 had improvement and 2 had no change
Dixon et al. 2006 [12]	Prospective cohort	AGB	60	30 (50%)	6 (10%)	29.5 ± 10 months	Low	
Esquivel et al. 2018 [13]	Prospective cohort	SG	43	21 (48.8%)	0 (0%)	12 months	Low	
Furuya et al. 2007 [14]	Prospective cohort	RYGB	18	12 (66.7%)	Exact number is not clear, maximum 3 (16.7%)	2 years	Low	No progression of fibrosis, fibrosis disappeared in 75%
Lassailly et al. 2015 [15]	Prospective cohort	RYGB, AGB, SG, BIB	82	82 (100%)	12 (14.6%)	12 months	Low	Fibrosis improved in 33.8%, patients with persistent NASH had lower weight loss, 30.4% of LAGB patients had persistent NASH versus 7.6% of RYGB patients
Liu et al. 2007 [16]	Retrospective cohort	RYGB	39	23 (59.0%)	0 (0%)	18 months	Very low	

(continued)

Table 20.2 (continued)

Study	Study type	Procedure type	# of patients with paired biopsies	n (%) of patients with NASH on pre-op biopsy	n (%) of patients with NASH on post-op biopsy	Post-op biopsy interval	Quality	Other findings
Luyckx et al. 1998 [17]	Retrospective cohort	VBG, AGB	69	10 (14.4%)	18 (26.1%)	27 ± 15 months	Very low	
Meinhardt et al. 2006 [18]	Retrospective cohort	JIB	30	13 of 41 originally biospied (31.7%)	7 (23.3%)	4.8 ± 4 years	Very low	No worsening of liver histopathology in any cases but pre-post changes are not specifically delineated
Moretto et al. 2012 [19]	Retrospective cohort	RYGB	78	45 (57.7%)	21 (26.9%)	Not reported	Very low	5 of 43 patients with no fibrosis at baseline developed fibrosis by 2nd biopsy, fibrosis resolved in 16 of 35 patients with fibrosis at baseline
Parker et al. 2017 [20]	Prospective cohort	RYGB	15	15 (100%)	2 (13.3%)	Not reported	Low	Reevaluated once 60% weight loss or weight loss plateaued
Raj et al. 2015 [21]	Prospective cohort	SG	20	10 (50%)	0 (0%)	7 months	Low	
		RYGB	10	3 (30%)	1 (10%)			
Schneck et al. 2016 [22]	Prospective cohort	RYGB	9	9 (100%)	0 (0%)	55 months	Low	
Schwenger et al. 2018 [23]	Prospective cohort	RYGB	42	9 (21.4%)	1 (2.4%)	12 months	Low	Fibrosis also improved
Stratopoulos et al. 2005 [24]	Prospective cohort	VBG	51	50 (98%)	42 (82.4%)	18 months	Low	Grading system not consistent with other studies, of 42 patients with persistent NASH, majority had improved grade

Taitano et al. 2015 [25]	Retrospective cohort	RYGB, AGB	160	42 (26.3%)	5 (3.1%)	31 ± 26 months	Very low	Fibrosis present in 43 patients at baseline, resolved in 53%, improved in 3%, did not worsen in any case
Weiner 2010 [26]	Prospective cohort	RYGB, AGB, BPD-DS	116	116 (100%)	2 (1.7%)	18.6 ± 8.3 months	Low	Both patients with persistent NASH underwent AGB
Vargas et al. 2012 [27]	Prospective cohort	RYGB	26	25 (96.1%)	4 (15.3%)	16 ± 3 months	Low	

often used in clinical trials, but the diagnosis of NASH requires specific components and must be evaluated separately [28]. The remaining 11 studies either examined steatosis alone or did not include enough histologic information to evaluate the presence of NASH before and after bariatric surgery.

No randomized clinical trials of the effect of bariatric surgery on NASH were found. Of the 19 observational studies reviewed in Table 20.2, 6 were retrospective cohort studies and 13 were prospective cohort studies. The overall quality of the evidence was low, relying on highly selected patient populations. Patients in the prospective studies had a high rate of dropout, which is likely due to the invasive nature of a second liver biopsy. For the majority of these studies, the postoperative biopsy (and therefore the entire included patient cohort) was obtained because the patient needed a second operation or had a lab abnormality prompting a biopsy, further increasing the risk of bias. In addition, for all of the included studies, the initial recruitment event was not the diagnosis of NASH but the planned bariatric operation. This makes the evidence difficult to interpret and apply to patients with NASH looking for treatment options, rather than to bariatric surgery candidates who happen to have NASH.

These observational cohort studies consistently report improvement in the degree of steatosis and a high proportion of patients with complete resolution of NASH after bariatric surgery. Of the studies using a consistent definition for the histologic diagnosis of NASH, NASH resolution was seen in 53–100% of patients, with 5 studies reporting NASH resolution in their entire patient cohort. Only one study reported an increase in NASH postoperatively [17].

Studies included patients undergoing most bariatric operations, including Roux-en-Y gastric bypass, adjustable gastric banding, sleeve gastrectomy, biliointestinal bypass, vertical banded gastroplasty, jejunoileal bypass, and biliopancreatic diversion with duodenal switch. Most of these operations are now quite rare, with the sleeve gastrectomy and Roux-en-Y gastric bypass most common. Both of these operations appear to have a high rate of NASH resolution in the limited cohorts available. There is no evidence to suggest either sleeve gastrectomy or Roux-en-Y is superior for treating NASH.

NASH resolution appears to be related to the degree of weight loss achieved. In one study, 30.4% of laparoscopic adjustable gastric band patients had persistent NASH versus just 7.6% of Roux-en-Y gastric bypass patients, with the patients in the Roux-en-Y group losing more weight over time [15]. A study of adolescents undergoing sleeve gastrectomy, intragastric balloon placement, or lifestyle modification found that only the sleeve gastrectomy improved NASH [34]. This appeared related to the degree of weight loss achieved; patients in the surgical group lost 21.5% of their body weight versus 3.4% for those with an intragastric balloon and 1.7% for those who underwent lifestyle modification alone. These findings are consistent with prior medical weight loss studies in NASH, which found that 7–10% total body weight loss was required to see histologic improvement [7].

While it is not one of the diagnostic criteria for NASH, fibrosis is the strongest predictor of NASH progression and long-term outcomes, including overall mortality [38–40]. Changes in fibrosis after bariatric surgery are reported in six of the included studies. Overall, most patients had stable or improved hepatic fibrosis, though a few isolated patients had worsening of fibrosis over time. The effects of bariatric surgery on fibrosis in NASH patients will need to be addressed by future trials.

In all of the included studies, the initial biopsy diagnosing NASH was obtained at the time of the bariatric operation. However, many patients who undergo bariatric surgery are required by their physician or insurance company to demonstrate some degree of weight loss prior to their operation; the degree of preoperative weight loss and potential for NASH improvement during this interval is not adequately accounted for in studies to date. Therefore, the actual degree of NASH in patients undergoing bariatric surgery may be underreported.

The existing literature is limited by significant heterogeneity in the histologic definitions used, types of bariatric procedures performed, time of follow-up, and baseline patient populations. The need for biopsy and lack of a specific medical comparator make clinical trial design for NASH and bariatric surgery difficult. However, there are randomized clinical trials planned in NASH patients to compare lifestyle therapy to bariatric surgery (NCT03472157, NCT03426111), pharmacologic therapy with liraglutide to bariatric surgery (NCT02654665), and the efficacy of the sleeve gastrectomy versus Roux-en-Y gastric bypass (NCT03524365). These trials may provide additional clarity and stronger evidence for bariatric surgery as a NASH therapy.

Data regarding the safety of bariatric surgery in patients with NASH and specifically NASH cirrhosis are limited. A study utilizing the Nationwide Inpatient Sample found that mortality in patients undergoing bariatric surgery was higher in those with cirrhosis (0.9% for compensated and 16.3% for patients with uncompensated) than those without cirrhosis (0.3%) [41]. The data in this analysis was from 1998 to 2007 and likely included more open surgery than is currently performed. More recent case series report similar complication rates between bariatric patients with and without liver disease [42, 43]. A meta-analysis of 122 cirrhotic patients undergoing bariatric surgery (97% with Child's Class A cirrhosis) found increased early and late mortality in these patients compared to the general population [44]. No patients undergoing sleeve gastrectomy had perioperative mortality. This study included patients with cirrhosis diagnosed at the time of surgery and is therefore difficult to generalize to the elective treatment of NASH.

Current studies utilize surrogates for liver sequelae, such as changes in histology, to assign benefit to therapies for NASH. However, the main concerns prompting the treatment of NASH are hepatocellular carcinoma, cirrhosis, and the need for liver transplantation. From a well-matched retrospective cohort analysis using insurance data, we found that patients with NAFLD/NASH who undergo bariatric surgery have a significantly decreased risk of progression to cirrhosis compared to patients who do not undergo surgery [45]. Future studies will need to prospectively evaluate these ultimate outcomes.

20.4 Recommendations

Given the lack of high-quality evidence regarding bariatric surgery as a treatment for NASH, it is difficult to make strong recommendations. The AASLD does not yet recommend bariatric surgery specifically for treatment of NASH or NAFLD [2]. However, the existing observational cohort studies have a substantial level of agreement supporting improvement in NASH after bariatric surgery for highly selected cohorts. For patients with NASH or suspected NASH who are otherwise eligible for bariatric surgery, either due to BMI or BMI and comorbidities, referral for bariatric surgery is reasonable, particularly when patients have tried and failed to lose weight through lifestyle modification (evidence quality moderate, strong recommendation). Awareness of bariatric surgery as a possible treatment for NASH should prompt primary care providers and hepatologists to discuss this option with otherwise eligible patients and refer them as appropriate. For patients with NASH who do not meet eligibility criteria for bariatric surgery, the current evidence is not adequate to support the procedure.

20.5 A Personal View of the Data

While the existing evidence for bariatric surgery as a NASH therapy is limited to observational studies with significant risk for bias, there is considerable and consistent research suggesting that weight loss of at least 7–10% is the best treatment for NASH that is currently available. Our experience and multiple clinical trials have shown that bariatric surgery is the most effective method for achieving and sustaining this level of weight loss. Thus, if a patient is known to have NASH based on biopsy or has hepatic steatosis on imaging studies with significant risk factors (obesity, dyslipidemia, type 2 diabetes) for NASH, it is entirely reasonable to refer these patients for bariatric surgery evaluation, particularly if they are unable to achieve weight loss with lifestyle changes and medical therapy. Many patients with this constellation of medical conditions will qualify for bariatric surgery regardless of their NASH status; however, some patients with borderline BMI and type 2 diabetes may have NASH but not qualify for bariatric surgery under the current guidelines. Every attempt should be made to help these patients access surgical weight loss. Currently, much of the focus on NASH treatment is on pharmaceuticals. However, results from ongoing clinical trials do not appear to demonstrate the effect sizes that have been observed after bariatric surgery. As higher quality evidence is made available from clinical trials, we suspect NASH (and likely NAFLD) will be incorporated into bariatric surgery eligibility guidelines and treatment algorithms from organizations such as the AASLD. While observational cohorts have provided the initial data, results from randomized trials of best medical therapy (currently lifestyle change) versus bariatric surgery, specifically for patients with NASH, will likely be required to tip the scales of evidence.

References

1. Younossi Z, Anstee QM, Marietti M, et al. Global burden of NAFLD and NASH: trends, risk factors and prevention. Nat Rev Gastroenterol Hepatol. 2018;15(1):11–20.
2. Chalasani N, Younossi Z, Lavine JE, et al. The diagnosis and management of nonalcoholic fatty liver disease: practice guidance from the American Association for the Study of Liver Diseases. Hepatology. 2018;67(1):328–57.
3. Ong JP, Elariny H, Collantes R, et al. Predictors of nonalcoholic steatohepatitis and advanced fibrosis in morbidly obese patients. Obes Surg. 2005;15(3):310–5.
4. Estes C, Razavi H, Loomba R, Younossi Z, Sanyal AJ. Modeling the epidemic of nonalcoholic fatty liver disease demonstrates an exponential increase in burden of disease. Hepatology. 2018;67(1):123–33.
5. Estes C, Anstee QM, Arias-Loste MT, et al. Modeling NAFLD disease burden in China, France, Germany, Italy, Japan, Spain, United Kingdom, and United States for the period 2016–2030. J Hepatol. 2018;69(4):896–904.
6. Matteoni CA, Younossi ZM, Gramlich T, Boparai N, Liu YC, McCullough AJ. Nonalcoholic fatty liver disease: a spectrum of clinical and pathological severity. Gastroenterology. 1999;116(6):1413–9.
7. Musso G, Cassader M, Rosina F, Gambino R. Impact of current treatments on liver disease, glucose metabolism and cardiovascular risk in non-alcoholic fatty liver disease (NAFLD): a systematic review and meta-analysis of randomised trials. Diabetoligia. 2012;55(4):885–904.
8. Vilar-Gomez E, Martinez-Perez Y, Calzadilla-Bertot L, et al. Weight loss through lifestyle modification significantly reduces features of nonalcoholic steatohepatitis. Gastroenterology. 2015;149(2):367–78.
9. Barker KB, Palekar NA, Bowers SP, et al. Non-alcoholic steatohepatitis: effect of Roux-en-Y gastric bypass surgery. Am J Gastroenterol. 2006;101(2):368–73.
10. de Almeida SR, Rocha PRS, Sanches MD, et al. Roux-en-Y gastric bypass improves the non-alcoholic steatohepatitis (NASH) of morbid obesity. Obes Surg. 2006;16(3):270–8.
11. Dixon JB, Bhathal PS, Hughes NR, et al. Nonalcoholic fatty liver disease: improvement in liver histologic analysis with weight loss. Hepatology. 2004;39(6):1647–54.
12. Dixon JB, Bhathal PS, O'Brien PE. Weight loss and non-alcoholic fatty liver disease: falls in gamma-glutamyl transferase concentrations are associated with histologic improvement. Obes Surg. 2006;16(10):1278–86.
13. Esquivel CM, Garcia M, Armando L, et al. Laparoscopic sleeve gastrectomy resolves NAFLD: another indication for bariatric surgery? Obes Surg. 2018;28(12):4022–33.
14. Furuya CK Jr, de Oliveira CP, de Mello ES, et al. Effects of bariatric surgery on nonalcoholic fatty liver disease: preliminary findings after 2 years. J Gastroenterol Hepatol. 2007;22(4):510–4.
15. Lassailly G, Caiazzo R, Buob D, et al. Bariatric surgery reduces features of non-alcoholic steatohepatitis in morbidly obese patients. Gastroenterology. 2015;149(2):379–88.
16. Liu X, Lazenby AJ, Clements RH, et al. Resolution of nonalcoholic steatohepatits after gastric bypass surgery. Obes Surg. 2007;17(4):486–92.
17. Luyckx FH, Desaive C, Thiry A, et al. Liver abnormalities in severely obese subjects: effect of drastic weight loss after gastroplasty. Int J Obes Relat Metab Disord. 1998;22(3):222–6.
18. Meinhardt NG, Souto KE, Ulbrich-Kulczynski JM, et al. Hepatic outcomes after jejunoileal bypass: is there a publication bias? Obes Surg. 2006;16(9):1171–8.
19. Moretto M, Kupski C, da Silva VD, et al. Effect of bariatric surgery on liver fibrosis. Obes Surg. 2012;22(7):1044–9.
20. Parker BM, Wu J, You J, et al. Reversal of fibrosis in patients with nonalcoholic steatohepatosis after gastric bypass surgery. BMC Obes. 2017;4:32.
21. Raj PP, Gomes RM, Kumar S, et al. The effect of surgically induced weight loss on nonalcoholic fatty liver disease in morbidly obese Indians: "NASHOST" prospective observational trial. Surg Obes Relat Dis. 2015;11(6):1315–22.

22. Schneck A, Anty R, Patouraux S, et al. Roux-en Y gastric bypass results in long-term remission of hepatocyte apoptosis and hepatic histological features of non-alcoholic steatohepatitis. Front Physiol. 2016;7:334.
23. Schwenger KJP, Fischer SE, Jackson T, et al. In nonalcoholic fatty liver disease, Roux-en-Y gastric bypass improves liver histology while persistent disease is associated with lower improvements in waist circumference and glycemic control. Surg Obes Relat Dis. 2018;14(9):1233–9.
24. Stratopoulos C, Papakonstantinou A, Terzis I, et al. Changes in liver histology accompanying massive weight loss after gastroplasty for morbid obesity. Obes Surg. 2005;15(8):1154–60.
25. Taitano AA, Markow M, Finan JE, et al. Bariatric surgery improves histological features of nonalcoholic fatty liver disease and liver fibrosis. J Gastrointest Surg. 2015;19(3):429–36.
26. Weiner RA. Surgical treatment of non-alcoholic steatohepatitis and non-alcoholic fatty liver disease. Dig Dis. 2010;28(1):274–9.
27. Vargas V, Allende H, Lecube A, et al. Surgically induced weight loss by gastric bypass improves non alcoholic fatty liver disease in morbid obese patients. World J Hepatol. 2012;4(12):382–8.
28. Brunt EM, Kleiner DE, Wilson LA, Belt P, Neuschwander-Tetri B. The NAS and the histopathologic diagnosis in NAFLD: distinct clinicopathologic meanings. Hepatology. 2011;53(3):810–20.
29. von Schönfels W, Beckman JH, Ahrens M, et al. Histological improvement of NAFLD in patients with obesity after bariatric surgery based on standardized NAS (NAFLD activity score). Surg Obes Relat Dis. 2018;14(10):1607–16.
30. Aldoheyan T, Hassanain M, Al-Mulhim A, et al. The effects of bariatric surgeries on nonalcoholic fatty liver disease. Surg Endosc. 2017;31(3):1142–7.
31. Caiazzo R, Lassailly G, Leteurtre E, et al. Roux-en-Y gastric bypass versus adjustable gastric banding to reduce nonalcoholic fatty liver disease: a 5-year controlled longitudinal study. Ann Surg. 2014;260(5):893–8.
32. Froylich D, Corcelles R, Daigle C, et al. Effect of Roux-en-Y gastric bypass and sleeve gastrectomy on nonalcoholic fatty liver disease: a comparative study. Surg Obes Relat Dis. 2015;12(1):127–31.
33. Garg H, Aggarwal S, Shalimar. Utility of transient elastography (fibroscan) and impact of bariatric surgery on nonalcoholic fatty liver disease (NAFLD) in morbidly obese patients. Surg Obes Relat Dis. 2018;14(1):81–91.
34. Manco M, Mosca A, de Peppo F, et al. The benefit of sleeve gastrectomy in obese adolescents on nonalcoholic steatohepatitis and hepatic fibrosis. J Pediatr. 2017;180:31–37.e2.
35. Mathurin P, Hollebecque A, Arnalsteen L, et al. Prospective study of the long-term effects of bariatric surgery on liver injury in patients without advanced disease. Gastroenterology. 2009;137(2):532–40.
36. Moschen AR, Molnar C, Wolf AM, et al. Effects of weight loss induced by bariatric surgery on hepatic adipocytokine expression. J Hepatol. 2009;51(4):765–77.
37. Tai C, Huang C, Hwang J, et al. Improvement of nonalcoholic fatty liver disease after bariatric surgery in morbidly obese Chinese patients. Obes Surg. 2012;22(7):1016–21.
38. Angulo P, Machado MV, Diehl AM. Fibrosis in nonalcoholic fatty liver disease: mechanisms and clinical implications. Semin Liver Dis. 2015;35(2):132–45.
39. Angulo P, Kleiner DE, Dam-Larsen S, et al. Liver fibrosis, but no other histologic feature, associated with outcomes of patients with nonalcoholic fatty liver disease. Gastroenterology. 2015;149(2):389–97.
40. Ekstedt M, Hagström H, Nasr P, et al. Fibrosis stage is the strongest predictor for disease-specific mortality in NAFLD after up to 33 years of follow-up. Hepatology. 2015;61(5):1547–54.
41. Mosko JD, Nguyen GC. Increased perioperative mortality following bariatric surgery among patients with cirrhosis. Clin Gastroenterol Hepatol. 2011;9(10):897–901.
42. Wolter S, Duprée A, Coelius C, et al. Influence of liver disease on perioperative outcome after bariatric surgery in a Northern German cohort. Obes Surg. 2017;27(1):90–5.

43. Singh T, Kochhar GS, Goh GB, et al. Safety and efficacy of bariatric surgery in patients with advanced fibrosis. Int J Obes. 2017;41(3):443–9.
44. Jan A, Narwaria M, Mahawar KK. A systematic review of bariatric surgery in patients with liver cirrhosis. Obes Surg. 2015;25(8):1518–26.
45. Wirth K, Sheka A, Kizy S, et al. Bariatric surgery is associated with decreased progression of nonalcoholic fatty liver disease to cirrhosis: a retrospective cohort analysis. Ann Surg. 2020;272(1):32–9.

Is Roux-en-Y Gastric Bypass Less Safe Than Sleeve Gastrectomy?

21

Mikhail Attaar and Stephen P. Haggerty

21.1 Introduction

The two most commonly performed weight loss procedures worldwide are the laparoscopic Roux-en-Y gastric bypass (LRYGB) and laparoscopic sleeve gastrectomy (LSG) [1]. The LRYGB was developed in the United States in 1994 and considered the gold-standard surgical treatment for morbid obesity due to substantial long-term weight loss and resolution of comorbidities [2–4]. However, the relative disadvantages include a steep learning curve and potential for more severe complications [5, 6]. In contrast, LSG, a relatively newer procedure that was previously performed as the first stage in a two stage biliopancreatic diversion with duodenal switch, has gained popularity in recent years due to its simplicity and satisfactory outcomes in terms of weight loss and resolution of comorbidities [7–9]. The purpose of this chapter is to review the published literature comparing LRYGB and LSG with a specific focus on safety and rates of complications.

21.2 Search Strategy

A Pub-med search was performed of the literature published in the English language using the following search terms, either alone or in combination in order to obtain the maximal number of articles: "sleeve gastrectomy", "vertical gastrectomy", "vertical sleeve gastrectomy", "gastric bypass", "Roux-en-Y gastric bypass",

M. Attaar
University of Chicago Medical Center, Chicago, IL, USA

S. P. Haggerty (✉)
Northshore University HealthSystem, Evanston, IL, USA
e-mail: shaggerty@northshore.org

© Springer Nature Switzerland AG 2021
J. Alverdy, Y. Vigneswaran (eds.), *Difficult Decisions in Bariatric Surgery*,
Difficult Decisions in Surgery: An Evidence-Based Approach,
https://doi.org/10.1007/978-3-030-55329-6_21

"bariatric surgery". The reference list of identified papers as well as topical reviews were checked for additional articles for inclusion. For studies in which multiple articles have been published at different time points on the same population, the most recently published article with the most complete follow-up was included. Individual trials are detailed in Tables 21.1 and 21.2 and meta-analyses and systematic reviews are detailed in Table 21.3.

21.3 Results

21.3.1 Early (<30 Days) Complications

The most common early (<30 days) complications after LSG and LRYGB include major issues like bleeding requiring transfusion, anastomotic or staple line leak, gastric or bowel obstruction, bowel perforation, intra-abdominal infection, deep vein thrombosis, myocardial infarction and minor complications such as pneumonia, dysphagia, dehydration, nausea and vomiting, ileus and superficial surgical site infections (SSI) [21, 26].

Guerrier and colleagues [30] analyzed NSQIP database records for 47,982 (42.0%) and 66,380 (58.0%) patients undergoing LSG and LRYGB, respectively. On univariate analysis, LSG patients had a lower rate of organ space infection (0.45% vs. 0.68%, $p < 0.001$), lower rate of bleeding requiring transfusions (1.00% vs. 1.60%, $p < 0.001$), lower rate of sepsis (0.34% vs. 0.49%, $p < 0.001$), and septic shock (0.12% vs. 0.22%, $p < 0.001$) and required fewer unplanned reoperations (1.34% vs. 2.56%, $p < 0.001$) than LRYGB patients. Both groups had similar rates of deep venous thrombosis (0.33% vs. 0.28%, $p = 0.15$) and pulmonary embolism (0.17% vs. 0.21%, $p = 0.15$). Mortality was lower among LSG patients (0.09% vs. 0.14%, $p = 0.01$). On multivariate analysis, RYGB was associated with higher risk-adjusted 30-day serious morbidity than LSG (odds ratio 1.61; 95% CI 1.52–1.71, $p < 0.001$). Older age, female gender, higher BMI, and insulin-dependent diabetes were also associated with risk of serious morbidity (C-statistic = 0.60). They concluded that serious morbidity following bariatric surgery is uncommon; however, LSG may be associated with modest protection from adverse 30-day outcomes in comparison to LRYGB. However, their conclusion was limited by a difference in baseline risk factors of the populations studied.

In their matched cohort study of 429 patients, Casillas et al. [21] found similar mortality rates between LSG and LRYGB, while complications requiring

Table 21.1 PICO table

P (Patients)	I (Intervention)	C (Comparator)	O (Outcomes)
Patients undergoing bariatric surgery	Roux-en-Y Gastric Bypass	Sleeve gastrectomy	Intraoperative complication rate, readmission rate, reoperation rate, 30-day mortality, long-term complication rate

Table 21.2 Individual studies

Study Study type	Study period		N	Early complications (<30 days)	Readmission rate	Reoperation rate	Late complications (>30 days)	Nutritional deficiencies	Study quality
Effect of Laparoscopic Sleeve Gastrectomy versus Laparoscopic Roux-en-Y Gastric Bypass on Weight Loss at 5 Years Among Patients With Morbid Obesity: The SLEEVEPASS Randomized Clinical Trial [10] Multicenter, multi-surgeon, open-label, randomized clinical equivalence trial	2008–2010	LSG	121	Minor = 9 patients (7.4%) Major = 7 patients (5.8%)	4.2%	10 patients (8.3%)	Minor = 13 patients (10.7%) Major = 10 patients (8.3%)	NR	High quality
		LRYGB	119	Minor = 20 patients (17.1%) p = 0.02 Major = 11 patients (9.4%) p = 0.29	2.7%	18 patients (15.1%) p = 0.10	Minor = 13 patients (10.9%) p = 0.96 Major = 18 patients (15.1%) p = 0.10	NR	
Laparoscopic Roux-en-Y Gastric Bypass Versus Laparoscopic Sleeve Gastrectomy for the Treatment of Morbid Obesity: A Prospective Study with 5 Years of Follow-Up [11] Prospective non-randomized trial	2008	LSG	42	1 patient (2.3%)	NR	NR	2 patients (7.4%)	14.8% (anemia)	Moderate quality
		LRYGB	75	4 patients (5.3%) p > 0.05	NR	NR	6 patients (12.7%) p > 0.05	4.2% (anemia)	

(continued)

Table 21.2 (continued)

Study Study type	Study period	N	Early complications (<30 days)	Readmission rate	Reoperation rate	Late complications (>30 days)	Nutritional deficiencies	Study quality
Effect of Laparoscopic Sleeve Gastrectomy versus Laparoscopic Roux-en-Y Gastric Bypass on Weight Loss in Patients With Morbid Obesity: The SM-BOSS Randomized Clinical Trial [12] Randomized Trial — LSG	2007–2017	107	1 patient (0.9%)		16 patients (15.8%)	15 patients (14.9%)	NR	High quality
LRYGB		110	5 patients (4.5%) Not statistically significant		23 patients (22.1%) p = 0.33	18 patients (17.3%) Not statistically significant	NR	
Short- and Midterm Results between Laparoscopic Roux-en-Y Gastric Bypass and Laparoscopic Sleeve Gastrectomy for the Treatment of Morbid Obesity [13] Observational retrospective study — LSG	2008–2011	34	3 patients (8.8%)	NR	3 patients	13 patients	7 patients	Low quality
LRYGB		36	9 patients (25%) p > 0.05	NR	8 patients	7 patients p > 0.05	11 patients	
Randomized trial of Roux-en-Y gastric bypass versus sleeve gastrectomy in achieving excess weight loss [14] Randomized Trial — LSG		55	NR	18%	2 patients (4%)	NR	NR	Moderate quality
LRYGB		45	NR	47% p = 0.002)	6 patients (13%) p = 0.08	NR	NR	

Effectiveness and Safety of Sleeve Gastrectomy, Gastric Bypass, and Adjustable Gastric Banding in Morbidly Obese Patients: a Multicenter, Retrospective, Matched Cohort Study [15] Multicenter, retrospective, matched cohort study	2007–2010	LSG	245	19 patients (7.6%)	4.5%	25 patients (10.2%)	12 patients (5%)	NR	Moderate quality
		LRYGB	245	14 patients (5.7%) p = 0.367	0.4% p = 0.003	10 patients (4.1%) p = 0.009	23 patients (9%) p = 0.054	NR	
Randomized Clinical Trial of Laparoscopic Roux-en-Y Gastric Bypass Versus Laparoscopic Sleeve Gastrectomy for the Management of Patients with BMI < 50 kg/m² [16] Randomized Trial	2005–2007	LSG	30	2 patients (7%)	NR	1 patient	1 patient	At 3 years, only b12 found to be deficient more often in LRYGB (7 vs. 1 pt., p = 0.05)	Moderate quality
		LRYGB	30	2 patients (7%)	NR	2 patients	1 patient		

(continued)

Table 21.2 (continued)

Study / Study type	Study period		N	Early complications (<30 days)	Readmission rate	Reoperation rate	Late complications (>30 days)	Nutritional deficiencies	Study quality
Comparison of Early and Late Complications after Various Bariatric Procedures: Incidence and Treatment During 15 Years at a Single Institution [17] Retrospective study	1994–2008	LSG	151	11 (7.28)	NR	NR	2 patients (1.32)	Rates reported but not compared directly	Low quality
		LRYGB	137	10 (7.3)			9 patients (6.57)		
A Randomized Clinical Trial of Laparoscopic Roux-en-Y Gastric Bypass and Sleeve Gastrectomy for the Treatment of Morbid Obesity in China: a 5-Year Outcome [18] Randomized Trial	2007–2008	LSG	32	4 patients (3 minor, 1 major)	NR	2 patients (1 early, 1 late)	0 patients	NR	Moderate quality
		LRYGB	32	2 patients (all major) $p > 0.05$	NR	2 patients (1 early, 1 late)	8 patients (5 minor, 3 major) $p > 0.05$	NR	
Safety of laparoscopic sleeve gastrectomy and Roux-en-Y gastric bypass in elderly patients—analysis of the MBSAQIP [19] Retrospective matched cohort	2015	LSG	3371	Anastomotic leak ($p = 0.011$), superficial SSI ($p = 0.001$) higher in LRYGB. Acute renal failure higher in LSG (0.019). No difference in other outcomes	3.74%	0.89% (30 day)	NR	NR	Moderate quality
		LRYGB	3371		6.08% $p < 0.001$	2.49% (30 day) $p < 0.001$	NR	NR	

Study	Years	Procedure	N					Quality
Laparoscopic Roux-en-Y gastric bypass is as safe as laparoscopic sleeve gastrectomy. Results of a comparative cohort study [20] Retrospective study	2010–2017	LSG	206	10 patients (4.85%)	7 patients (3.40%)	3 patients (1.45%)	NR	Low quality
		LRYGB	279	13 patients (4.66%) p = 0.920	7 patients (2.51%) p = 0.593	5 patients (1.79%) p = 0.366	NR	
Comparative effectiveness of sleeve gastrectomy versus Roux-en-Y gastric bypass for weight loss and safety outcomes in older adults [21] Multicenter retrospective propensity matched study	2010–2015	LSG	252	Minor: 12 patients Major: 6 patients	NR	1.6%	Minor: 11 patients Major: 10 patients	Low quality
		LRYGB	177	Minor: 12 patients (p = NS) Major: 11 patients (p = 0.005)	NR	5.6%	Minor: 11 patients Major: 20 patients	
Early morbidity and mortality of laparoscopic sleeve gastrectomy and gastric bypass in the elderly: a NSQIP analysis [22] Retrospective study	2010–2011	LSG	155	14 patients (9%)	NR	5 patients (3.2%)	NR	Low quality
		LRYGB	850	77 patients (9.1%) (p = 0.992)	NR	33 patients (3.9%) (p = 0.693)	NR	

(continued)

Table 21.2 (continued)

Study Study type	Study period		N	Early complications (<30 days)	Readmission rate	Reoperation rate	Late complications (>30 days)	Nutritional deficiencies	Study quality
Laparoscopic Roux-en-Y gastric bypass versus laparoscopic sleeve gastrectomy: a case-control study and 3 years of follow-up [23] Retrospective case-control study	2006–2009	LSG	811	24 patients (2.9)	NR	6 patients (0.7)	27 patients (3.3)	NR	Moderate quality
		LRYGB	786	56 patients (7.1) p < 0.001	NR	8 patients (1.0) P = 0.118	96 patients (12.2) p < 0.001	NR	

Table 21.3 Meta-analyses

Study	Date	Early complications	Readmission	Reoperation	Late complications (>30 days)	Nutritional Deficiencies
Is laparoscopic sleeve gastrectomy a lower risk bariatric procedure compared with laparoscopic Roux-en-Y gastric bypass? A meta-analysis [24]	2014	Significant difference in bleeding (p = 0.001) and stenosis (0.001) between the 2 groups. No difference in leak, of DVT/PE rates	NR	No difference in rate of reoperation between procedures (p = 0.184)	NR	NR
Laparoscopic Sleeve Gastrectomy Versus Laparoscopic Roux-En-Y Gastric Bypass for Morbid Obesity and Related Comorbidities: A Meta-Analysis of 21 Studies [25]	2015	LRYGB has more major complications than LSG (OR 1.98, 95% CI = 1.22–3.22, P <0.01)	NR	NR	NR	NR
Postoperative Early Major and Minor Complications in Laparoscopic Vertical Sleeve Gastrectomy (LVSG) Versus Laparoscopic Roux-en-Y Gastric Bypass (LRYGB) Procedures: A Meta-Analysis and Systematic Review [26]	2016	Major: favored LSG (OR 0.49; 95% CI 0.24, 1.0; p = 0.05). Minor: No difference but favored LSG (OR = 0.71; 95% CI 0.31, 1.67; p = 0.4)	No enough studies reporting to perform statistical analysis	No difference but favored LSG (OR 0.58; 95% CI 0.23, 1.51; p = 0.3)	NR	NR
Safety and efficacy of laparoscopic sleeve gastrectomy versus laparoscopic Roux-en-Y gastric bypass: A systematic review and meta-analysis [27]	2019	Lower in LSG group (RR = 0.55; 95% CI, 0.36–0.84; P = 0.005)	No significant difference (RR = 0.57; 95% CI, 0.21–1.54; P = 0.27)	No significant difference (RR = 0.43; 95% CI, 0.14–1.27; P = 0.13)	NR	NR

(continued)

Table 21.3 (continued)

Study	Date	Early complications	Readmission	Reoperation	Late complications (>30 days)	Nutritional Deficiencies
Comparative analysis for the effect of Roux-en-Y gastric bypass versus sleeve gastrectomy in patients with morbid obesity: Evidence from 11 randomized clinical trials (meta-analysis) [28]	2019	LRYGB had significantly more early complications than LSG (RR 2.14; 95% CI: 1.26–3.64; P = 0.005)	NR	LRYGB may experience higher rate of reoperation (RR 1.73; 95% CI: 1.14–2.62; P = 0.01)	No significant difference in late complications (RR 1.29; 95% CI: 0.88–1.88; P = 0.19)	NR
A Comprehensive Comparison of LRYGB and LSG in Obese Patients Including the Effects on QoL, Comorbidities, Weight Loss, and Complications: a Systematic Review and Meta-Analysis [29]	2020	Occurred significantly more often after LRYGB than after LSG (OR = 2.11, 95% CI = 1.53–2.91, P < 0.001).	NR	NR	LRYGB was associated with more late complications than LSG (OR = 2.60, 95% CI = 1.93–3.49, P < 0.001)	NR

re-intervention or reoperation occurred in 1.6% after LSG and 5.6% after LRYGB for 1 year after the bariatric procedure. LRYGB had significantly higher early (p = 0.015) major complication rates compared with SG. Minor complication rates did not differ significantly between procedures. However, in a review of 485 patients, Lynn et al. [20] found no significant difference in early complications, re-admissions or re-operations between the two procedures.

Several meta-analyses have been performed to analyze early complications (Table 21.3). Most recently, Zhao and Jiao [28] performed a meta-analysis of 11 RCTs in 2019 and found a significant difference in early complications, favoring LSG, with pooled RR of 2.14 (95% CI: 1.26–3.64; P = 0.005). In addition, the reoperation rate was higher in the RYGB group with a pooled RR of 1.73 (95% CI: 1.14–2.62; P = 0.01). The analysis was performed using a fixed-effect model, as no significant heterogeneity among the studies was found. Likewise, Hu et al. [29] found a much higher early complication rate after RYGB compared to LSG, OR = 2.11, 95% CI = 1.53–2.91, p < 0.001). In contrast, Zellmer et al. [24] found that leak rate and mortality was similar between the two. In a meta-analysis of 28 studies (10,906 patients) undergoing LRYGB compared to 33 studies (4816 patients) undergoing LSG, they found significantly higher rates of bleeding (3.1% vs. 2.0%, p = 0.001) and stricture or stenosis (3.4% vs. 1.3%, p = 0.001) after LRYGB. Deep vein thrombosis and re-operation rates were also similar between the two. Another meta-analysis and systematic review of six and five randomized controlled trials by Osland et al. reported on early major and minor complications respectively [26]. The relative odds of an early major complication were significantly reduced for LSG versus LRYGB (OR 0.49; 95% CI 0.24, 1.0; p = 0.05). A non-statistically significant reduction in relative odds of 29% favoring the LSG procedure was observed for minor complications within 30 days (OR = 0.71; 95% CI 0.31, 1.67; p = 0.4) [26].

In summary, there is abundant high quality evidence showing that while major early complication rates are low for both procedures, the LSG is associated with significantly fewer early major surgical complications compared to LRYGB.

21.3.2 Late (>30 Days) Complications

The most common and frequently reported late complications (>30 days) after LRYGB are internal hernia, anastomotic stricture, incisional hernia, small bowel obstruction, marginal ulcer gastroesophageal reflux disease (GERD) and nutrient deficiencies. LSG has relatively fewer long term complications, although small bowel obstruction, incisional hernia and nutrient deficiencies can occur. However, a commonly reported late complication that has gained the most attention is gastroesophageal reflux, either worsening or de novo, which often leads to revisional surgery. Comparisons of overall late complication rates between LRYGB and LSG can be found in Table 21.2. Each complication is analyzed in further depth below.

21.3.3 Internal Hernia

Internal hernia (IH) is a complication that is unique to RYGB and has increased with the shift toward laparoscopic versus open surgery [31]. There are two potential spaces that are created after RYGB; when the alimentary limb is brought up to the gastric pouch, a mesenteric defect called Petersen's space if formed between the mesentery of the alimentary limb and the mesocolon. A separate space between the biliary limb and the common limb is created due to the jejunojejunal anastomosis. Small bowel can herniate into either of those spaces [32]. IH can lead to intermittent abdominal pain or present with late bowel obstruction [33]. Multiple studies reported on rates of internal hernia, ranging from 1.6 to 14.3% [10–15, 18].

21.3.4 Gastrojejunal Stenosis/Anastomotic Stricture

Stricture of stenosis at the anastomosis site also unique to RYGB and is commonly treated with endoscopic dilation but can sometimes require revision. Only two studies reported on the rate of stricture and found that between 4.32 and 6.3% of patients suffered from this complication [18, 23].

21.3.5 Incisional Hernia

Incisional hernia can occur after any surgery and multiple studies reported on their rates after bariatric surgery. Generally, rates of incisional hernia are similar between LRYGB and LSG and no study had enough power to compare rates of incisional hernia directly. Rates after LRYGB were between 0.8 and 5.11% and between 0.8 and 2.5% after LSG [10, 12, 17, 21].

21.3.6 Small Bowel Obstruction

Small bowel obstruction (SBO), or obstructive ileus, can be either an early or late compilation and occur for a variety of reasons including stenosis of the anastomosis, torsion of the biliopancreatic limb, or due to herniation of small bowel through trocar sites. Internal hernia is also a well-recognized cause of SBO, discussed previously [33]. Late small bowel obstruction can occur after any surgery and is most commonly due to adhesions. In studies that reported rates of late small bowel obstruction not through to be caused by incisional hernia or internal hernia, the range was between 1.46 and 3.3% with insufficient power in all studies to determine significant differences between LRYGB and LSG [12, 16, 17, 21, 23].

21.3.7 Intestinal Ulcer

Ulcers can occur after both sleeve gastrectomy and RYGB, however the most commonly recognized complication is marginal ulceration at the anastomotic site in RYGB. It usually occurs within the first 2 months postoperatively and presents with symptoms such as abdominal pain, vomiting and occasionally with bleeding. Treatment includes cessation of NSAIDs, proton pump inhibitor therapy and Carafate. While medical management is usually successful, surgical options includes revision of the anastomosis [33]. In studies that reported rates of ulceration, they were found to be relatively low at 0.38–5% of patients, with the true rate likely on the lower end of that range as studies with a larger number of patients commonly reported lower rates [10, 15, 21, 23].

21.3.8 GERD

There are a number of studies that show that LRYGB is associated with a decrease in GERD postoperatively [34, 35]. Indeed, the American College of Gastroenterology clinical practice guidelines for GERD recommend gastric bypass as the preferred method of surgically managing reflux in the obese population [36]. On the other hand, LSG may predispose patients to de novo GERD due to the increased intraluminal pressure in the sleeve and is frequently cited as a relative contraindication to the procedure [37–41].

Many individual studies reported only on rates of de novo reflux after LSG, which ranged from 3.6 to 9.1% of patients [10, 11, 14]. In those studies which analyzed reflux in more detail, Peterli et al. [12] found in a relatively large randomized trial that after 5 years, remission of reflux symptoms was seen in 25% of patients in the LSG group and 60.4% of patients in the LRYGB group (absolute difference, -0.36%; 95% CI, -0.57% to -0.15%; P = 0.002) and worsening of symptoms was more often seen in the sleeve gastrectomy group (31.8% vs. 6.3%; absolute difference, 0.36%; 95% CI, 0.13%–0.59%; P = 0.006). Additionally, 31.6% of patients who had no GERD at baseline reported de novo reflux symptoms 5 years LSG, whereas this was the case only in 10.7% of patients who underwent LRYGB (absolute difference, 0.31%; 95% CI, 0.08–0.54%; P = 0.01). In a separate study that focused on acid-related symptoms after bariatric surgery, Elias et al. [42] found that after RYGB, a noticeable reduction in acid-related symptoms was seen at 2 years when compared to baseline (9.9–6.4%, P = 0.001); however, there was no significant difference at 5 years. In SG, the prevalence of acid related symptoms doubled at 2 and 5 years (5.9–14.1% and 15.4%, respectively, P < 0.001 for both). In a meta-analysis by Zhao and Jiao [28], they found that LRYGB led to greater improvements in GERD symptoms compared to LSG (RR 1.48; 95% CI: 1.07–2.04; P = 0.02). They also found that LSG leads to worsening of GERD symptoms (RR 0.16; 95% CI: 0.06–0.44; P = 0.0004) and is associated with development of de novo GERD (RR 0.33; 95% CI: 0.15–0.68; P = 0.003). In summary, the evidence indicates that in patients with a preoperative diagnosis of GERD, most frequently defined in studies as a need for daily PPI therapy, LSG results in worsening of GERD symptoms significantly more often than after LRYGB. In patients with no preoperative diagnosis of GERD, LSG leads to the de novo development of GERD in a significantly greater number of patients than LRYGB.

21.3.9 Nutrient Deficiencies

Nutrient deficiencies, most commonly iron, calcium/vitamin D, protein and vitamin B12, occur relatively frequently after bariatric surgery, the majority occurring after malabsorptive operations. It has also been recognized in prospective studies and through general practice that many patients who suffer from morbid obesity have nutrient deficiencies preoperatively [43, 44].

A prospective study found that nutrient deficiencies including Vitamin B12 ($p < 0.0001$) and Vitamin D ($p < 0.02$) were more common after LRYGB than after LSG [44]. Kehagias studied nutrient deficiencies in detail up to 3 year postoperatively and found that iron and vitamin B12 deficiencies were most commonly encountered, with vitamin B12 deficits, but not iron deficits, significantly more frequent in the LRYGB group ($p = 0.05$) [16]. Another study was underpowered to detect a difference but found anemia to be more common after LRYGB [14]. In contrast, Leyba et al. found that 4.2% patients in the LRYGB group and 14.8% in the LSG group suffered from anemia, which was not significant however [11]. Finally, Albeladi et al. found that 20.6% of patients after LSG and 28.9% of patients after LRYGB developed a vitamin deficiency, although what they considered to be a vitamin deficiency was not detailed [13].

Summary of Late Complications
In summary, when analyzing each complication individually or in studies with smaller sample sizes, there is generally insufficient power to detect a difference or investigators found no difference between operations [10–13, 15–18, 21, 23]. Boza et al. [23] were the only group to find a significant difference in late complications favoring LSG (12.2% vs. 3.3%, $p < 0.001$), likely due to their large numbers; though, their study is older, published in 2012. When specifically considering nutrient deficiencies [14, 16, 44], however, there is evidence to suggest that LSG is safer than LRYGB. On the other hand, in terms of worsening and development of GERD, rates are lower after LRYGB [12, 28, 42]. When considering all late complications together, in their meta-analysis, Hu et al. [29] found that LRYGB was associated with more late complications than LSG (OR = 2.60, 95% CI = 1.93–3.49, $P < 0.001$). Yet, in their meta-analysis, Zhao and Jiao [28] did not find a difference between rates of late complications (RR 1.29; 95% CI: 0.88–1.88; $P = 0.19$). Thus, the data is mixed but trends toward more late complications after LRYGB with the exception of development and worsening of GERD, which is more frequent after LSG.

21.4   Recommendations Based on the Data

Both LRYGB and LSG have been found to lead to significant weight loss with resolution of comorbidities. In capable hands, both procedures are safe with an extremely
low mortality rate and a low morbidity rate. However, based on review of the literature, we conclude the LSG is slightly but safer than the LRYGB (evidence quality
high; strong recommendation).

21.5   A Personal View of the Data

Since 2011 the United States has seen a steady increase in the proportion of weight
loss surgery cases done using the LSG (17.8% in 2011 up to 61.4% in 2018) and
steady decrease in the LRYGB (36.7% in 2011 to 17% in 2018). There are several
reasons for this, including the LSG being technically less demanding, having a
shorter learning curve, taking less time to perform and potentially having lower
early and late complications. We have thoroughly reviewed a large amount of moderate and high quality evidence substantiating the concept that LRYGB does in fact
have higher associated complications and is therefore less safe than LSG. However,
this may need to be taken with a grain of salt.

Shauer and colleagues found the learning curve to be 100 for LRYGB, while
Carandina found it to be 60 cases for the LSG [5, 45]. In a systematic review of the
literature, Wehrtmann and colleagues found that proficiency was achieved after
70–150 LRYGB compared to 60–100 LSG [46]. Because the learning curves are
different, analyzing data on complication rates may lead to bias depending on where
the surgeons are on the learning curve. In addition, the retrospective unmatched
studies may include patients with more comorbidities in the gastric bypass group.
As a bariatric and minimally invasive surgeon, I perform both procedures on a regular basis. In my personal experience, I have found that anecdotally, LRYGB to be a
longer operation but have similar recovery to the LSG and have similar early and
late complication and re-operation rates. Furthermore, the data on new onset and
worsening of GERD after LSG should not be taken lightly as we have had to revise
patients from sleeve to gastric bypass due to intractable reflux. Aside from GERD,
there are potentially greater and more severe early and late complications with the
LRYGB such as bleeding, infection, ulcers, internal hernia and small bowel obstruction. However, most of these can be prevented or lessened by strict surgical and
medical protocols. These include: strict anti-smoking and NSAID policies to prevent ulcers as well as strict adherence to technical principles such as closing the
mesenteric defects and avoiding tension and ischemia at the anastomosis. When
these are followed, and the surgeon is over the learning curve, the difference in
safety becomes very small and therefore we may base the choice of procedure on
patient factors such as BMI, diabetes, and gastroesophageal reflux disease with
esophagitis. We also factor in patient preference, which should not be understated.

Ultimately, the choice of bariatric procedures must take into account a combination of factors including patient BMI and comorbidities as well as surgeon experience, and patients should be well informed of the success rates, safety profile and possible complications of their chosen procedure.

> **Recommendations**
> 1. Both LRYGB and LSG are very safe operations. LSG has a slightly better safety profile than the LRYGB, but ultimately the operation chosen should be based on patient factors and surgeon experience (evidence quality high; strong recommendation).

References

1. Angrisani L, Santonicola A, Iovino P, Formisano G, Buchwald H, Scopinaro N. Bariatric Surgery Worldwide 2013. Obes Surg. 2015;25:1822–32.
2. Wittgrove AC, Clark GW, Tremblay LJ. Laparoscopic gastric bypass, Roux-en-Y: preliminary report of five cases. Obes Surg. 1994;4:353–7.
3. Attiah MA, Halpern CH, Balmuri U, Vinai P, Mehta S, Baltuch GH, Williams NN, Wadden TA, Stein SC. Durability of Roux-en-Y gastric bypass surgery: a meta-regression study. Ann Surg. 2012;256:251–4.
4. Edholm D, Svensson F, Näslund I, Karlsson FA, Rask E, Sundbom M. Long-term results 11 years after primary gastric bypass in 384 patients. Surg Obes Relat Dis. 2013;9:708–13.
5. Schauer P, Ikramuddin S, Hamad G, Gourash W. The learning curve for laparoscopic Roux-en-Y gastric bypass is 100 cases. Surg Endosc. 2003;17:212–5.
6. Franco JVA, Ruiz PA, Palermo M, Gagner M. A review of studies comparing three laparoscopic procedures in bariatric surgery: sleeve gastrectomy, Roux-en-Y gastric bypass and adjustable gastric banding. Obes Surg. 2011;21:1458–68.
7. Himpens J, Dobbeleir J, Peeters G. Long-term results of laparoscopic sleeve gastrectomy for obesity. Ann Surg. 2010;252:319–24.
8. Rawlins L, Rawlins MP, Brown CC, Schumacher DL. Sleeve gastrectomy: 5-year outcomes of a single institution. Surg Obes Relat Dis. 2013;9:21–5.
9. Abbatini F, Capoccia D, Casella G, Soricelli E, Leonetti F, Basso N. Long-term remission of type 2 diabetes in morbidly obese patients after sleeve gastrectomy. Surg Obes Relat Dis. 2013;9:498–502.
10. Salminen P, Helmiö M, Ovaska J, Juuti A, Leivonen M, Peromaa-Haavisto P, Hurme S, Soinio M, Nuutila P, Victorzon M. Effect of laparoscopic sleeve gastrectomy vs laparoscopic Roux-en-Y gastric bypass on weight loss at 5 years among patients with morbid obesity: the SLEEVEPASS randomized clinical trial. JAMA. 2018;319:241.
11. Leyba JL, Llopis SN, Aulestia SN. Laparoscopic Roux-en-Y gastric bypass versus laparoscopic sleeve gastrectomy for the treatment of morbid obesity. A prospective study with 5 years of follow-up. Obes Surg. 2014;24:2094–8.
12. Peterli R, Wölnerhanssen BK, Peters T, et al. Effect of laparoscopic sleeve gastrectomy vs laparoscopic Roux-en-Y gastric bypass on weight loss in patients with morbid obesity: the SM-BOSS randomized clinical trial. JAMA. 2018;319:255.
13. Albeladi B, Bourbao-Tournois C, Huten N. Short- and midterm results between laparoscopic Roux-en-Y gastric bypass and laparoscopic sleeve gastrectomy for the treatment of morbid obesity. J Obes. 2013;2013:1–6.

14. Ignat M, Vix M, Imad I, D'Urso A, Perretta S, Marescaux J, Mutter D. Randomized trial of Roux-en-Y gastric bypass *versus* sleeve gastrectomy in achieving excess weight loss. Br J Surg. 2017;104:248–56.
15. Dogan K, Gadiot RPM, Aarts EO, Betzel B, van Laarhoven CJHM, Biter LU, Mannaerts GHH, Aufenacker TJ, Janssen IMC, Berends FJ. Effectiveness and safety of sleeve gastrectomy, gastric bypass, and adjustable gastric banding in morbidly obese patients: a multicenter, retrospective, matched Cohort study. Obes Surg. 2015;25:1110–8.
16. Kehagias I, Karamanakos SN, Argentou M, Kalfarentzos F. Randomized clinical trial of laparoscopic Roux-en-Y gastric bypass versus laparoscopic sleeve gastrectomy for the management of patients with BMI < 50 kg/m2. Obes Surg. 2011;21:1650–6.
17. Skroubis G, Karamanakos S, Sakellaropoulos G, Panagopoulos K, Kalfarentzos F. Comparison of early and late complications after various bariatric procedures: incidence and treatment during 15 years at a single institution. World J Surg. 2011;35:93–101.
18. Zhang Y, Zhao H, Cao Z, Sun X, Zhang C, Cai W, Liu R, Hu S, Qin M. A randomized clinical trial of laparoscopic Roux-en-Y gastric bypass and sleeve gastrectomy for the treatment of morbid obesity in china: a 5-year outcome. Obes Surg. 2014;24:1617–24.
19. Janik MR, Mustafa RR, Rogula TG, Alhaj Saleh A, Abbas M, Khaitan L. Safety of laparoscopic sleeve gastrectomy and Roux-en-Y gastric bypass in elderly patients—analysis of the MBSAQIP. Surg Obes Relat Dis. 2018;14:1276–82.
20. Lynn W, Ilczyszyn A, Rasheed S, Davids J, Aguilo R, Agrawal S. Laparoscopic Roux-en-Y gastric bypass is as safe as laparoscopic sleeve gastrectomy. Results of a comparative cohort study. Ann Med Surg. 2018;35:38–43.
21. Casillas RA, Kim B, Fischer H, Zelada Getty JL, Um SS, Coleman KJ. Comparative effectiveness of sleeve gastrectomy versus Roux-en-Y gastric bypass for weight loss and safety outcomes in older adults. Surg Obes Relat Dis. 2017;13:1476–83.
22. Spaniolas K, Trus TL, Adrales GL, Quigley MT, Pories WJ, Laycock WS. Early morbidity and mortality of laparoscopic sleeve gastrectomy and gastric bypass in the elderly: a NSQIP analysis. Surg Obes Relat Dis. 2014;10:584–8.
23. Boza C, Gamboa C, Salinas J, Achurra P, Vega A, Pérez G. Laparoscopic Roux-en-Y gastric bypass versus laparoscopic sleeve gastrectomy: a case-control study and 3 years of follow-up. Surg Obes Relat Dis. 2012;8:243–9.
24. Zellmer JD, Mathiason MA, Kallies KJ, Kothari SN. Is laparoscopic sleeve gastrectomy a lower risk bariatric procedure compared with laparoscopic Roux-en-Y gastric bypass? A meta-analysis. Am J Surg. 2014;208:903–10.
25. Zhang Y, Ju W, Sun X, Cao Z, Xinsheng X, Daquan L, Xiangyang X, Qin M. Laparoscopic sleeve gastrectomy versus laparoscopic Roux-En-Y gastric bypass for morbid obesity and related comorbidities: a meta-analysis of 21 studies. Obes Surg. 2015;25:19–26.
26. Osland E, Yunus RM, Khan S, Alodat T, Memon B, Memon MA. Postoperative early major and minor complications in laparoscopic vertical sleeve gastrectomy (LVSG) versus laparoscopic Roux-en-Y gastric bypass (LRYGB) procedures: a meta-analysis and systematic review. Obes Surg. 2016;26:2273–84.
27. Zhao K, Liu J, Wang M, Yang H, Wu A. Safety and efficacy of laparoscopic sleeve gastrectomy versus laparoscopic Roux-en-Y gastric bypass: a systematic review and meta-analysis. J Eval Clin Pract. 2020;26:290–8.
28. Zhao H, Jiao L. Comparative analysis for the effect of Roux-en-Y gastric bypass vs sleeve gastrectomy in patients with morbid obesity: evidence from 11 randomized clinical trials (meta-analysis). Int J Surg. 2019;72:216–23.
29. Hu Z, Sun J, Li R, Wang Z, Ding H, Zhu T, Wang G. A comprehensive comparison of LRYGB and LSG in obese patients including the effects on QoL, comorbidities, weight loss, and complications: a systematic review and meta-analysis. Obes Surg. 2020;30:819–27.
30. Guerrier JB, Dietch ZC, Schirmer BD, Hallowell PT. Laparoscopic sleeve gastrectomy is associated with lower 30-day morbidity versus laparoscopic gastric bypass: an analysis of the American College of Surgeons NSQIP. Obes Surg. 2018;28:3567–72.

31. Higa KD, Ho T, Boone KB. Internal Hernias after Laparoscopic Roux-en-Y Gastric Bypass: Incidence, Treatment and Prevention. Obes Surg. 2003;13:350–4.
32. Kristensen SD, Naver L, Jess P, Floyd AK. Effect of closure of the mesenteric defect during laparoscopic gastric bypass and prevention of internal hernia. Dan Med J. 2014;61(6):A4854.
33. Marmuse J-P, Parenti LR. Gastric bypass. Principles, complications, and results. J Visc Surg. 2010;147:e31–7.
34. De Groot NL, Burgerhart JS, Van De Meeberg PC, De Vries DR, Smout AJPM, Siersema PD. Systematic review: the effects of conservative and surgical treatment for obesity on gastro-oesophageal reflux disease. Aliment Pharmacol Ther. 2009;30:1091–102.
35. Madalosso CAS, Gurski RR, Callegari-Jacques SM, Navarini D, Thiesen V, Fornari F. The impact of gastric bypass on gastroesophageal reflux disease in patients with morbid obesity: a prospective study based on the montreal consensus. Ann Surg. 2010;251:244–8.
36. Katz PO, Gerson LB, Vela MF. Guidelines for the diagnosis and management of gastroesophageal reflux disease. Am J Gastroenterol. 2013;108:308–28.
37. Chang P, Friedenberg F. Obesity and GERD. Gastroenterol Clin N Am. 2014;43:161–73.
38. Khan A. Impact of obesity treatment on gastroesophageal reflux disease. World J Gastroenterol. 2016;22:1627.
39. Lazoura O, Zacharoulis D, Triantafyllidis G, Fanariotis M, Sioka E, Papamargaritis D, Tzovaras G. Symptoms of gastroesophageal reflux following laparoscopic sleeve gastrectomy are related to the final shape of the sleeve as depicted by radiology. Obes Surg. 2011;21:295–9.
40. DuPree CE, Blair K, Steele SR, Martin MJ. Laparoscopic sleeve gastrectomy in patients with preexisting gastroesophageal reflux disease: a national analysis. JAMA Surg. 2014;149:328.
41. Sheppard CE, Sadowski DC, de Gara CJ, Karmali S, Birch DW. Rates of reflux before and after laparoscopic sleeve gastrectomy for severe obesity. Obes Surg. 2015;25:763–8.
42. Elias K, Hedberg J, Sundbom M. Prevalence and impact of acid-related symptoms and diarrhea in patients undergoing Roux-en-Y gastric bypass, sleeve gastrectomy, and biliopancreatic diversion with duodenal switch. Surg Obes Relat Dis. 2019;16(4):520–7.
43. Davies DDJ, Baxter DJM, Baxter JN. Nutritional deficiencies after bariatric surgery. Obes Surg. 2007;17(9):1150–8.
44. Gehrer S, Kern B, Peters T, Christoffel-Courtin C, Peterli R. Fewer nutrient deficiencies after laparoscopic sleeve gastrectomy (LSG) than after laparoscopic Roux-Y-gastric bypass (LRYGB)—a prospective study. Obes Surg. 2010;20:447–53.
45. Carandina S, Montana L, Danan M, Zulian V, Nedelcu M, Barrat C. Laparoscopic sleeve gastrectomy learning curve: clinical and economical impact. Obes Surg. 2019;29:143–8.
46. Wehrtmann FS, de la Garza JR, Kowalewski KF, et al. Learning curves of laparoscopic Roux-en-Y gastric bypass and sleeve gastrectomy in bariatric surgery: a systematic review and introduction of a standardization. Obes Surg. 2020;30:640–56.

The National Shift to Sleeve Gastrectomy: Long-Term Disappointment and Recidivism or Patient Preference?

Randal Zhou and John M. Morton

22.1 Introduction

Obesity has reached a world-wide epidemic and more than a third of the United States adult population is obese. Since 2012, laparoscopic sleeve gastrectomy (SG) has been accepted as a primary procedure by the American Society of Metabolic and Bariatric Surgery (ASMBS) and accepted by all major insurers. Currently, SG is being performed with increasing frequency, bypassing laparoscopic Roux-en-Y gastric bypass (GB) as the most commonly performed bariatric procedure in the United States. The long-term outcomes studies of SG among patients of advanced obesity are limited. This chapter will analyze the available data of SG compared to GB in regards to weight recidivism and its effects on diabetes mellitus (DM) and GERD resolution by analyzing evidence in the following 6 categories: comparative outcomes, special populations, weight loss outcomes, weight regain/lack of treatment effect, GERD complications, and patient and surgeon preference/resource utilization.

22.2 Search Strategy

We conducted our search using the following search terms from in PubMed: sleeve gastrectomy long-term follow up; sleeve gastrectomy and super morbid obesity, GERD or Barrett's Esophagus, diabetes resolution; sleeve gastrectomy/bariatric surgery in special populations, inflammatory bowel disease, immunosuppression, prior abdominal surgery; sleeve gastrectomy compared to gastric bypass long-term follow

R. Zhou · J. M. Morton (✉)
Yale University, School of Medicine, New Haven, CT, USA

Division of Bariatric and Minimally Invasive Surgery, New Haven, USA
e-mail: John.Morton@Yale.edu

© Springer Nature Switzerland AG 2021
J. Alverdy, Y. Vigneswaran (eds.), *Difficult Decisions in Bariatric Surgery*,
Difficult Decisions in Surgery: An Evidence-Based Approach,
https://doi.org/10.1007/978-3-030-55329-6_22

Table 22.1 PICO Terms

P (Patients)	I (Intervention)	C (Comparator)	O (Outcomes)
Patients with severe/ morbid obesity, type 2 diabetes, GERD, morbidity after bariatric surgery	Sleeve gastrectomy	Roux-en-Y gastric bypass	Weight loss, lack of treatment effect, type 2 diabetes remission, GERD resolution/ progression, and cost

up, patient preference and bariatric surgery, sleeve gastrectomy, morbidity, readmission, operative time, and cost (Table 22.1). The results were narrowed by the following criteria: English language and published within the last 5 years.

22.3 Results

In order to better characterize the available literature, we summarized the results in 6 sub-categories.

22.3.1 Comparative Outcomes Between Sleeve Gastrectomy and Gastric Bypass (Table 22.2)

Mixed evidence exists in comparing the outcomes of these 2 procedures, however both SG and GB are superior to medication alone for inducing remission of type 2 DM, especially in the non-severely obese population. In the STAMPEDE trial, Schauer et al. randomized 150 patients who had type 2 diabetes to receive either intensive medical therapy alone or intensive medical therapy plus GB or SG. 90% of the patients completed 5 year follow up. They found that patients who underwent surgery had a greater mean percentage reduction from baseline in HgbA1c (2.1% vs. 0.3% p = 0.003). At 5 years, changes from baseline body weight were superior in post bariatric surgery patients compared to medical therapy (−23%, −19%, and −5% in GB, SG, and medical therapy, respectively). Changes in TG levels were superior in the bariatric surgery group (−40%, −29%, and −8%), HDL level (32%, 30%, and 7%), use of insulin (−35%, −34%, and −13%), and quality-of-life (general health score increases of 17, 16, and 0.3) [1].

Another study further substantiates SG in its effects in DM. Nedelcu et al. looked at the effect of SG on type 2 DM at 5 years. In 52 patients with diabetes, the mean duration was 10.8 ±10.8 years before operation. The preoperative HgbA1c was 8 ± 2% in 45 patients; >/=9% in 17 patients (38%). Prolonged DM remission at 5 years was found in 9 patients (17%). No patient who required insulin preoperatively went into remission. Improvement of diabetes was found in 27 patients (52%) at 5 years [2].

Several studies compared the rate of DM remission/improvement between SG and GB, and most studies demonstrated that GB was superior both in the short and

Table 22.2 Comparative outcomes

Study	Patients	Outcome classification	Sleeve gastrectomy	Gastric bypass	Quality of evidence
Schauer et al. [1]	150 Randomized to intensive medical therapy or bariatric surgery plus medical therapy at 5 years	Weight change Triglycerides Use of insulin Quality of life All comparisons showed bariatric (SG/GB) superior compared to medical therapy ($p < 0.05$)	−23% −40% −35% 17	−19% −29% −34% 16	High
Nedelcu et al. [2]	52 retrospective	Type 2 DM after SG at 5 years	Remission 17%. None in patients who required insulin preoperatively. Improvement in 52%.		Low
Dang et al. [3]	207 retrospective	Type 2 DM remission at 1 year	38.1%	57.7% (OR 6.58, 95% CI 2.79–15.5)	Low
Sha et al. [4]	Meta-analysis of RCTs of 296 patients	DM remission in non-severely obese patients (BMI < 35)	DM remission rate and %EWL were of no difference between GB and SG	High	High
Salminen et al. [5]	Randomization of 240 to SG or GB	Complete or partial DM remission after 5 years follow up	37% (15/41)	51% (24/40) ($p = 0.99$)	Moderate
Celio et al. [6]	50,987 Retrospective	Co-morbidity resolution at 1 year: Diabetes mellitus (DM), hypertension (HTN), gastroesophageal reflux disease (GERD), hyperlipidemia (HL), and obstructive sleep apnea (OSA)	DM 50.8% HTN 34.5% GERD 32.5% HL 32.5% OSA 40.6%	DM 61.6% ($p < 0.001$) HTN 43.1% ($p < 0.001$) GERD 53.9% ($p < 0.001$) HL 39.7% ($p < 0.001$) OSA 42.8% ($p = 0.058$)	Low

(continued)

Table 22.2 (continued)

Study	Patients	Outcome classification	Sleeve gastrectomy	Gastric bypass	Quality of evidence
Lager et al. [7]	714 retrospective	Total weight (TW) and excess weight loss (EWL), hemoglobin A1c (HgbA1c) in all patients, HgbA1c in diabetics, and total cholesterol (TC) at 4 years	TW 18.6% EWL 38.5% HgbA1c decrease 0.45 to 0.73% DM HgbA1c decrease 0.45% (±0.15%) TC increase 12.7 ± 3.6 mg/dL	TW 25.6% (p < 0.0001) EWL 57.6% (p < 0.0001) HbA1c decrease 0.91–1.12% (p = 0.004) DM HgbA1c decrease 1.28% (±0.21%) (p = 0.002) TC decrease 0.3 ± 5.4 mg/dL (p = 0.01)	Low

long-term. Dang et al. conducted a retrospective review of 207 diabetic patients who underwent SG or GB and reported their 1 year remission rates to be 38.1% and 57.7% for SG and GB, respectively. GB was associated with higher odds ratio of DM remission (OR 6.58, 95% CI 2.79–15.5) [3].

In patients who are non-severely obese, SG may be equivalent in comparison to GB in regards to DM remission. Sha et al. performed a meta-analysis of RCTs evaluating GB vs SG for type 2 DM in non-severely obese patients (BMI < 35). At mid-term follow up, in the 296 patients included, DM remission rate and %EWL were of no difference between GB and SG. GB was associated with lower BMI, waist circumference, LDL, and higher HDL; however HgbA1c, fasting plasma glucose, total cholesterol, and TG were not significantly different [4]. There was no significance difference in DM remission between GB and SG in another study. Salminen et al. randomized 240 patients to SG or GB and followed them for 5 years. Complete or partial remission of type 2 DM was seen in 37% (n = 15/41) after sleeve gastrectomy and 51% (n = 24/40) after gastric bypass (P = 0.99) [5].

However, when evaluating obesity-related comorbidities resolution, several studies demonstrated GB superiority compared to SG, especially in advanced obesity at medium-term follow up. Celio et al. found that in 50,987 class 5 obesity patients (BMI >/=50), at 1 years compared to SG, GB patients had increased resolution of all measured co-morbidities: DM (61.6 vs 50.8%, p < 0.001), hypertension (43.1 vs 34.5%, p < 0.001), GERD (53.9 vs 32.5%, p < 0.001), hyperlipidemia (39.7 vs. 32.5%, p < 0.001), and obstructive sleep apnea (42.8 vs. 40.6%, p = 0.058) [6].

Lager et al. found that in 714 patients, at 4 years follow-up, GB patients lost 34.4 kg of total weight, 25.7% of total weight, and 57.6% EWL as compared to SG patients who lost 26.7 kg, 18.6%, and 38.5% (p < 0.0001 for all measures). In GB patients, HgbA1c decreases were consistent over time with range of 0.91 to 1.12%

at 4 years. On the other hand, in SG patients, improvements in HgbA1c decreased over time from a reduction of 0.73% at 1 year to 0.45% at 4 years (p = 0.004). Among patients with DM, HgbA1c improvements at 4 years were 1.28% (±0.21%) vs. 0.45% (±0.15%) for GB vs SG patients (p = 0.002). Total cholesterol decreased in the GB patients at 4 years by 0.3 ± 5.4 mg/dL, but increased in SG patients by 12.7 ± 3.6 mg/dL (p = 0.01). There was only a significant difference at 3 years in systolic blood pressure in favor of GB (12.6 vs 6.5 mmHg, p = 0.001) [7].

22.3.2 Special Populations (Table 22.3)

In special populations, i.e. patients with immunosuppression, inflammatory bowel disease (IBD), and prior abdominal operations, SG appears to be safer. Hefler et al. utilized the MBSAQIP data to study the effects of chronic corticosteroid and immunosuppressant after bariatric surgery. 430,936 patients were included, of these 7214 (1.7%) were chronically immunosuppressed. Their analyses found statistically higher odds of 30-day major complication rates (OR 1.39, 95% CI 1.25–1.55;

Table 22.3 Special populations

Study	Patients	Outcome classification	Sleeve gastrectomy	Gastric bypass	Quality of evidence
Hefler et al. [8]	430,936 MBSAQIP retrospective	7214 (1.7%) chronically immunosuppressed	30-day major complication OR 1.39, 95% CI 1.25–1.55 (p < 0.001) Bleed OR 1.49, 95% CI 1.24–1.8 (p < 0.001) Anastomotic leak OR 1.38, 95% CI 1.02–1.87 (p = 0.037)		Low
Major et al. [9]	Retrospective 2413 Group 1 no prior abdominal surgery, Group 2 at least 1 abdominal surgery.	Operation time. Intra-operative adverse events. Length of stay.	Group 2 prolonged median operation time for GB (p = 0.012). Such correlation was not found in SG patients (p = 0.396). Group 1 and 2 similar intraoperative adverse events and post operative complications. Group 2 longer length of stay (p = 0.034). Readmissions were similar.		Low
Heshmati et al. [10]	Retrospective 1 year follow up of 54 patients (SG N = 35, GB N = 19)	Increased severity of IBD post-op Post-op complication	4% 3%	37.5% (p = 0.016) 26% (p = 0.02)	Low

p < 0.001), bleed (OR 1.49, 95% CI 1.24–1.8; p < 0.001) and anastomotic leak (OR 1.38, 95% CI 1.02–1.87; p = 0.037) amongst the immunosuppressed. Their secondary analysis found higher rates of 30-day major complications for immunosuppressed patients undergoing GB (9.6% vs 5%; p < 0.001) [8].

Major et al. conducted a retrospective analysis of 2413 patients and evaluated if previous abdominal surgery affected the course and outcomes after bariatric surgery. Group 1 had no history of abdominal surgery and group 2 patients had undergone at least 1 abdominal surgery. Group 2 had a significantly prolonged median operation time for GB (p = 0.012). Such correlation was not found in SG patients (p = 0.396). Group 1 and 2 had similar intraoperative adverse events and postoperative complications. Group 2 had a longer median length of stay (p = 0.034), while readmissions were similar [9].

In a retrospective study conducted by Heshmati et al., examined 54 Crohn's Disease (CD, N = 31) or ulcerative colitis (UC, N = 23) patients and followed them for 1 year. 19 patients underwent GB and 35 underwent SG. There was a significant difference in the proportion of patients who had worsened CD after GB compared with SG (37.5% vs. 4%; p = 0.016). In addition, there was a greater rate of postoperative complication after GB vs SG (26% vs. 3%; p = 0.02). GB was associated with a greater number of patients with an increased requirement of IBD-medications. SG resulted in less weight loss however had a lower rate of severe complications. SG may be a safer surgery in this patient population [10].

22.3.3 Weight Loss Outcomes (Table 22.4)

Laparoscopic sleeve gastrectomy is well established as a primary bariatric surgery with durable long-term weight loss. Arman et al. analyzed 110 consecutive SG patients with >11-year follow up and looked at progression of weight, satisfaction, evolution of co-morbidities, and GERD. For the 47 patients who maintained the sleeve construction, the excess body mass index loss (EBMIL) was 62.5% vs 81.7% (p = 0.015) for the 16 patients who underwent conversion procedure. None of the 7 patients preoperatively suffering from GERD had remission after SG. Patient satisfaction score remains good despite unfavorable GERD outcomes [11]. In addition, Noel et al. found that for 116 patients with long-term follow up (8 years), the mean EWL was 67% and that 70.7% of patients had >50% EWL. Comorbidity resolution were: hypertension, 59.4%; diabetes 43.4%; OSA 72.4% [12].

However, when compared to GB, some studies have showed inferiority of SG. Sharples et al. performed a systematic review and meta-analysis of randomized controlled trials comparing long-term outcomes of GB and SG. GB demonstrated greater %EWL compared with SG (65.7% vs 57.3%, P < 0.0001). Resolution of HL was more common after GB (69.6% vs. 55.2%, p = 0.0443). Remission of GERD was more common after GB (60.4% vs. 25%, p = 0.002) [13]. In addition, Ahmed et al. conducted a longitudinal long-term (7 years) study comparing weight change and comorbidities in patients who underwent SG vs. GB. At year 7, mean weight loss was 23.6% for SG and 30.4% for GB, P = 0.001) [14].

Table 22.4 Weight loss outcomes

Study	Patients	Outcome classification	Sleeve gastrectomy	Gastric bypass	Quality of evidence
Arman et al. [11]	110 prospective SG patients	Weight, satisfaction, evolution of GERD with 11+ years follow up	N = 47 EBMIL 62.5% 0/7 cured from GERD. Patient satisfaction equivalent vs GB.	Conversion N = 16 EBMIL 81.7% (p = 0.015)	Low
Noel et al. [12]	116 Retrospective	Mean EWL, >50% EWL, and comorbidity resolution: HTN, DM, and OSA at 8 years after SG	Mean EWL 67%, >50% EWL 70.7%, HTN 59.4% DM 43.4% OSA 72.4%		Low
Sharples et al. [13]	Systematic review and meta-analysis of 5 RCTs	EWL at 5 years.	57.3%	65.7% (p < 0.0001)	High
Ahmed et al. [14]	116 (SG = 59) (GB = 57) Retrospective	Mean WL after 7 years	23.6%	30.4% (p = 0.001)	Low

22.3.4 Weight Regain/Lack of Treatment Effect (Table 22.5)

The lack of treatment effect seems to higher in SG compared to GB. Morton et al. found that at 12 months, weight loss results followed a normal bell-curve distribution for laparoscopic adjusted gastric band (LAGB), SG, and GB. However, at 24 and 36 months, percent excess weight loss (%EWL), both LAGB and SG appeared to follow a flatter distribution. At 1 year, the odds ratio of a lack of a successful treatment of SG compared to GB was 6.305 (2.125–19.08; P = 0.0004) and at 3 years, the OR for SG compared to GB was 32.4 (7.31–43.4; P < 0.0001) [15].

The lack of treatment effect phenomenon is further exemplified in advanced obesity and GBB may be superior in weight loss in this population. Ece et al. performed a retrospective analysis of 186 SG patients with follow up for 41.2 ± 7.3 months after SG. 83 patients (50.9%) were class 4 (BMI 40–49), 52 (31.9%) were of the class 5 obesity (BMI 50–59), and 28 (17.2%) were also class 5+ obese, with BMI >/= 60. The mean %TWL at 12, 24, 36, and 41.2 months was 34.7, 34.4, 31.4, and 29.6%, respectively. The most heavy group of patients (class 5+) experienced significantly lower %EWL (48.6) compared to class 4 and class 5 obese groups (65.6 and 59.8) at 41.2 months [16].

Table 22.5 Weight regain

Study	Patients	Outcome classification	Sleeve gastrectomy	Gastric bypass	Quality of evidence
Morton et al. [15]	1331 SG (N = 243) GB (N = 963) Prospective	Weight loss failure at 1 and 3 years odds ratio (OR)	1 year OR: 6.305 3 years OR: 32.4	1 year: 1 (p = 0.0004) 3 years: 1 (p = 0.0001)	Moderate
Ece et al. [16]	186 retrospective	TWL for morbidly obese (MO, BMI 40–49), super-obese (SO, BMI 50–59), super-super obese (SSO, BMI >/= 60), and %EWL at 12, 24, 36, and 41.2 months (Mos) after SG.	SSO TWL at 12 Mos 34.7%, 24 Mos 34.4%, 36 Mos 31.4%, 41.2 Mos 29.6%. SSO EWL at 41.2 Mos 48.6% SO EWL 65.6% MO EWL 59.8%		Low
Jain et al. [17]	4932 SG (N = 1699), GB (N = 3236) Retrospective	EWL in BMI 45 to 55 at 5 years	BMI >/=45 EWL 56.5% BMI >/=55 EWL 53.5%	BMI >/=45 EWL 66.6 (p < 0.001) BMI >/=55 EWL 63.8% (p < 0.001)	Low
Guan et al. [18]	Meta-analysis, 32 studies: 3 RCTs, 29 observational studies with 6665 patients.	Revision rate after SG after >/= 3 years.	>/= 3 years 10.4% >10 years 22.6%		High
Toolabi et al. [19]	120, GB (N = 64) and SG (N = 56), prospective	WL, EWL and weight regain (WR) after 5 years.	WL 24.6% EWL 61.9% WR 32%	WL 30.4% (p = 0.005) EWL 79.4% (p = 0.001) WR 9.3% (p = 0.004)	Low
Sepulvada et al. [20]	148 SG retrospective	Weight loss failure (%EWL < 50) after 7 years	33.3% fail at 5 years and 50% fail at 7 years.		Low
Bhandari et al. [21]	306, GB (N = 154) and SG (N = 152) retrospective	EWL and weight loss failure (%EWL < 50) after 6 years	EWL 50% WL failure 46.9%	EWL 61% (p = 0.0001) WL failure 11.5% (no p value)	Low

Jain et al. conducted a retrospective review of 4935 patients who underwent SG (N = 1699) or GB (N = 3236) with follow-up up to 5 years and found that patients in the BMI 45 to 55, there a significant higher %EWL in GB vs. SG [17].

Lack of treatment effect in SG is associated with conversions to GB. Guan et al. found that in mid-long-term outcomes (>/=3 years) after SG the overall revision rate was 10.4%. In patients with >10 years follow-up, the rate increased to 22.6%. Lack of effect of treatment was the most common indication for revision [18].

The higher lack of effect of SG compared to GB is further represented in the following observational studies. Toolabi et al. performed a prospective study on 120 patients who underwent GB (N = 64) and SG (N = 56). At 5 years, %WL (30.4 ± 1.3% vs 24.6 ± 1.3%, P = 0.005), and %EWL (79.4 ± 3.6% vs. 61.9 ± 3.5%, P = 0.001) were significantly higher in GB vs. SG respectively. Weight regain occurred in 9.3% in GB and 32% in SG (P = 0.004) [19]. This is based on the definition proposed by Baig et al.: 1. 25% increase in lost weight from the first 1 year postop, OR 2. weight regain more than 10 kg from weight at 1 year after surgery [22].

Sepulvada et al. performed a 7 year retrospective study of 148 SG patients. They found that up to one third of patients experience lack of treatment effect at the fifth year and 50% endure treatment failure in the seventh year. Lack of effect was defined as %EWL <50% [20]. Bhandari et al. performed a retrospective review on 154 GB and 152 SG patients. After 6 years the %EWL for SG was 50% and GB 61% (p = 0.0001). The lack of treatment effect (%EWL <50) for SG was 46.9% and GB 11.5% [21].

22.3.5 GERD Complications (Table 22.6)

Studies consistently demonstrate the association of SG with GERD development/progression and its inferiority in inducing remission of GERD compared to GB. This has potential correlation with development of pre-cancerous lesions, reason for conversion to GB, and/or weight-loss treatment lack of effect.

Peterli et al. found that in 217 patients randomized to SG and GB, GERD remission was observed more frequently after GB (60.4%) than after SG (25%). GERD worsened more often after SG (31.8%) than GB (6.3%) [23]. In addition, Chuffart et al. found that after 6 years follow-up in 41 SG patients, de novo GERD occurred in 22%, persistent GERD in 22%, and 5% required conversion to GB due to reflux [24].

In a multicenter study by Sebastianelli et al., systematic endoscopy was conducted at least 5 years after SG, the prevalence of Barrett's Esophagus (BE) in 90 patients was 18.8%. Lack of treatment effect was significantly associated with BE (p < 0.01). 36.8% of patients experienced weight loss failure and among patients with BE, it was 70.6% (P < 0.01). GERD symptoms were present in 21% of patients before surgery and rose to 76% at the time of follow up (p < 0.01). Half of the patients in this study complained of de novo GERD that were mild in 12 (18%) and severe in the remaining 56 (82%). The use of PPIs increased from 22% (20 patients) to 52% (46 patients) at the follow-up (p < 0.0001). Esophagitis on endoscopy at

Table 22.6 GERD complications

Study	Patients	Outcome classification	Sleeve gastrectomy	Gastric bypass	Quality of evidence
Peterli et al. [23]	217 randomization to SG and GB	GERD remission/progression after 5 years	Remission 25% Progression 31.8%	60.4% 6.3%	Moderate
Chuffart et al. [24]	41 after SG retrospective	GERD after 6 years	De novo GERD 22% Persistent GERD 22% GERD requiring conversion to GB 5%		Low
Sebastianelli et al. [25]	90 after SG retrospective	Prevalence of Barrett's esophagus (BE), WL failure association with BE, GERD progression, PPI use, and esophagitis after at least 5 years.	Prevalence of BE 18.8%, WL failure 70.6% in patients with BE. GERD before SG 21% to 76% at follow up (p < 0.01). PPI use 22% before SG to 52% at follow up (p < 0.0001). Esophagitis 10% before SG to 41% 5 years post op.		Low
Genco et al. [26]	110 prospective	Visual analogue scale (VAS) of GERD, PPI consumption, and endoscopy before SG and after with mean 58 months	After surgery vs before: VAS score 3 vs 1.8 (p = 0.018) GERD symptoms 68.1% vs 33.6% (p < 0.0001) PPI intake 57.2% vs. 19.1% (p < 0.0001). Endoscopy upward migration Z-line 73.6%, biliary-like reflux 74.5%. New non-dysplastic BE 17.2%.		Moderate
Sorcicelli et al. [27]	144 prospective	GERD symptoms, PPI intake, pre and post SG endoscopy with mean follow up 66 months. Diagnosis of GERD post SG was not reliable based on symptoms.	GERD 70.2% PPI 63.9% Post op endoscopy 72.9% pathological findings: EE 59.8%, non-dysplastic BE 13.1%.		Low

increased from 10% (9 patients) pre-operatively, to 41% (37 patients) 5 years post-operatively [25].

Genco et al. examined 162 patients who underwent preoperative visual analogue scale (VAS) evaluation of GERD symptoms, recording of PI consumption, and upper endoscopy. 110 patients (69.1%) participated in follow up at a mean of 58 months. VAS score, GERD symptoms, and PPI intake significantly increased compared to before surgery (3 vs. 1.8, p = 0.018; 68.1% vs. 33.6%, P < 0.0001; 57.2% vs. 19.1%, p < 0.0001). On endoscopy, an upward migration of the Z-line was found in 73.6% and a biliary-like esophageal reflux was found in 74.5%. A significant increase in incidence and severity of EE was discovered. Non-dysplastic BE was newly diagnosed in 19 patients (17.2%) [26].

A GERD diagnosis after SG is often based on symptoms and PPI consumption as objective tests are performed less often. Sorcicelli et al. conducted a prospective study of 144 patients with a mean follow-up of 66 months and found that GERD symptoms and PPI intake was present in 70.2% and 63.9% of patients, respectively. Post-operative upper endoscopy revealed pathological esophageal findings in 105 of 144 patients (72.9%), significantly increased compared to preoperative endoscopy. Erosive esophagitis was found in 86 patients post-operatively (59.8%). Nondysplastic BE was found in 13.1% (19 patients). After a logistic regression analysis, it was discovered that the probability of suffering from GERD symptoms did not change significantly among different degrees of EE or in case of BE diagnosis (OR 0.4–1.29). Even after adjustment based on PPI usage, the results were similar. The authors conclude that the diagnosis of GERD post SG was not reliable based on symptoms [27].

22.3.6 Patient and Surgeon Preference/Resource Utilization
(Table 22.7)

Several reasons may persuade patients and/or surgeons to pursue SG over GB; these reasons include: decreased overall morbidity/mortality, easier and quicker operation, and lower cost. Young et al. performed a retrospective analysis of the American College of Surgeons NSQIP data of 24,117 patients who underwent SG or GB. They found that SG had a shorter mean operative time (101 vs. 133 min, p < 0.01), a lower rate of deep wound infections (0.06% vs. 0.20%, p = 0.05), lower serious morbidity rate (3.8% vs. 5.8%, p < 0.01), and a 30-day reoperation rate (1.6% vs. 2.5%, p < 0.01) [28].

In addition, Alizadeh et al. retrospectively reviewed MBSAQIP data of 29,588 patients and found that SG was associated with significantly shorter operative time compared to GB (78 ± 39 *vs* 122 ± 54 min, *P* < 0.01), lower overall morbidity (2.3% *vs* 4.4%, AOR 0.53, CI 0.46–0.60, *P* < 0.01), lower serious morbidity (1.5% *vs* 2.3%, AOR 0.64, CI 0.53–0.76, p < 0.01), lower 30-day reoperation (1.2% *vs* 2.3%, AOR 0.52, CI 0.43–0.63, p < 0.01), and lower 30-day readmission (4.2% *vs* 6.6%,

Table 22.7 Patient and surgeon preference/resource utilization

Study	Patients	Outcome classification	Sleeve gastrectomy	Gastric bypass	Quality of evidence
Young et al. [28]	24,117 retrospective NSQIP	Operative time Deep wound infection Serious morbidity 30-day reoperation	101 min 0.06% 3.8% 1.6%	133 min (p < 0.01) 0.20% (p = 0.05) 5.8% (p < 0.01) 2.5% (p < 0.01)	Low
Alizadeh et al. [29]	29,588 retrospective MBSAQIP	Operative time Overall morbidity Serious morbidity 30-day reoperation 30-day readmission	79 min 2.3% 1.5% 1.2% 4.2%	122 min (p < 0.01) 4.4% (AOR 0.53 CI 0.46–0.60, $P < 0.01$) 2.3% (AOR 0.64, CI 0.53–0.76, p < 0.01) 2.3% (AOR 0.52, CI 0.43–0.63, p < 0.01) 6.6% (AOR 0.62, CI 0.55–0.69, $P < 0.01$)	Moderate
Berger et al. [30]	Retrospective review of MBSAQIP of 130,007 patients (LAGB N = 7378; SG N = 80,646; GB N = 41,983)	30-day readmission rates	2.8% OR 1.89 (95% CI 1.52–2.33)	4.9% OR 3.06 (95% CI 2.46–3.81)	Moderate

AOR 0.62, CI 0.55–0.69, $P < 0.01$). The authors conclude that, SG's popularity may in part be related to its improved perioperative safety profile [29].

Lastly, Berger et al. evaluated the national readmission rates of 130,007 patients from the MBSAQIP data. Of those, 7378 were laparoscopic adjusted gastric banding (LAGB) (5.7%), 80,646 were SG (62%), and 41,983 were GB (32.3%). The overall 30-day readmission rate was 4.4% and the most common causes were nausea, vomiting, electrolyte, and nutrition depletion. LAGB had the lowest rate of 1.4%, followed by SG (2.8%), and then GB (4.9%). When compared with LABG, SG had a readmission odds ratio (OR) of 1.89; 95% CI 1.52–2.33 and GB had the highest, with an OR of 3.06; 95% CI 2.46–3.81 [30].

22.4 Recommendations Based on the Data

22.4.1 Comparative Outcomes Between Sleeve Gastrectomy and Gastric Bypass

SG has a moderate effect on DM in the medium term, especially in the non-severely obese patients. In addition, when compared to medical therapy alone, the addition of bariatric surgery, whether it may be sleeve gastrectomy or gastric bypass, is superior in inducing type 2 DM remission and/or cure in short and medium-term. This is supported by high quality of evidence. However, when in studies comparing GB to SG, GB almost unanimously demonstrate higher efficacy for inducing DM improvement or remission in the short and medium-term. This is supported by moderate quality of evidence (QoE).

Either SG or GB plus medical therapy is more effective than medical therapy alone for the management of type 2 diabetes and hypertriglyceridemia. QoE high.

For the non-severely obese patients, compared to GB, SG may have equivalent efficacy in inducing DM remission. QoE high.

When comparing resolution of obesity-related comorbidities (DM, HTN, GERD, HL, and OSA), GB is superior to SG at short and medium-term but may or may not be superior at long-term. QoE moderate.

22.4.2 Special Populations

Although both SG and GB are nearly equivalent in overall morbidity and mortality, certain patient factors may disproportionately increase the risk of GB due to the need for multiple anastomoses and bowel manipulation. Literature review demonstrated increased risk in patients with inflammatory bowel disease, with immunosuppression, and those with multiple intra-abdominal surgeries. All of the evidence are retrospective, therefore the quality of evidence is low.

SG may be safer in special populations: inflammatory bowel disease, immunosuppressed, and patients with prior abdominal operation. QoE low.

22.4.3 Weight Loss Outcomes

Centers have established with long-term follow up that sleeve gastrectomy is durable in maintaining weight loss, therefore its long-term efficacy should not be discredited. The quality of evidence is moderate. However, when compared to GB, some studies have demonstrated inferiority in weight loss of SG in medium and long-term. The quality of evidence is also high in this aspect.

SG has durable weight-loss efficacy in the long-term. QoE moderate.

When discussing SG and GB long-term weight loss outcomes, patients should be informed that GB is superior and has less lack of treatment effect. QoE high.

22.4.4 Weight Regain/Lack of Treatment Effect

When compared to SG, literature demonstrates less lack of treatment effect of GB and higher weight-loss potential. This is most common reason for conversion of SG to GB. The quality of evidence ranges from moderate to high. There is also suggestion that SG is inferior in weight loss in class 5 obesity (BMI > 50) when compared to GB. In addition, when comparing resolution of co-morbidities at short and medium-term, GB is superior and SG's effects are variable in the long-term, especially in class 5 obesity. The above evidence ranges from moderate to low as they are mainly observational.

Long-term weight loss outcomes for SG is variable across studies and may be worse especially for Class 5+ obesity (BMI=/>60). QoE low.

Weight regain or lack of treatment effect is significantly higher after SG compared to GB after medium and long-term follow up. QoE moderate.

In Class 5 obesity (BMI > 50), weight loss potential is significantly larger after GB compared to SG. QoE moderate.

Revisional rates after SG increased with long-term follow up. QoE moderate.

22.4.5 GERD Complications

SG is associated with development of de novo GERD and the progression of disease in medium follow up. It has been associated with the sole or main reason for conversion to GB. When compared to GB, SG induces more GERD progression and less GERD remission. In-turn, this is associated with development of Barrett's Esophagus which has ramification in not just disease progression but also lack of effect in weight loss after medium follow up. These statements are supported by moderate to low quality evidence.

In comparing GERD remission or progression after medium-term follow up, GB is superior. SG has direct correlation to de novo GERD development, subjective and objective worsening, and increased PPI intake. Therefore, in bariatric patients with symptomatic GERD, GB should be recommended. QoE moderate.

Barret's esophagus is correlated with weight loss failure. QoE low.

22.4.6 Patient and Surgeon Preference/Resource Utilization

Several reasons may persuade patients and/or surgeons to pursue SG rather than GB. Supported by moderate quality of evidence, these reasons include: lower morbidity, readmission, operative duration, and overall cost.

Surgeon/patient preference for SG may be due to: lower operative time, morbidity, readmission, and overall cost. QoE moderate.

22.5 Personal View of the Data

While the sleeve gastrectomy has grown tremendously over the past decade, further delineation of its appropriate utilization needs to be determined. The safety profile of the sleeve gastrectomy is superior to the gastric bypass while the benefits of the gastric bypass exceeds sleeve gastrectomy. Future investigation should be undertaken to determine if sleeve gastrectomy benefits may be enhanced by standardization and/or adjuvant pharmaceutical intervention.

References

1. Schauer PR, Bhatt DL, Kirwan JP, Wolski K, Aminian A, Brethauer SA, et al. Bariatric surgery versus intensive medical therapy for diabetes – 5-year outcomes. N Engl J Med. 2017;376(7):641–51.
2. Nedelcu M, Loureiro M, Skalli M, Galtier F, Jaussent A, Deloze M, et al. Laparoscopic sleeve gastrectomy: effect on long-term remission for morbidly obese patients with type 2 diabetes at 5-year follow up. Surgery. 2017;162(4):857–62.
3. Dang JT, Sheppard C, Kim D, Switzer N, Shi X, Tian C, et al. Predictive factors for diabetes remission after bariatric surgery. Can J Surg. 2019;62(5):315–9.
4. Sha Y, Huang X, Ke P, Wang B, Yuan H, Yuan W, et al. Laparoscopic roux-en-Y gastric bypass versus sleeve Gastrectomy for type 2 diabetes mellitus in nonseverely obese patients: a systematic review and meta-analysis of randomized controlled trials. Obes Surg. 2020;30:1660–70.
5. Salminen P, Helmiö M, Ovaska J, Juuti A, Leivonen M, Peromaa-Haavisto P, et al. Effect of laparoscopic sleeve Gastrectomy vs laparoscopic roux-en-Y gastric bypass on weight loss at 5 years among patients with morbid obesity: the SLEEVEPASS randomized clinical trial. JAMA. 2018;319(3):241–54.
6. Celio AC, Wu Q, Kasten KR, Manwaring ML, Pories WJ, Spaniolas K. Comparative effectiveness of roux-en-Y gastric bypass and sleeve gastrectomy in super obese patients. Surg Endosc. 2017;31(1):317–23.
7. Lager CJ, Esfandiari NH, Luo Y, Subauste AR, Kraftson AT, Brown MB, et al. Metabolic parameters, weight loss, and comorbidities 4 years after roux-en-Y gastric bypass and sleeve Gastrectomy. Obes Surg. 2018;28(11):3415–23.
8. Hefler J, Dang J, Modasi A, Switzer N, Birch DW, Karmali S. Effects of chronic corticosteroid and immunosuppressant use in patients undergoing bariatric surgery. Obes Surg. 2019;29(10):3309–15.
9. Major P, Droś J, Kacprzyk A, Pędziwiatr M, Małczak P, Wysocki M, et al. Does previous abdominal surgery affect the course and outcomes of laparoscopic bariatric surgery? Surg Obes Relat Dis. 2018;14(7):997–1004.
10. Heshmati K, Lo T, Tavakkoli A, Sheu E. Short-term outcomes of inflammatory bowel disease after Roux-en-Y gastric bypass vs sleeve gastrectomy. J Am Coll Surg. 2019;228(6):893–901.e1.
11. Arman GA, Himpens J, Dhaenens J, Ballet T, Vilallonga R, Leman G. Long-term (11+years) outcomes in weight, patient satisfaction, comorbidities, and gastroesophageal reflux treatment after laparoscopic sleeve gastrectomy. Surg Obes Relat Dis. 2016;12(10):1778–86.
12. Noel P, Nedelcu M, Eddbali I, Manos T, Gagner M. What are the long-term results 8 years after sleeve gastrectomy? Surg Obes Relat Dis. 2017;13(7):1110–5.

13. Sharples AJ, Mahawar K. Systematic review and meta-analysis of randomised controlled trials comparing long-term outcomes of Roux-En-Y gastric bypass and sleeve gastrectomy. Obes Surg. 2019;30(2):664–72.
14. Ahmed B, King WC, Gourash W, Belle SH, Hinerman A, Pomp A, et al. Long-term weight change and health outcomes for sleeve gastrectomy (SG) and matched roux-en-Y gastric bypass (RYGB) participants in the longitudinal assessment of bariatric surgery (LABS) study. Surgery. 2018;164(4):774–83.
15. Azagury D, Mokhtari TE, Garcia L, Rosas US, Garg T, Rivas H, et al. Heterogeneity of weight loss after gastric bypass, sleeve gastrectomy, and adjustable gastric banding. Surgery. 2019;165(3):565–70.
16. Ece I, Yilmaz H, Alptekin H, Yormaz S, Colak B, Yilmaz F, et al. Comparative effectiveness of laparoscopic sleeve Gastrectomy on morbidly obese, super-obese, and super-super obese patients for the treatment of morbid obesity. Obes Surg. 2018;28(6):1484–91.
17. Jain D, Sill A, Averbach A. Do patients with higher baseline BMI have improved weight loss with roux-en-Y gastric bypass versus sleeve gastrectomy? Surg Obes Relat Dis. 2018;14(9):1304–9.
18. Guan B, Chong TH, Peng J, Chen Y, Wang C, Yang J. Mid-long-term Revisional surgery after sleeve Gastrectomy: a systematic review and meta-analysis. Obes Surg. 2019;29(6):1965–75.
19. Toolabi K, Sarkardeh M, Vasigh M, Golzarand M, Vezvaei P, Kooshki J. Comparison of laparoscopic roux-en-Y gastric bypass and laparoscopic sleeve Gastrectomy on weight loss, weight regain, and remission of comorbidities: a 5 years of follow-up study. Obes Surg. 2019;30(2):440–5.
20. Sepúlveda M, Alamo M, Saba J, Astorga C, Lynch R, Guzmán H. Long-term weight loss in laparoscopic sleeve gastrectomy. Surg Obes Relat Dis. 2017;13(10):1676–81.
21. Bhandari M, Reddy M, Kosta S, Mathur W, Fobi M. Laparoscopic sleeve gastrectomy versus laparoscopic gastric bypass: a retrospective cohort study. Int J Surg. 2019;67:47–53.
22. Baig SJ, Priya P, Mahawar KK, Shah S, Group IBSORI. Weight regain after bariatric surgery-a multicentre study of 9617 patients from Indian bariatric surgery outcome reporting group. Obes Surg. 2019;29(5):1583–92.
23. Peterli R, Wölnerhanssen BK, Peters T, Vetter D, Kröll D, Borbély Y, et al. Effect of laparoscopic sleeve Gastrectomy vs laparoscopic roux-en-Y gastric bypass on weight loss in patients with morbid obesity: the SM-BOSS randomized clinical trial. JAMA. 2018;319(3):255–65.
24. Chuffart E, Sodji M, Dalmay F, Iannelli A, Mathonnet M. Long-term results after sleeve Gastrectomy for Gastroesophageal reflux disease: a single-center French study. Obes Surg. 2017;27(11):2890–7.
25. Sebastianelli L, Benois M, Vanbiervliet G, Bailly L, Robert M, Turrin N, et al. Systematic endoscopy 5 years after sleeve Gastrectomy results in a high rate of Barrett's esophagus: results of a multicenter study. Obes Surg. 2019;29(5):1462–9.
26. Genco A, Soricelli E, Casella G, Maselli R, Castagneto-Gissey L, Di Lorenzo N, et al. Gastroesophageal reflux disease and Barrett's esophagus after laparoscopic sleeve gastrectomy: a possible, underestimated long-term complication. Surg Obes Relat Dis. 2017;13(4):568–74.
27. Soricelli E, Casella G, Baglio G, Maselli R, Ernesti I, Genco A. Lack of correlation between gastroesophageal reflux disease symptoms and esophageal lesions after sleeve gastrectomy. Surg Obes Relat Dis. 2018;14(6):751–6.
28. Young MT, Gebhart A, Phelan MJ, Nguyen NT. Use and outcomes of laparoscopic sleeve Gastrectomy vs laparoscopic gastric bypass: analysis of the American College of Surgeons NSQIP. J Am Coll Surg. 2015;220(5):880–5.
29. Alizadeh RF, Li S, Gambhir S, Hinojosa MW, Smith BR, Stamos MJ, et al. Laparoscopic sleeve Gastrectomy or laparoscopic gastric bypass for patients with metabolic syndrome: an MBSAQIP analysis. Am Surg. 2019;85(10):1108–12.
30. Berger ER, Huffman KM, Fraker T, Petrick AT, Brethauer SA, Hall BL, et al. Prevalence and risk factors for bariatric surgery readmissions: findings from 130,007 admissions in the metabolic and bariatric surgery accreditation and quality improvement program. Ann Surg. 2018;267(1):122–31.

Single-Stage Duodenal Switch is Better than Two-Stage

23

L. Kasey Welsh and Ranjan Sudan

23.1 Introduction

Biliopancreatic diversion with duodenal switch (BPD/DS) as described by Hess and Hess [1] and Marceau et al. [2] over two decades ago remains a less commonly performed operation and has been primarily reserved for patients with a body mass index (BMI) ≥ 50 kg/m^2 or those with severe obesity-related comorbidities [3]. Despite providing the most effective long-term weight loss and resolution of conditions such as diabetes mellitus [4–6], BPD/DS represents less than 1% of the total bariatric operations performed in the United States [7]. Potential reasons are that it is considered a more technically challenging bariatric procedure, with higher short and long-term morbidity and mortality compared to the Roux-en-Y gastric bypass or the sleeve gastrectomy [4].

A two-stage approach with the first-stage consisting of a vertical sleeve gastrectomy (SG), followed by a second-stage duodenal switch after initial weight loss has been advocated in an attempt to decrease perioperative complications and minimize the complexity and technical challenge of the malabsorptive portion of the operation [6, 8, 9].

The theoretical advantages of performing BPD/DS with a staged approach also allows for the opportunity to identify patients who might achieve acceptable results with SG alone, thus avoiding the morbidity linked to the malabsorption operation, and as a vetting process for patients who possess the required level of compliance necessary follow-up visits and supplementation. The data are limited regarding any benefit or superiority of a two-stage approach. Several reports confirm that a single-stage BPD/DS can be safely performed, including in patients with higher BMIs and that a two-step approach is not necessarily superior [6, 8, 10–13].

L. K. Welsh · R. Sudan (✉)
Department of Surgery, Duke University Medical Center, Durham, NC, USA
e-mail: ranjan.sudan@duke.edu

© Springer Nature Switzerland AG 2021
J. Alverdy, Y. Vigneswaran (eds.), *Difficult Decisions in Bariatric Surgery*,
Difficult Decisions in Surgery: An Evidence-Based Approach,
https://doi.org/10.1007/978-3-030-55329-6_23

23.2 Search Strategy

A literature search of English language publications from 2000 to 2020 was performed to identify published data on single and two-stage BPD/DS using PubMed. Terms used in the search included "duodenal switch, single- and one-stage," "second-stage duodenal switch," "duodenal switch after failed sleeve gastrectomy," "revision bariatric surgery," "duodenal switch outcomes," "super morbidly obese," in addition to "perioperative complications," and "long-term outcomes." An emphasis on safety and postoperative outcomes was employed (Table 23.1).

Seven studies including two retrospective matched cohort studies, one retrospective cohort study, and three retrospective observational studies were included in our summary (Table 23.2). The data was classified using the GRADE system (Table 23.3).

23.3 Results

23.3.1 Clinical Relevance

The prevalence of obesity has been increasing steadily over the last two decades [14, 15] and severe obesity is increasing at an alarming rate [16]. Surgery remains the most effective solution and BPD/DS provides the best long-term weight loss maintenance and complete or near complete resolution of obesity-related comorbidities such as diabetes, hypertension, and asthma with a mortality rate of 1.1% [4].

SG as a stand-alone operation emerged from the restrictive portion of BPD/DS and was endorsed in 2011 by the American Society for Metabolic and Bariatric Surgery (ASMBS) for the treatment for morbid obesity [17]. This operation has quickly become the most popular weight loss operation due in part to a lower technical difficulty and favorable complication profile [18]. The option for a staged approach to a BPD/DS appears to be a logical option for certain higher-risk candidates.

Earlier reports have emphasized the higher risks of a single-stage BPD/DS operation as compared to a two-stage approach in heavier patients with BMI $\geq$ 50 kg/m^2 [19]. Two studies have directly compared single and two-stage BPD/DS using retrospective matched cohorts. Iannelli et al. [20] found that when a two-stage approach

Table 23.1 PICO table

P (Patients)	I (Intervention)	C (Comparator)	O (Outcomes)
patients with morbid obesity	single-stage BPD/DS	two-stage BPD/DS	morbidity and mortality, conversion rates, operative time, LOS, %EWL, SG revision, insurance benefits, costs, technical aspects, robotic application, BMI disparities

BPD/DS biliopancreatic diversion with duodenal switch, *LOS* length of stay, *SG* sleeve gastrectomy, *%EWL*, percentage excess weight loss, *BMI* body mass index in kg/m^2

Table 23.2 Summary of reviewed studies

Author	Year	Design	Country	n	Quality	Conclusions
Sudan	2007	retrospective observational	USA	47	Low	A robotic surgical approach to BPD/DS is safe, feasible, and reproducible.
Buchwald	2008	retrospective observational	USA	190	Low	BPD/DS can be performed relatively safely in the morbidly and super morbidly obese and does not require a two-stage procedure.
Topart	2009	retrospective observational	France	86	Low	Laparoscopic single-stage BP-DS can be performed safely in the morbidly and super morbidly obese. SG should be considered in higher risk populations.
Iannelli	2013	retrospective matched cohort	France	220	Moderate	Two-stage BPD/DS has similar results as single-stage.
Rezvani	2013	retrospective cohort	USA	226	Low	BPD/DS outcomes not significantly different for BMI $\geq$ 50 compared to <50.
Antanavicius	2014	retrospective observational	USA	179	Low	One-stage robot-assisted BPD/DS is feasible and well-tolerated, and effective.
Biertho	2018	retrospective matched cohort	Canada	118	Moderate	Second-stage BPD/DS is an effective option for the management of suboptimal outcomes after SG. 3 years outcomes did not significantly differ from single-stage.

BPD/DS biliopancreatic diversion with duodenal switch, *SG* sleeve gastrectomy, *BMI*, body mass index in kg/m^2

is employed, 73% of patients experienced acceptable weight loss and were able to avoid the second-stage completion biliopancreatic diversion. The 3-year excess body weight loss (EWL) and resolution or obesity-related co-morbidities were equivocal for the 37% of the patient in that series and required a second-stage completion BPD/DS [20]. Interestingly, no significant difference was seen in the rate of postoperative complications and the composite hospital stay duration was the same. One patient in the second-stage group died of aspiration pneumonia after a leak at the esophagogastric junction after SG.

Table 23.3 Summary of study data

Author	n		Age (mean)		Preop BMI (mean)		% Male		Approach	Conversion %		P	Operative time (mins)		P	LOS		P	Morbidity % (30 d)		P	Mortality % (30 d)		%EWL		Follow up
	TS	SS	TS	SS	TS	SS	TS	SS		TS	SS		TS	SS		TS	SS		TS	SS		TS	SS	TS	SS	
Biertho (2018)	59	59	44	43.4	53.8	52.7	37.3	37.3	Lap	2.0	0	–	111+175	206	<0.005[a] <0.001[b]	4.2+4.6	4.9	0.02[a] 0.1[b]	2+3	3	0.8[a] 0.8[b]	0	0	81	81	2 years
Iannelli (2013)	110	110	41	38.7	55.3	54.9	26.4	10.0	Lap	0	5.0	<0.05	NR	NR		7	6.8	0.8	8.2	15.5	0.1	0.9	0	72.7	73.3	3 years
Antanavicius (2014)	179	–	44.2	–	50.3	–	23.5	–	Robotic	0.	–		249	–		2.7	–		5	–		0	–	79.9	–	2 years
Rezvani (2013)	99	–	44.9	–	50.2	–	26.1	–	Lap	3.0	–		287	–		3.6	–		11	–		0	–	NR	–	30 days
Topart (2009)	49	–	38.2	–	55	–	6.1	–	Mixed	2.1	–		193	–		6.2	–		16.3	–		0	–	NR	–	NR
Buchwald (2008)	190	–	43	–	53.4	–	21.6	–	Mixed	NR	–		337	–		6	–		37	–		0	–	NR	–	30 days
Sudan (2007)	47	–	38	–	45	–	4.3	–	Robotic	6.4	–		514	–		NR	–		8.5[c]	–		0	–	NR	–	NR

BMI body mass index in kg/m², *LOS* length of stay, *%EWL* percent excess weight loss, *SS* single-stage, *TS* two-stage, *NR* not reported, *lap* laparoscopic

[a]P comparing SG with single-stage BPD/DS

[b]P comparing second-stage BPD/DS with single-stage BPD/DS

[c]Only anastomotic leaks reported

Using a different design, Biertho et al. [21] examined patients that underwent BPD/DS for weight loss failure after previous SG. Patients were matched to those that underwent a single-stage BPD/DS and retrospectively compared for various parameters. They concluded that at 3 years, global outcomes including EWL, early and late complications, and nutritional deficiencies did not significantly differ between the two groups.

In regards to the efficacy and feasibility of BPD/DS as a primary operations, Rezvani et al. [11] specifically analyzed data from single-stage laparoscopic BPD/DS stratified by BMI. They concluded that 30-day outcomes are not significantly different for BMI $\geq$ 50 kg/m^2 compared to < 50 kg/m^2 supporting that a single-stage BPD/DS can be safely performed in the super morbidly obese patient. The findings of Topart et al. further support that BPD/DS is safe and effective for BMI between 50 and 60 kg/m^2, but that a two-stage approach can be considered for patients with BMI > 60 kg/m^2 and especially in male patients who historically exhibit higher risks of complication [8, 22].

The safety of BPD/DS in extreme BMI patients is further supported by Buchwald et al. [23] which supports that BPD/DS can be performed in the morbidly and super morbidly obese, and does not require a two-stage procedure as long as attention to meticulous surgical technique is maintained. Intuitively, it would seem that as the BMI increases, a trend toward greater mortality rate would be expected. However, for super obese patients (BMI between 50 and 60 kg/m^2) the postoperative mortality rate has remained relatively low and is not significantly different from those with a BMI between 35 and 50 kg/m^2 [4, 5]. BMI is not the only contributing factor for the increased technical challenge during any bariatric operations. Male gender is one known factor to contribute to higher rates of morbidity and mortality after bariatric procedures [22]. Other factors making the BPD/DS more difficult include intra-abdominal adiposity, large liver, and high amounts of abdominal torque [12]. Understandably, the decision-making algorithm for operation selection is more nuanced than BMI and the complexities of weighing the constellation of each individual's comorbidities is beyond the limitations of this chapter.

The rising popularity and utilization of robotic platforms deserve to be mentioned due to the purported benefits in simplifying some of the more technically challenging aspects of BPD/DS. Antanavicius et al. [10] published data on single-stage robotically assisted BPD/DS as a feasible, well-tolerated, and effective approach to the technically challenging aspects of the operation with favorable results, similar to our own robotic experience [12, 13]. The robotic platform offers superior optics and allows for multiple-axis articulation for increased precision in performing hand-sewn anastomoses that are critical in BPD/DS. Robotic arms also reduce transmission of tissue torque related to abdominal wall thickness and provide improved surgeon ergonomics. Effective laparoscopic suturing is a viable option, the robotic system offers some advantage in performing the complex gastro-intestinal anastomoses required in BPD/DS. Our first BPD/DS was performed in 2000 and are first series of robotic BPD/DS cases was published in 2007. The results demonstrated favorable outcomes and no mortality in 47 patients. Prolonged operative times were related to overcoming a steep learning curve [13]. Our subsequent analysis demonstrated a decreased operative duration utilizing a totally robotic technique with each successive case and no technical complications were experienced, including anastomotic leaks [12]. Noted disadvantages of robotic assisted surgery include increased costs, longer operating times, and lack of tactile feedback.

We recognize that there are contradictory reports from experienced surgeons, including that of Kim et al. who cite higher complication and mortality rates for BPD/DS [6]. Our experience and that of others is that BPD/DS does not require a two-stage procedure [23]. We are hesitant to support SG as a planned first stage of a scheduled two-stage BPD/DS for all cases based on the limited data and our personal experience. While the individual operative times and hospital length of stay of SG and second-stage BDP/DS are slightly less compared to the single-stage approach, the combined values are arguably much more. Two separate operations expose patients additional time under general anesthesia and an additional hospitalization. We recognize that the data to support one approach over another is limited and that in certain situations and two-stage approach may be warranted. To better understand those situations and conditions further investigation such as a randomized controlled trial would need to be done. Considering the low volume and selective indications for BPD/DS, such a study would be very difficult to perform.

A large portion of patients may lose a significant amount of weight after initial SG and will no longer meet criteria for a second operation, but still have unresolved obesity-related comorbidities that could have been better addressed with BPD/DS from the start. Many insurance providers will only cover one bariatric surgery per lifetime, unless a subsequent operation is deemed necessary to treat a complication, further limiting access to a definitive operation with the highest likelihood of success. Cost is a frequently mentioned, but poorly understood, as figures are often not disclosed. It is safe to assume that a second operation with an additional hospital stay would understandably equate to higher costs for both the patient and the payor.

23.4 Approval of SADI

In 2011, Sanchez-Pernaute and Torres [24] described the single-anastomosis duodeno-ileostomy (SADI) as a way to simplify the surgical technique and limit risks of deficiencies after traditional BPD/DS. Implementation of this technique is growing as an easier and possibly safer alternative to traditional BPD/DS and was recently approved by the ASMBS as an endorsed procedure [25]. It is too early to know for sure, but it will be interesting to see how SADI versus traditional single and two-stage BPD/DS plays out in the near future.

23.5 Recommendations

- BPD/DS is a safe and effective operation for the appropriately selected patient and is a viable and safe option for individual with a higher BMI (>60 kg/m^2).

- The data comparing single-stage to two-stage operations are limited and the quality is restricted to retrospective cohort studies at best. The current literature fails to identify a clear superiority of a two-stage approach compared to a single-stage.
- The lack of high-quality data support the continued practice of single-stage BPD/DS by qualified and experienced surgeons with the appropriate multidisciplinary follow up support.

23.6   Personal View

The BPD/DS is a technically demanding operation that takes longer to perform than the RYGB or the SG. The two-stage operation was conceived when surgeons encountered a higher morbidity and mortality rate early in their learning curve. This was an attempt to reduce perioperative complications and the duration of the operation. Since that time, the skill set of surgeons has improved greatly and complication rates and duration of the operation have decreased considerably. Further, the use of the robot has also reduced ergonomics strain on the surgeon. Therefore, patients with higher complexity can undergo a single-stage BPD/DS operation with very acceptable morbidity and mortality in experienced centers and has been my preferred approach. However, this operation should not be offered casually to the patients due to its long-term nutritional consequences. If surgeons are not comfortable with their technique or if a patient is high-risk for a longer operation then a two-stage operation is a good alternative to reduce risk.

References

1. Hess DS, Hess DW. Biliopancreatic diversion with a duodenal switch. Obes Surg. 1998 Jun;8(3):267–82.
2. Marceau P, Biron S, Bourque RA, Potvin M, Hould FS, Simard S. Biliopancreatic diversion with a new type of gastrectomy. Obes Surg. 1993 Feb;3(1):29–35.
3. Mechanick JI, Kushner RF, Sugerman HJ, et al. American association of clinical endocrinologists, the obesity society, and American society for metabolic & bariatric surgery medical guidelines for clinical practice for the perioperative nutritional, metabolic, and nonsurgical support of the bariatric surgery patient. Surg Obes Relat Dis. 2008 Sep–Oct;4(5 Suppl):S109–84.
4. Buchwald H, Avidor Y, Braunwald E, et al. Bariatric surgery: a systematic review and meta-analysis. Jama. 2004 Oct 13;292(14):1724–37.
5. Buchwald H, Estok R, Fahrbach K, Banel D, Sledge I. Trends in mortality in bariatric surgery: a systematic review and meta-analysis. Surgery. 2007 Oct;142(4):621-632. discussion 32-5.
6. Kim WW, Gagner M, Kini S, et al. Laparoscopic vs. open biliopancreatic diversion with duodenal switch: a comparative study. J Gastrointest Surg. 2003 May–Jun;7(4):552–7.
7. Estimate of Bariatric Surgery Numbers, 2011–2018. Available at: https://asmbs.org/resources/estimate-of-bariatric-surgery-numbers. Accessed Jan 2020.
8. Topart P, Becouarn G, Ritz P. Should biliopancreatic diversion with duodenal switch be done as single-stage procedure in patients with BMI > or = 50 kg/m^2? Surg Obes Relat Dis. 2010 Jan–Feb;6(1):59–63.

9. Cottam D, Qureshi FG, Mattar SG, et al. Laparoscopic sleeve gastrectomy as an initial weight-loss procedure for high-risk patients with morbid obesity. Surg Endosc. 2006 Jun;20(6):859–63.
10. Antanavicius G, Rezvani M, Sucandy I. One-stage robotically assisted laparoscopic biliopancreatic diversion with duodenal switch: analysis of 179 patients. Surg Obes Relat Dis. 2015 Mar–Apr;11(2):367–71.
11. Rezvani M, Sucandy I, Klar A, Bonanni F, Antanavicius G. Is laparoscopic single-stage biliopancreatic diversion with duodenal switch safe in super morbidly obese patients? Surg Obes Relat Dis. 2014 May–Jun;10(3):427–30.
12. Sudan R, Bennett KM, Jacobs DO, Sudan DL. Multifactorial analysis of the learning curve for robot-assisted laparoscopic biliopancreatic diversion with duodenal switch. Ann Surg. 2012 May;255(5):940–5.
13. Sudan R, Puri V, Sudan D. Robotically assisted biliary pancreatic diversion with a duodenal switch: a new technique. Surg Endosc. 2007 May;21(5):729–33.
14. Katzmarzyk PT, Mason C. Prevalence of class I, II and III obesity in Canada. Cmaj. 2006 Jan 17;174(2):156–7.
15. Hales CM, Carroll MD, Fryar CD, Ogden CL. Prevalence of obesity among adults and youth: United States, 2015–2016. NCHS Data Brief. 2017 Oct;288:1–8.
16. Wang Y, Beydoun MA, Liang L, Caballero B, Kumanyika SK. Will all Americans become overweight or obese? estimating the progression and cost of the US obesity epidemic. Obesity (Silver Spring). 2008 Oct;16(10):2323–30.
17. Ali M, El Chaar M, Ghiassi S, Rogers AM. American society for metabolic and bariatric surgery updated position statement on sleeve gastrectomy as a bariatric procedure. Surg Obes Relat Dis. 2017 Oct;13(10):1652–7.
18. Kizy S, Jahansouz C, Downey MC, Hevelone N, Ikramuddin S, Leslie D. National trends in bariatric surgery 2012–2015: demographics, procedure selection, readmissions, and cost. Obes Surg. 2017 Nov;27(11):2933–9.
19. Ren CJ, Patterson E, Gagner M. Early results of laparoscopic biliopancreatic diversion with duodenal switch: a case series of 40 consecutive patients. Obes Surg. 2000 Dec;10(6):514-523; discussion 24.
20. Iannelli A, Schneck AS, Topart P, Carles M, Hebuterne X, Gugenheim J. Laparoscopic sleeve gastrectomy followed by duodenal switch in selected patients versus single-stage duodenal switch for superobesity: case-control study. Surg Obes Relat Dis. 2013 Jul-Aug;9(4):531–8.
21. Biertho L, Theriault C, Bouvet L, et al. Second-stage duodenal switch for sleeve gastrectomy failure: a matched controlled trial. Surg Obes Relat Dis. 2018 Oct;14(10):1570–9.
22. DeMaria EJ, Portenier D, Wolfe L. Obesity surgery mortality risk score: proposal for a clinically useful score to predict mortality risk in patients undergoing gastric bypass. Surg Obes Relat Dis. 2007 Mar–Apr;3(2):134–40.
23. Buchwald H, Kellogg TA, Leslie DB, Ikramuddin S. Duodenal switch operative mortality and morbidity are not impacted by body mass index. Ann Surg. 2008 Oct;248(4):541–8.
24. Sanchez-Pernaute A, Rubio MA, Perez Aguirre E, Barabash A, Cabrerizo L, Torres A. Single-anastomosis duodenoileal bypass with sleeve gastrectomy: metabolic improvement and weight loss in first 100 patients. Surg Obes Relat Dis. 2013 Sep–Oct;9(5):731–5.
25. Endorsed Procedures and Devices. Available at: https://asmbs.org/resources/endorsed-procedures-and-devices?/resources/approved-procedures. Accessed Jan 2020.

Part VI

Complications

Stenting for Leaks After Sleeve Gastrectomy

Betty Li and Uzma D. Siddiqui

24.1 Introduction

In the past decade, laparoscopic sleeve gastrectomy (LSG) has gained significant popularity as a treatment for obesity. In comparison to other restrictive bariatric procedures, sleeve gastrectomy has proven effective in achieving considerable weight loss without increased risk of complications. However there has been significant morbidity and mortality associated with post-operative anastomotic leaks. The reported incidence of LSG leaks range between 0.1 and 7% and can be higher in re-operative surgery [1–3]. Within the literature, the causes of a staple line leak are broadly grouped into either ischemic or mechanical causes. Leaks commonly occur in the proximal third of the anastomosis: large majority (>80%) at the angle of His or at the gastroesophageal junction (GEJ) and to a lesser degree the mid-aspect of the gastric body or distal third [3–5].

The management of leaks following sleeve gastrectomy is challenging and controversial. There is no uniform guideline regarding the optimal treatment strategy and often vary depending on the size of the disruption, the extent of the abdominal infection, and the location. A range of leak management options have been investigated, including medical management with intravenous antibiotics and parenteral nutrition, reoperation, and percutaneous drainage. More recently, endoluminal interventions, including the use of temporary stents to exclude the anastomotic defect and divert GI contents has become recognized as an effective treatment of LSG leaks. In a recent systematic analysis on the management of acute staple-line leaks, studies that solely described stent placement as a treatment strategy had a pooled initial success rate of 62% [6]. The use of endoscopic stents has a number of notable advantages compared to other options including avoiding the need for

B. Li (✉) · U. D. Siddiqui
Center for Endoscopic Research and Therapeutics (CERT), Chicago, IL, USA
e-mail: Betty.Li@uchospitals.edu; usiddiqui@bsd.uchicago.edu

© Springer Nature Switzerland AG 2021
J. Alverdy, Y. Vigneswaran (eds.), *Difficult Decisions in Bariatric Surgery*,
Difficult Decisions in Surgery: An Evidence-Based Approach,
https://doi.org/10.1007/978-3-030-55329-6_24

surgical revision, preventing the risks of prolonged parenteral nutrition, and rapid healing while allowing for oral nutrition [7]. However, stent placement poses its own unique difficulties and complications. In this chapter we discuss the literature available on endoscopic stenting in LSG leaks, review the difficult decisions in using this modality and finally the management of refractory cases.

24.2   Search Strategy

A literature search for publications from 2000 to 2020 was used to identity data on endoscopic stent placement after laparoscopic sleeve gastrectomy leaks. Four online electronic databases were searched (PubMed/Medline). The search was performed utilizing MeSH search terms and key words, these included "laparoscopic sleeve gastrectomy", "sleeve gastrectomy", "laparoscopic bariatric surgery", "staple line leak", "stents", "endoscopic stents", "treatment" and "management". Boolean operators (AND or OR) were integrated into the search in order to maximize article capture. The end search result was further supplemented by hand searching the reference lists from included and excluded articles.

24.3   Results

24.3.1 Patient Presentation

Staple line leaks can cause significant mortality and morbidity if not diagnosed quickly. Patients can present with a range of symptoms including shoulder pain, severe food intolerance, fevers, chills, worsening abdominal pain or hemodynamic instability [1]. However, symptoms may be non-specific and is often extremely difficult to separate from normal variants in postoperative patients. Early leaks tend to present with sudden onset left upper quadrant pain radiating to the left shoulder while late leaks may be more insidious in onset with gradual increasing discomfort and nausea, with or without a fever [1, 8]. Tachycardia is reported to be the most sensitive indicator of a leak [9]. A diagnostic workup should be considered in any patient who develops tachycardia, fever, or abdominal pain after sleeve gastrectomy [10].

24.3.2 Leak Diagnosis/Imaging Studies

There are two main imaging modalities to diagnose a sleeve leak: upper GI (UGI) contrast studies or abdominal computed tomography (CT) scan. In stable patients, the study of choice is a CT scan with oral and IV contrast because it has higher sensitivity (83–93%) than UGI contrast studies (0–25%) and it allows for better evaluation of undrained fluid collections [2, 8, 11]. It is important to note however that CT scans have a high rate of false negatives because it often fails to detect small staple line leaks, making an UGI study more helpful in this respect. Occasionally, ingestion of methylene blue can be used to help assess for a leak that is difficult to diagnose with other techniques; this is only helpful when postoperative surgical drains remain in place [8]. If there is high suspicion for gastric leak, despite negative imaging, early surgical exploration should be considered.

24.3.3 Peri-procedural Considerations

The mainstay of treatment relies on medical support, drainage of leaked material and facilitated repair of the wall defect. Over the last 15 years, the cornerstone of endoscopic intervention of sleeve leaks has been placement of removable stents to bypass the wall defect to allow healing. The success rate of complete healing after treatment with endoluminal stents can be as high as 70–100% [3, 11–14]. However, stent placement while effective, is not exempt of complications. There are a multitude of factors that affect the success of endoscopic management of leaks and include: patient selection, time to leak diagnosis, sleeve characteristic, and stent selection.

24.3.3.1 Patient Assessment and Stability

Patient stability is an important primary consideration when assessing candidates for temporary stent placement. According to expert opinion, an unstable patient with a symptomatic leak requires immediate reoperation [10]. Patients with signs of septic shock or generalized peritonitis require timely initiation of broad-spectrum antibiotics and warrant prompt surgical exploration (open or laparoscopic) [2, 15, 16]. Drainage of any leaked content or fluid collection should be completed prior to endoscopic stent placement.

24.3.3.2 Leak Presentation and Concomitant Strictures/Stenosis

The duration of leak is an essential consideration in choosing the appropriate treatment.

According to the best practice guidelines from the International Sleeve Gastrectomy Expert Panel Consensus, leaks can be categorized according to their time of presentation from the operative procedure (acute<7 days, early: 1–6 weeks, late: 6–12 weeks, and chronic: >12 weeks) [10]. Overall, stents have shown excellent results in the treatment of early leaks but the success of stent placement for late/chronic leaks are less consistent [3, 10, 17]. Martin del Campo and colleagues found that success rates decreased in proportion to the duration of the leak [18]. In another study, nine patients treated for chronic leak after LSG had a failure rate of 84%, one third of whom eventually required total gastrectomy. This is in contrast to a reported 87% success rate of leak closure by Puli et al. in patients with primarily acute and early leaks. In recent years, some surgeons have advocated an expanded role of surgery in the management of even acute leaks especially in the setting of peritonitis due to the high suspicion that the leak is likely caused by mechanical faults or tissue injury and that would resolve more quickly with surgical repair [19].

Furthermore, the location of the defect can impact the difficulty and feasibility of the endoscopic intervention. Leaks at the gastroesophageal junction, proximal or mid-aspect of the sleeve are more amenable to stenting than distal anastomotic defects [20]. This is in part due to the incisura and the difficulty of adequate sealing of the defect in the distal third of the gastric sleeve with regular esophageal stents, new long stents are often required [21]. When assessing the integrity of the gastric sleeve either with direct visualization or UGI study, it is important to also evaluate for twists or strictures and where these irregularities are located. This may be a cause of persistent increase intraluminal pressure would impact the choice of stent, whether an adjunct therapy should be performed, and the duration of treatment.

24.3.4　Choosing the Right Stent

24.3.4.1　Traditional Esophageal Stents

Esophageal stents have evolved significantly since their initial use in the management of post-LGS leaks. There are now an exhaustive variety of options available; different sizes, lengths, materials, and choice of custom-tailored stents. There is unfortunately very limited data available to validate use of one specific type of stent. Various stent materials have not shown a statistically significant difference in the success rate of treating esophageal leaks, but no similar studies have been done to directly compare different stents for the management of staple line leaks following sleeve gastrectomy [22]. It is important to note that the use of endoscopic esophageal stent for management of LSG leaks is an off-label use, as most stents are US Food and Drug Administration (FDA)-approved for malignant esophageal strictures or fistulas. The overall quality of evidence is poor as published data is predominantly retrospective case series. Many articles include either insufficient details or significant heterogeneity among patient population and leak characteristic to allow for a comparison of different types of stent.

Currently, the most widely used traditional esophageal stents in post-LSG leaks are self-expandable stents. These stents typically consist of cross-hatched rows of material that expand after deployment and remain in position with radial force and luminal friction. There is one available self-expandable plastic stent (SEPS) (Polyflex, Boston Scientific) that is FDA approved for esophageal fistula and removability. However, due to its cumbersome nature and large caliber, rigid introducer catheter, SEPS are not wide used in the United States. There are a multitude of self-expandable metal (SEMS) available in the United States including those manufactured by Boston Scientific, Cook Medical, EndoChoice, Merit-Endotek, and Taewoong Medical Co [23]. There is no significant difference in success rate of leak resolution between metal and plastic stents [12, 24, 25]. Therefore, due to ease of passage and low profile, flexible catheters, SEMS are commonly used off-label for treatment of sleeve leaks.

SEMS used for post-LSG leaks are either fully covered (FCSEMS), or partially covered (PCSEMS). Manufacturers have developed various coating materials, usually silicone or a polymer, to prevent tissue ingrowth. In general, fully covered metal stents (FCSEMS) have been advocated for the treatment of benign disease given the relative ease of subsequent removal and are the most commonly used type of stent employed for closure of leaks and fistulae. However, FCSEMS are associated with higher rates of migration than other stents. Stent migration can result in unsuccessful leak closure, mucosal erosions, and rarely intestinal obstruction requiring stent repositioning, retrieval, or replacement [26]. A recent retrospective review of 24 patients after sleeve gastrectomy (SG), demonstrated a 66.7% success rate of healing leaks with fully covered nitinol esophageal stent (Wallflex; Boston Scientific, Natick, MA). Notably, this study found a migration rate of 22%, with all migrated stents successfully retrieved endoscopically [18]. In another larger multicenter retrospective study of 110 patients treated for post-LSG leaks, stent migration was most frequently observed with FCSEMS (46.1%), but was also seen to a lesser extent with PCSEMS (15.4%) and SEPS (25.0%) [24]. In the study, perforation from stent migration occurred 4.5% of stents placed and was only reported with FCSEMS.

Endoscopists have explored using stent anchoring techniques to minimize stent migration. Endoscopic sutures have demonstrated better results than clips [27]. In a systematic review and meta-analysis, suture fixation decreased stent migration rates to 15.9% [28] (Figs. 24.1, 24.2 and 24.3). Other studies have also reports similar improvement in rates of migration [29, 30]. Additionally, a comparative multicenter study showed that, only patients with a prior history of stent migration were less likely to experience recurrent stent migration with endoscopic suturing [27]. However, the degree of decline in migration rates is not consistently demonstrated throughout the current literature; some cohorts have continued to experience migration rate as high as 47% despite using sutures anchoring techniques [31, 32]. Inconsistent and poor guidance on the technical aspects of suture fixation is the limiting aspect of this endoscopic technique. Information regarding the number of sutures placed, the tension of the sutures, and the location are often excluded in case

Fig. 24.1 LSG anastomotic leak

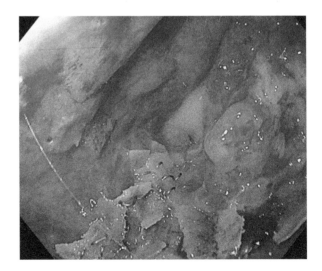

Fig. 24.2 LSG
anastomotic leak (close
up view)

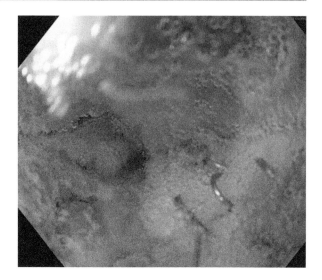

Fig. 24.3 Fully covered
self-expandable metal stent
(FCSEMS) with
suturing device

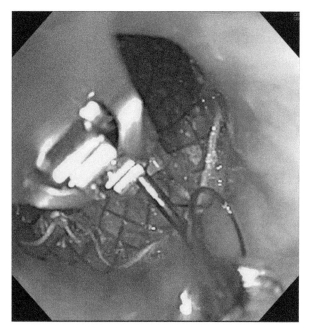

reports or are extremely variable [30, 31]. More recently, a new over the scope clip specially designed for stent fixation has been developed that allows for easier deployment (Stentfix OTSC, Ovesco, Tuebingen, Germany). However, there is no comparative data to date on this new device.

Partially covered stents are an alternative choice to fully covered stent, although their use in post-LSG leaks are more limited. PCSEMS are designed with metal exposed at the proximal and distal ends to allow for greater traction, decrease leak between stent and luminal wall, and decrease incidence of stent displacement. However, tissue ingrowth causing the stent to be embedded into the esophageal wall is an important reported limitation affecting the safety of stent removal in up to 25% of patients [33, 34]. Very few studies have evaluated partially covered stents solely in the treatment post-LSG leaks and a majority of case series pool experience for all patients treated after bariatric surgery. In Roux-en-Y gastric bypass leaks, the use of partially covered stents prevented major migration but at the cost of significant mucosal injury and difficult removal. In a series of 8 patients, Wei et al. identified significant mucosal injury (erosion, ulceration, and granulation tissue) at the proximal uncovered portion in 79% of stents placed [35]. In one retrospective analysis, 3 of 5 patients treated for early leak post-LSG with partially covered metallic stent had no significant stent migrations however due to tissue ingrowth on either end of the partially covered stents, the median intervention time for removal was 23 min longer [5]. To address the complication of embedded partially covered stents, endoscopists have developed a stent-in-stent technique. This method consists of a fully covered SEMs or SEPs be placed inside the lumen of the embedded stent to induce ischemia and pressure necrosis. To ensure success, stents diameter should at least equal to the embedded stent and the length of the fully covered stent should completely overlap the reactive tissue ingrowth. Studies report that extractions done in this fashion had a successful removal rate of 91–100% with a SIS dwell time of 1–3 weeks [33, 34]. Nonetheless, the decision to use partially covered stents should weigh the lower risk of stent migration with the increase risk of embedded stent and need for additional endoscopic interventions.

24.3.4.2   Large Bariatric Stents

In recent years, new bariatric stents have been developed specifically for the treatment of post- LSG leaks to address the shortcomings of traditional esophageal stents. There is a tendency for stent migration with shorter stent length. These novel stents are designed with longer lengths and with larger diameters to theoretically decrease the risk of stent migration and increase mucosal coaptation. Manufacturers have also developed flared ends/larger flanges to help anchor the stent in place. The flared proximal end is also thought to provide a tight mucosal seal which is important to prevent ongoing contamination. These ultra-large stents are positioned from the distal esophagus to either the prepyloric or postpyloic position, completely bypassing the entire gastric sleeve. Available bariatric stents include Megastent (Taewoong Medical Industries, Kangseo-GuSongjung-Dong, South Korea), Niti-S Beta stent (Taewoong Medical Industries), and the Hanarostent (M.I.Tech, Seoul, South Korea). Unfortunately, many of the studies related to these novel stents included a heterogeneous population, including leaks after different types of surgery (Roux-en-Y gastric bypass and LSG), different duration of leak (acute and chronic), previous endoscopic treatment, and combined techniques (CSEMS and over-the-scope-clips).

The largest retrospective series to date was conducted by de Moura and colleagues. Thirty-seven patients with acute and early leaks post-LSG, were treated with one of two novel large bariatric stents. Both stents have a length of 24 cm and a body diameter of 28 mm, with either 32 or 36 mm proximal and distal flanges. Overall, 78% of leaks resolved with stent placement. A trend toward higher success rates were noted in stents that were placed in a pre-pyloric rather than a post-pyloric position, largely due to less displacement in the former rather than any adverse events [36]. Of note, neither the size of the leak nor the stent dwell time was statistically significant in stent success. The most common adverse events were patient reported symptoms including abdominal pain, nausea, reflux (89%), followed by stent migration (21%) with two requiring surgery for removal, 10 ulcerations, and 2 esophageal perforations. The writers concluded that the longer stent design with large flanges did not seem to decrease migration rates significantly but unfortunately may contribute to higher rates of serious adverse events. Other studies also report that the success rate of bariatric stents were comparable to that of traditional fully covered stents [37–39]. Similar to De Moura et al., these studies showed that stent migration continued to be a complication despite the longer length with higher rates of additional associated adverse events: intolerance necessitating removal, esophageal strictures, bleeding, perforation [14, 38–40].

Another area of interest is the development of stents that naturally decompose into non-toxic chemical over time, called biodegradable stents (BDS). The design of an absorbable stent is appealing for the treatment of postsurgical leaks because it would obviate the need for endoscopic stent removal. While there are a number of stents available in the market, majority have been used in treatment of esophageal/gastric strictures. They are not FDA-approved for treatment of post-LSG leaks.

24.3.5 Post Procedure Follow-Up and Stent Removal

After initial placement of a stent, it is important to assess reflux from the distal end or lack of tight seal at the proximal end, as both of these would lead to persistent leakage. If either are seen, it may be important to reposition the stent or to add a second overlapping stent. Oral intake is usually restricted for the first 24–48 h to allow for full stent expansion. Most authors liberated oral diet stepwise from liquid to semi-solid and finally to regular diet over the course of days to weeks [41]. A proton pump inhibitor is often prescribed for the duration of stenting [18]. Stent intolerance is frequent and can occur in over 50% of patient with nausea and/or vomiting during the first week, requiring IV antiemetics, and intolerance leading to stent removal occurs in about 10–15% of patients [42].

The approach of stent surveillance during the stenting period can vary depending on institutional practices. Majority of interventionalists complete a UGI study or CT with oral contrast routinely after initial stent placement to ensure appropriate placement. However, re-imaging to assess for migration or persistence of leakage is much more variable; some endoscopists have completed abdominal x-rays at regular intervals to survey stent positioning while others obtain studies whenever there is a clinical suspicion of persistent leakage or stent displacement [18, 38]. When stent migration was suspected, endoscopy was usually performed to adjust the stent position or to exchange the stent. Healing is defined as the absence of leakage of contrast agent as shown by various imaging techniques (barium swallow, CT scan).

Regarding the duration in which stents should remain in situ, several studies have suggested that stents should not be kept in place for longer than 6–8 weeks [18, 26, 43]. The decision is a balance between allowing enough time for leak closure while decreasing the risk of stent migration or tissue hyperplasia. Factors associated with a shorter time to healing: small size (≤1 cm) of fistula, interval between LSG and fistula diagnosis ≤3 days and a short interval (≤21 days) between fistula diagnosis and first endoscopy [9, 24]. Blackmon and colleagues did not have difficulty with extraction of fully covered nor partially covered SEMs if the attempted within a 30-days [7]. However, interventionalists have noted that stent removal earlier than 4 weeks showed persistent leak and required additional endoscopic therapy (glue injection with clipping or stent re-insertion) [44]. With partially covered stents embedding can occur as early as 2–3 weeks after stent placement with [34].

Healing of the leak should be confirmed on imaging or endoscopically by contrast injection prior to stent removal. In cases with persistent leakage, repeat endoscopic therapy could be explored. Most common reasons for failed endoscopic extraction are stent migration and mucosal hypertrophy.

24.3.5.1 Failure of Initial Stent Placement, Is It Worth Re-Stenting

In an international expert panel consensus statement on best practice guidelines, 88% of expert bariatric surgeons believed that if GI stenting has not lead to healing of a chronic proximal leak or fistula after SG within 12 weeks, surgical intervention is indicated [45]. A systematic review by Hughes and colleagues showed that patients solely treated with endoscopic stent placement had a pooled initial success rate of 62% [6]. Fourteen percent of patients in this study required further endoscopic treatment. Overall, conventional SEMs achieves an efficacy of about 70–80% with a median of 1–3 endoscopies, and a mean time for healing that varies between 43 and 82 days [6, 32, 46–48]. In case of persistent leak despite stent placement for 6–8 weeks, placement of a second SEM may achieve leak closure success rate of up to 80–90% [48]. Adjunct or alternative endoscopic therapies can also be explored. However, in a large multicenter study that reviewed outcomes of 110 post-LSG leak patients found that the chance of healing was greater following surgery than endoscopic treatment if treatment duration exceeded 6 month (50.0% vs. 41.7% respectively) following surgery than following endoscopic treatment when duration of treatment exceeded 6 months [24].

24.3.6 Adjunct/Alternative Techniques

When peri-esophageal fluid collections or strictures are identified, adjunct therapies such as drainage and/or dilation can be completed with stenting. Endoscopic internal drainage (EID) consists of inserting one or two double-pigtail plastic stents into the fluid-filled cavity to facilitate drainage into the digestive lumen. This endoscopic intervention has gained popularity as a stand-alone treatment of post-SG [36, 49]. In the largest series reporting on EID, 78% of patients were cured by EID alone after a mean of 58 days without the need for further interventions [49]. A study by Nedeleu et al. suggests that pigtail drainage without stents should be reserved for freely draining fistulae smaller than 10 mm [42]. However, those with larger leaks, would likely benefit from a combination of EID and stent placement. The combination of covered stent and double pigtail drainage for the treatment of leaks (>2 cm in diameter) associated with significantly fewer endoscopic procedures and a shorter treatment duration [50].

Stenosis and strictures after LSG occur with a prevalence of 0.1–3.9% [51]. These lesions often cause higher pressures in the gastric sleeve and can precipitate anastomotic leaks. Dilation of a stenotic region is usually done with through the scope (TTS) balloons or achalasia pneumatic balloons. TTS dilations have a reported efficacy of about 40% and may require multiple sessions [9]. Pneumatic dilations have an efficacy of up to 70% but is a challenging technique and is not without risks as it requires serial dilations with high inflating pressures [52, 53]. Pneumatic dilations in conjunction with a septotomy technique to drain walled-off peri-gastric collections have had notable efficacy in the management of late and chronic leaks following sleeve gastrectomy [54, 55]. However, only short-segment stenotic lesions are amenable to dilation [56].

Methods to directly close the wall defect including fibrin glues, suturing, or clips have also been proposed and can sometimes be used to augment endoscopic stenting [36]. The use of sealant materials for post-LSG leaks have not demonstrated consistent efficacy as stand-alone therapy. Some studies have shown that sealants have better outcomes when used after stent placement [57] While generally well tolerated frequently multiple applications are often required. Small-capacity through-the-scope clips (TTSC) have also been used sequentially to close leaks. However, TTSC have fallen out of favor since the development of newer and larger over-the-scope clips (OTSC) [58]. OTSCs allow for full-thickness bites, bringing a bigger region of tissue into approximation. OTSC placement have been reported be safe and effective for the treatment chronic GI fistulas after LSG [59]. However, the data regarding its utility in early leaks are not clear. A systematic analysis done in 2017 noted that only 73 cases of post-LSG leaks/fistulas had been treated with over-the-scope clips (OTSC) and a total of 24 was done with concomitant stent placement [60]. The overall closure success rate was 85%. Of note about half of the leaks sized less than 10 mm [60]. Importantly, the tissue surrounding the leak or fistula must be robust enough to be held within the jaws of the clips.

Endoscopic suturing is technically more challenging than the application of clipping devices or sealants, however, it is capable of closing larger defects. Small case series have demonstrated its potential usefulness as either a primary treatment or as an adjunct to other therapeutic interventions for leaks after LSG [61]. However, this modality struggles with durability of closure, with high rates of reopening especially with defects >20 mm [62].

24.4   Recommendations Based on the Data

- Surgical/percutaneous drainage coupled with self-expandable metal stent (SEMS) is appropriate first-line modality for the management of leaks after sleeve gastrectomy, especially those not classified as chronic (low quality evidence, strong recommendation).
- We recommend the use of fully covered stents with endoscopic suturing as opposed to partially covered stents in post-LSG leaks to prevent stent embedding (low quality evidence, strong recommendation).
- Embedded stents are more common with partially covered SEMS and a stent-in-stent technique should be used for removal of the embedded stents (low quality evidence, strong recommendation).
- No specific time to stent removal can be recommended and the duration of stenting should be individualized.
- Data on the use of biodegradable stents are limited and cannot be recommended at this time.

24.4.1 A Personal View of the Data

The data, although low quality in general, suggests that endoscopic stent placement should be considered for stable patients who develop early post-LSG leaks. While a number of factors influence the rate of successful leak resolution and the rate of complications over 60% of patients with primary leaks can avoid the morbidity and mortality of reoperation. Despite the fact that temporary stent placement is fraught complications and stent design has a long way to go, we still believe, this technique should become the method of choice in treatment of early post-LSG leaks. Prospective studies with larger samples sizes should be undertaken to better evaluate and compare the variety of techniques available. More research is also needed to clearly identify the appropriate treatment of chronic leak after LSG.

References

1. Deitel M, Gagner M, Erickson AL, Crosby RD. Third international summit: current status of sleeve gastrectomy. Surg Obes Relat Dis. 2011;7(6):749–59. https://doi.org/10.1016/j.soard.2011.07.017.
2. Kim J, Azagury D, Eisenberg D, DeMaria E, Campos GM. ASMBS position statement on prevention, detection, and treatment of gastrointestinal leak after gastric bypass and sleeve gastrectomy, including the roles of imaging, surgical exploration, and nonoperative management. Surg Obes Relat Dis. 2015;11(4):739–48. https://doi.org/10.1016/j.soard.2015.05.001.
3. Moszkowicz D, et al. Sleeve gastrectomy severe complications: is it always a reasonable surgical option? Obes Surg. 2013;23(5):676–86. https://doi.org/10.1007/s11695-012-0860-4.
4. Baker RS, Foote J, Kemmeter P, Brady R, Vroegop T, Serveld M. The science of stapling and leaks. Obes Surg. 2004;14(10):1290–8. https://doi.org/10.1381/0960892042583888.

5. Garofalo F, Noreau-Nguyen M, Denis R, Atlas H, Garneau P, Pescarus R. Evolution of endoscopic treatment of sleeve gastrectomy leaks: from partially covered to long, fully covered stents. Surg Obes Relat Dis. 2017;13(6):925–32. https://doi.org/10.1016/j.soard.2016.12.019.
6. Hughes D, Hughes I, Khanna A. Management of staple line leaks following sleeve gastrectomy—a systematic review. Obes Surg. 2019;29(9):2759–72. https://doi.org/10.1007/s11695-019-03896-3.
7. Blackmon SH, Santora R, Schwarz P, Barroso A, Dunkin BJ. Utility of removable esophageal covered self-expanding metal stents for leak and fistula management. Ann Thorac Surg. 2010;89(3):931–7. https://doi.org/10.1016/j.athoracsur.2009.10.061.
8. Tan JT, Kariyawasam S, Wijeratne T, Chandraratna HS. Diagnosis and management of gastric leaks after laparoscopic sleeve gastrectomy for morbid obesity. Obes Surg. 2010;20(4):403–9. https://doi.org/10.1007/s11695-009-0020-7.
9. Souto-Rodríguez R. Endoluminal solutions to bariatric surgery complications: a review with a focus on technical aspects and results. World J Gastrointest Endosc. 2017;9(3):105–26. https://doi.org/10.4253/wjge.v9.i3.105.
10. Rosenthal RJ, et al. International sleeve gastrectomy expert panel consensus statement: best practice guidelines based on experience of >12,000 cases. Surg Obes Relat Dis Off J Am Soc Bariatr Surg. 2012;8(1):8–19. https://doi.org/10.1016/j.soard.2011.10.019.
11. Spyropoulos C, Argentou M-I, Petsas T, Thomopoulos K, Kehagias I, Kalfarentzos F. Management of gastrointestinal leaks after surgery for clinically severe obesity. Surg Obes Relat Dis. 2012;8(5):609–15. https://doi.org/10.1016/j.soard.2011.04.222.
12. Alazmi W, Al-Sabah S, Ali DA, Almazeedi S. Treating sleeve gastrectomy leak with endoscopic stenting: the Kuwaiti experience and review of recent literature. Surg Endosc. 2014;28(12):3425–8. https://doi.org/10.1007/s00464-014-3616-5.
13. Murino A, Arvanitakis M, Le Moine O, Blero D, Devière J, Eisendrath P. Effectiveness of endoscopic management using self-expandable metal stents in a large cohort of patients with post-bariatric leaks. Obes Surg. 2015;25(9):1569–76. https://doi.org/10.1007/s11695-015-1596-8.
14. Simon F, Siciliano I, Gillet A, Castel B, Coffin B, Msika S. Gastric leak after laparoscopic sleeve gastrectomy: early covered self-expandable stent reduces healing time. Obes Surg. 2013;23(5):687–92. https://doi.org/10.1007/s11695-012-0861-3.
15. Aydın MT, et al. Endoscopic stenting for laparoscopic sleeve gastrectomy leaks. Turk J Surgery Ulusal Cerrahi Derg. 2016;32(4):275–80. https://doi.org/10.5152/UCD.2016.3122.
16. Nimeri A, Ibrahim M, Maasher A, Al Hadad M. Management algorithm for leaks following laparoscopic sleeve gastrectomy. Obes Surg. 2016;26(1):21–5. https://doi.org/10.1007/s11695-015-1751-2.
17. Puig CA, Waked TM, Baron TH, Song LMWK, Gutierrez J, Sarr MG. The role of endoscopic stents in the management of chronic anastomotic and staple line leaks and chronic strictures after bariatric surgery. Surg Obes Relat Dis. 2014;10(4):613–7. https://doi.org/10.1016/j.soard.2013.12.018.
18. Martin del Campo SE, Mikami DJ, Needleman BJ, Noria SF. Endoscopic stent placement for treatment of sleeve gastrectomy leak: a single institution experience with fully covered stents. Surg Obes Relat Dis. 2018;14(4):453–61. https://doi.org/10.1016/j.soard.2017.12.015.
19. Musella M, Milone M, Bianco P, Maietta P, Galloro G. Acute leaks following laparoscopic sleeve gastrectomy: early surgical repair according to a management algorithm. J Laparoendosc Adv Surg Tech. 2015;26(2):85–91. https://doi.org/10.1089/lap.2015.0343.
20. Nguyen NT, Nguyen X-MT, Dholakia C. The use of endoscopic stent in management of leaks after sleeve gastrectomy. Obes Surg. 2010;20(9):1289–92. https://doi.org/10.1007/s11695-010-0186-z.
21. Mathus-Vliegen EMH. The cooperation between endoscopists and surgeons in treating complications of bariatric surgery. Best Pract Res Clin Gastroenterol. 2014;28(4):703–25. https://doi.org/10.1016/j.bpg.2014.07.011.
22. Abulfaraj M, Mathavan V, Arregui M. Therapeutic flexible endoscopy replacing surgery: part 1—leaks and fistulas. Tech Gastrointest Endosc. 2013;15(4):191–9. https://doi.org/10.1016/j.tgie.2013.08.001.

23. Hindy P, Hong J, Lam-Tsai Y, Gress F. A comprehensive review of esophageal stents. Gastroenterol Hepatol. 2012;8(8):526–34.
24. Christophorou D, et al. Endoscopic treatment of fistula after sleeve gastrectomy: results of a multicenter retrospective study. Endoscopy. 2015;47(11):988–96. https://doi.org/10.105 5/s-0034-1392262.
25. Spaander M, et al. Esophageal stenting for benign and malignant disease: European society of gastrointestinal endoscopy (ESGE) clinical guideline. Endoscopy. 2016;48(10):939–48. https://doi.org/10.1055/s-0042-114210.
26. Puli SR, Spofford IS, Thompson CC. Use of self-expandable stents in the treatment of bariatric surgery leaks: a systematic review and meta-analysis. Gastrointest Endosc. 2012;75(2):287–93. https://doi.org/10.1016/j.gie.2011.09.010.
27. Ngamruengphong S, et al. Endoscopic suturing for the prevention of stent migration in benign upper gastrointestinal conditions: a comparative multicenter study. Endoscopy. 2016;48(09):802–8. https://doi.org/10.1055/s-0042-108567.
28. Law R, Prabhu A, Fujii-Lau L, Shannon C, Singh S. Stent migration following endoscopic suture fixation of esophageal self-expandable metal stents: a systematic review and meta-analysis. Surg Endosc. 2018;32(2):675–81. https://doi.org/10.1007/s00464-017-5720-9.
29. Krishnan V, Hutchings K, Godwin A, Wong JT, Teixeira J. Long-term outcomes following endoscopic stenting in the management of leaks after foregut and bariatric surgery. Surg Endosc. 2019;33(8):2691–5. https://doi.org/10.1007/s00464-018-06632-7.
30. Sharaiha RZ, et al. Esophageal stenting with sutures: time to redefine our standards? J. Clin. Gastroenterol. 2014;49(6):e57–60. https://doi.org/10.1097/MCG.0000000000000198.
31. Fujii LL, Bonin EA, Baron TH, Gostout CJ, Song LMWK. Utility of an endoscopic suturing system for prevention of covered luminal stent migration in the upper GI tract. Gastrointest Endosc. 2013;78(5):787–93. https://doi.org/10.1016/j.gie.2013.06.014.
32. Smith ZL, et al. Outcomes of endoscopic treatment of leaks and fistulae after sleeve gastrectomy: results from a large multicenter U.S. cohort. Surg Obes Relat Dis. 2019;15(6):850–5. https://doi.org/10.1016/j.soard.2019.04.009.
33. DaVee T, et al. Stent-in-stent technique for removal of embedded partially covered self-expanding metal stents. Surg Endosc. 2016;30(6):2332–41. https://doi.org/10.1007/s00464-015-4475-4.
34. Hirdes MMC, Siersema PD, Houben MHMG, Weusten BLAM, Vleggaar FP. Stent-in-stent technique for removal of embedded esophageal self-expanding metal stents. Am J Gastroenterol. 2011;106(2):286–93. https://doi.org/10.1038/ajg.2010.394.
35. Wei W, Ramaswamy A, de la Torre R, Miedema BW. Partially covered esophageal stents cause bowel injury when used to treat complications of bariatric surgery. Surg Endosc. 2013;27(1):56–60. https://doi.org/10.1007/s00464-012-2406-1.
36. de Moura DTH, et al. Outcomes of a novel bariatric stent in the management of sleeve gastrectomy leaks: a multicenter study. Surg Obes Relat Dis. 2019;15(8):1241–51. https://doi.org/10.1016/j.soard.2019.05.022.
37. Klimczak T, Klimczak J, Szewczyk T, Janczak P, Jurałowicz P. Endoscopic treatment of leaks after laparoscopic sleeve gastrectomy using MEGA esophageal covered stents. Surg Endosc. 2018;32(4):2038–45. https://doi.org/10.1007/s00464-017-5900-7.
38. Shehab H, Abdallah E, Gawdat K, Elattar I. Large bariatric-specific stents and over-the-scope clips in the management of post-bariatric surgery leaks. Obes Surg. 2018;28(1):15–24. https://doi.org/10.1007/s11695-017-2808-1.
39. van Wezenbeek MR, de Milliano MM, Nienhuijs SW, Friederich P, Gilissen LPL. A specifically designed stent for anastomotic leaks after bariatric surgery: experiences in a tertiary referral hospital. Obes Surg. 2016;26(8):1875–80. https://doi.org/10.1007/s11695-015-2027-6.
40. Serra C, et al. Treatment of gastric leaks with coated self-expanding stents after sleeve gastrectomy. Obes Surg. 2007;17(7):866–72. https://doi.org/10.1007/s11695-007-9161-8.
41. Eubanks S, et al. Use of endoscopic stents to treat anastomotic complications after bariatric surgery. J Am Coll Surg. 2008;206(5):935–938. https://doi.org/10.1016/j.jamcollsurg.2008.02.016. discussion 938–939

42. Nedelcu M, Manos T, Cotirlet A, Noel P, Gagner M. Outcome of leaks after sleeve gastrectomy based on a new algorithm adressing leak size and gastric stenosis. Obes Surg. 2015;25(3):559–63. https://doi.org/10.1007/s11695-014-1561-y.
43. Southwell T, Lim TH, Ogra R. Endoscopic therapy for treatment of staple line leaks postlaparoscopic sleeve gastrectomy (LSG): experience from a large bariatric surgery centre in New Zealand. Obes Surg. 2016;26(6):1155–62. https://doi.org/10.1007/s11695-015-1931-0.
44. Guzaiz N, et al. Gastroesophageal stenting for the management of post sleeve gastrectomy leak. Saudi Med. J. 2016;37(12):1339–43. https://doi.org/10.15537/smj.2016.12.15761.
45. Kichler K, Rosenthal RJ, DeMaria E, Higa K. Reoperative surgery for nonresponders and complicated sleeve gastrectomy operations in patients with severe obesity. An international expert panel consensus statement to define best practice guidelines. Surg Obes Relat Dis. 2019;15(2):173–86. https://doi.org/10.1016/j.soard.2018.11.006.
46. Bashah M, Khidir N, El-Matbouly M. Management of leak after sleeve gastrectomy: outcomes of 73 cases, treatment algorithm and predictors of resolution. Obes Surg. 2020;30(2):515–20. https://doi.org/10.1007/s11695-019-04203-w.
47. Okazaki O, et al. Efficacy and safety of stents in the treatment of fistula after bariatric surgery: a systematic review and meta-analysis. Obes Surg. 2018;28(6):1788–96. https://doi.org/10.1007/s11695-018-3236-6.
48. Quezada N, et al. Effect of early use of covered self-expandable endoscopic stent on the treatment of postoperative stapler line leaks. Obes Surg. 2015;25(10):1816–21. https://doi.org/10.1007/s11695-015-1622-x.
49. Donatelli G, et al. Treatment of leaks following sleeve gastrectomy by endoscopic internal drainage (EID). Obes Surg. 2015;25(7):1293–301. https://doi.org/10.1007/s11695-015-1675-x.
50. Rebibo L, Hakim S, Brazier F, Dhahri A, Cosse C, Regimbeau J-M. New endoscopic technique for the treatment of large gastric fistula or gastric stenosis associated with gastric leaks after sleeve gastrectomy. Surg Obes Relat Dis. 2016;12(8):1577–84. https://doi.org/10.1016/j.soard.2016.04.026.
51. Peterson RM, Scott JD. Managing complications of bariatric surgery. Adv Surg. 2019;53:55–68. https://doi.org/10.1016/j.yasu.2019.04.004.
52. Vargas EJ, Abu Dayyeh BK. Keep calm under pressure: a paradigm shift in managing postsurgical leaks. Gastrointest Endosc. 2018;87(2):438–41. https://doi.org/10.1016/j.gie.2017.09.016.
53. Deslauriers V, et al. Endoscopic management of post-laparoscopic sleeve gastrectomy stenosis. Surg Endosc. 2018;32(2):601–9. https://doi.org/10.1007/s00464-017-5709-4.
54. Shnell M, Gluck N, Abu-Abeid S, Santo E, Fishman S. Use of endoscopic septotomy for the treatment of late staple-line leaks after laparoscopic sleeve gastrectomy. Endoscopy. 2017;49(01):59–63. https://doi.org/10.1055/s-0042-117109.
55. Campos JM, et al. Septotomy and balloon dilation to treat chronic leak after sleeve gastrectomy: technical principles. Obes Surg. 2016;26(8):1992–3. https://doi.org/10.1007/s11695-016-2256-3.
56. Parikh A, et al. Management options for symptomatic stenosis after laparoscopic vertical sleeve gastrectomy in the morbidly obese. Surg Endosc. 2012;26(3):738–46. https://doi.org/10.1007/s00464-011-1945-1.
57. Vilallonga R, Himpens J, Bosch B, van de Vrande S, Bafort J. Role of percutaneous glue treatment after persisting leak after laparoscopic sleeve gastrectomy. Obes Surg. 2016;26(7):1378–83. https://doi.org/10.1007/s11695-015-1959-1.
58. Winder JS, Pauli EM. Novel endoscopic modalities for closure of perforations, leaks, and fistula in the gastrointestinal tract. Tech Gastrointest Endosc. 2019;21(2):109–14. https://doi.org/10.1016/j.tgie.2019.04.004.
59. Mercky P, et al. Usefulness of over-the-scope clipping system for closing digestive fistulas. Dig Endosc. 2015;27(1):18–24. https://doi.org/10.1111/den.12295.
60. Shoar S, et al. Efficacy and safety of the over-the-scope clip (OTSC) system in the management of leak and fistula after laparoscopic sleeve gastrectomy: a systematic review. Obes Surg. 2017;27(9):2410–8. https://doi.org/10.1007/s11695-017-2651-4.

61. Lamb LC, et al. Use of an endoscopic suturing platform for the management of staple line dehiscence after laparoscopic sleeve gastrectomy. Obes Surg. 2019;30:895–900. https://doi.org/10.1007/s11695-019-04344-y.
62. Willingham FF, Buscaglia JM. Endoscopic management of gastrointestinal leaks and fistulae. Clin Gastroenterol Hepatol. 2015;13(10):1714–21. https://doi.org/10.1016/j.cgh.2015.02.010.

Reoperation for Repair of Anastomotic Leaks and Staple Line Disruptions

Andres Felipe Sanchez, Emanuele Lo Menzo, Samuel Szomstein, and Raul J. Rosenthal

25.1 Introduction

The worldwide prevalence of obesity continues to exhibit upward statistical trends. Between 2015 and 2016, the Centers for Disease Control and Prevention (CDC) reports 93.3 million or 39.8% of adults in the United States with obesity [1]. According to the 2013 AHA/ACC/TOS Guidelines for the Management of Overweight and Obesity in Adults, 64.5% of American adults are recommended for weight loss treatment [2]. With a high safety profile, bariatric surgery is recognized as the most effective treatment for morbid obesity. Based on its highly effective weight loss and improvement of comorbidities associated with obesity [3–5], it is not surprising that the total number of bariatric operations worldwide continue to increase [6]. Although uncommon, perioperative complications related to the technical aspect of bariatric surgery includes hemorrhaging, leak, and stenosis. This chapter reviews the etiologies of AL and SLD, as well as common presenting signs and symptoms, diagnostic evaluation, and operative and non-operative managements.

25.2 Etiology

An AL or SLD is a known, potentially severe complication following gastrointestinal surgery. Considered the most concerning operative complication after bariatric surgery, it can lead to significant morbidity and mortality if missed or mishandled. Leaks can occur either from an anastomosis or a staple-line. The causes of postoperative leak depend on patient and technical factors involved.

A. F. Sanchez · E. Lo Menzo · S. Szomstein · R. J. Rosenthal (✉)
The Bariatric and Metabolic Institute, Cleveland Clinic Florida, Weston, FL, USA
e-mail: SANCHEA8@ccf.org; lomenze@ccf.org; szomsts@ccf.org; rosentr@ccf.org

© Springer Nature Switzerland AG 2021
J. Alverdy, Y. Vigneswaran (eds.), *Difficult Decisions in Bariatric Surgery*,
Difficult Decisions in Surgery: An Evidence-Based Approach,
https://doi.org/10.1007/978-3-030-55329-6_25

25.2.1 Patient Dependent Factors

Patient related factors associated with higher incidence of developing anastomotic leak after bariatric surgeries are similar for all bariatric procedures. In particular, male patients, age > 55 years, those with super morbid obesity (body mass index >50 kg/m^2), those with obesity-associated comorbidities, and those with delayed wound healing are at significantly higher risk of developing a leak [7–9]. Various studies have reported the male sex is an independent risk factor for developing leaks. This is most likely attributed to males' tendency to develop more central than peripheral obesity and consequently a greater amount of intraperitoneal fat, increasing the technical difficulty of bariatric surgery. Studies have also found a correlation with medical history of diabetes, liver cirrhosis, renal failure, current or recent smoking history, and the presence of poor nutrition as risk factors for leak [10, 11]. Consequently, special consideration should be given to the elderly, male, diabetic, and smoking populations during postoperative surveillance.

25.2.2 Technical Factors

The optimal anastomosis is sealed, tension-free, with good vascular supply. Technical factors involved in developing a leak include issues such as poor technique and tissue apposition when constructing the anastomosis, excess tension, the presence of staple-line hemorrhaging, and tissue ischemia. The timing of a leak is strictly connected to its etiology. SLD secondary to issues such as poor technique in construction of the anastomosis most frequently occur within the first 48 hours postoperatively, whereas AL present 5–7 days postoperatively and are the result of tension that will ultimately create ischemia. Leaks due to distal narrowing can manifest chronically as a non-healing fistula [12, 13]. Also, the requirement of high dose vasopressors for hemodynamic instability secondary to other causes (i.e. hypovolemia, pulmonary embolisms, sepsis of other origin, etc.), can determine local ischemia of the anastomosis and determine a leak.

Technical factors involving poor technique in construction of the anastomosis include issues such as stapler misfiring due to stapler height, excessive tissue within the jaws of the stapler, and malformed staples at the staple-crotch [14]. When selecting the appropriate staple height and size, consideration should be given to the thickness of the gastric wall. However, there is no method to definitively measure the thickness of the gastric tissue. Experts agree that it would not be appropriate to use staples with closed height less than 1.5 mm on any part of the gastric wall [13]. Bunching of tissue or thickened tissue can lead to stapler misfiring. Adequate tissue mobilization to attain complete visualization and symmetrical lateral retraction avoiding rotation of the staple-line, are key factors to achieve proper staple formation. Oversewing staple-lines, buttressing materials, and fibrin glue have been used to provide staple-line reinforcement. Improper oversewing of the staple line has been reported to increase the risk of tearing at the point of suture penetration in sleeve gastrectomy [15, 16]. However, several international experts recommend providing staple-line reinforcement of the long staple line of the sleeve in order to minimize postoperative bleeding [13, 17, 18]. In fact, no definitive evidence exists on the advantage of staple-line reinforcement in postoperative sleeve leaks. The utilization of small bougie sizes less than 38-French is associated with increased risk of stricture and leak [8, 19].

This chapter will review the most common bariatric surgeries and the individual factors involved in the development of a postoperative leak.

Roux-en-Y Gastric Bypass Roux-en-Y gastric bypass (RYGB) induces weight loss by utilizing restrictive and hypoabsorptive strategies, where the jejunum is anastomosed to a 15–30 cc gastric pouch, and the biliopancreatic limb is then connected to the distal jejunum at a variable distance between 100 and 200 cm. Leaks are the second leading cause of mortality following RYGB surgery [7]. A review of the published literature reported the mean incidence of anastomotic leaks after RYGB to be at 0.8% [11]. They most commonly occur at the gastrojejunostomy (GJ); possibly due to excess tension and/or tissue ischemia at the anastomosis. Leaks at this location are likely to close spontaneously when managed nonoperatively (unless distal obstruction is present). Other potential sites for leaks include the gastric pouch, the gastric remnant, and the jejunojejunostomy (JJ) [10, 20].

Laparoscopic Sleeve Gastrectomy Laparoscopic sleeve gastrectomy (LSG) induces weight loss by utilizing restrictive and enterohormonal strategies, determined by the resection of approximately 80% of the stomach in a vertical fashion along the lesser curvature. Although LSG does not involve any anastomosis, the use of a long staple line increases the risk for technical SLD. A review of the published literature reported the mean incidence of anastomotic leaks after LSG to be at 0.7% [11], with the majority of cases presenting 5–7 days postoperatively. Leaks after LSG most commonly occur along the proximal staple line at the level of the gastroesophageal junction (GEJ) (near the gastric angle of His), most likely due to multiple factors including poor tissue apposition, ischemia, and hematomas. In addition and due to the high intraluminal gastric pressure associated with the newly formed narrow lumen of the stomach, these SLDs are difficult to heal without endoscopic or surgical intervention. The increased intraluminal gastric pressure can be exacerbated by the presence of distal narrowing, such as by torsion of the staple line resulting in a fixed stenosis or by poor technique when firing the first staple load. Also the presence of an intact pylorus contributes to this functional distal obstruction. Leaving at least 2 cm of width at the level of the incisura angularis, the narrowest portion of the stomach, prevents narrowing or obstruction [21]. Other factors that contribute to proximal leaks include tissue ischemia due to stapled transection of the fundus too close to the angle of His.

25.3   Leaks Presentation

25.3.1 Intraoperative Setting

The anastomosis or staple line should be examined intraoperatively to ensure proper sealing. This can be done visually and by performing an intraoperative leak test. During an intraoperative leak test, a dye and/or air is injected intraluminally at the anastomosis while the distal bowel/stomach is gently occluded. In the methylene blue test, presence of blue dye around the anastomosis is a positive test, indicative of a leak. In the air test, the anastomosis is submerged in saline solution, the tissue is insufflated using an endoscope, and the presence of air bubbles in the solution around the anastomosis is a positive test, indicative of a leak. Although useful in detecting leaks requiring immediate repair, these techniques have not been reported to decrease the postoperative risk of leak [22].

25.3.2 Postoperative Setting

Recognition of postoperative leaks can be particularly difficult in the morbidly obese population. Additionally, the clinical presentation can vary from asymptomatic to peritonitis, septic shock, multisystem organ failure, and death. Consequently, a high index of suspicion is important for the prompt recognition of a postoperative leak. The clinical assessment for postoperative anastomotic leaks requires a thorough analysis of the patient's vital signs and physical examination; making sure to highlight the abdominal examination. A rapid heart rate in the early postoperative setting should raise suspicion for possible leak [23]. Studies report early sustained tachycardia without oscillations and resistant to beta-blockers the principle indicator of an intra-abdominal leak (not to be confused with, early oscillating tachycardia responsive to fluid resuscitation and beta-blockers, the principle indicator of an acute hemorrhage). Tachycardia more than 120 beats per minute and/or respiratory compromise can be the most useful clinical indicators of leak [22–26]. Other clinical findings include fever and abdominal pain, which may radiate to the left shoulder or scapular region.

Leaks may have difficulty spontaneously resolving. If chronic, a leak can collect into an abscess and can form fistulous communications into adjacent structures. Gastrogastric, gastrocolic gastropleural, and gastrobronchial fistulous communications have been described in the literature [27, 28]. They can present clinically as asymptomatic or present with weight recidivism and/or non-specific symptoms related to the nearby viscera. Persistent cough, left-sided pleuritic pain, and physical examination compatible with left pleural effusion are indicative of left diaphragmatic erosion with contamination of the pleural cavity and pulmonary parenchyma [28]. Left shoulder and back pain are clinical symptoms of a possible anastomotic leak. Of course, the presence of left shoulder pain, as the only symptom, needs to be differentiated by other common etiologies, such as phrenic nerve irritation from CO_2, polar splenic infarcts determined by short gastric division, diaphragmatic irritation from the presence of a surgical drain, and pre-existing chronic back conditions.

25.4 Diagnostic Approach

Once a leak is suspected clinically, prompt diagnosis and treatment are essential. The diagnostic approach for leaks is based on clinical presentation. In early postoperative leaks presenting with signs and symptoms of hemodynamic compromise, the diagnosis is primarily clinical and emergency surgical re-exploration should be initiated, even in the absence of radiographic evidence, whereas in hemodynamically stable patients, diagnostic workup includes laboratory studies, UGI contrast studies, and CT scan to confirm the physician's clinical suspicion. Upper endoscopy can define the character-istics of a leak and can be an appropriate therapeutic option for certain situations.

Laboratory studies are often nonspecific. An early postoperative leak can present with significant leukocytosis with a left shift and elevated C-reactive protein levels >229 mg/l [29, 30]. Adjunct elevated drain amylase levels can also help identify anastomotic leaks, yielding a high sensitivity and specificity in cases using closed suction drain [22, 31]. Similarly, a methylene blue swallow test can evaluate for anastomotic leak by observing effluence of the dye through the closed suction drains after its oral administration [32]. Radiographic confirmation can be obtained by fluoroscopic studies and/or CT scan. Among the imaging studies, CT scan of the abdomen and pelvis using oral and intravenous (IV) contrast is the most sensitive and specific to diagnose leaks, and thus is the modality of choice for detecting leaks. Not only can it demonstrate contrast extravasation through the leak site and the presence of intra-abdominal collections, it can also identify potential indirect signs of leak, including surrounding tissue inflammation, fat stranding, intra-abdominal free air, and pleural effusions (see Fig. 25.1). Fluoroscopic studies, such as UGI studies using water-soluble contrast medium gastrograffin, can also identify

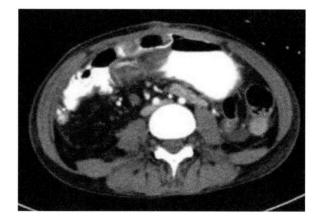

Fig. 25.1 Computed tomography (CT) scan of the abdomen and pelvis demonstrating the gastrojejunostomy following RYGB surgery and a large quantity of enteric contrast throughout the abdomen consistent with anastomotic leak

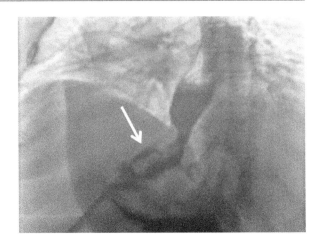

Fig. 25.2 Upper gastrointestinal contrast study demonstrating small amount of contrast extravasation (*arrow*) in region of gastrojejunostomy following RYGB surgery

contrast extravasation (see Fig. 25.2). UGI contrast studies are frequently performed routinely during the early postoperative period despite its low sensitivity (22–75% after RYGB, 0–25% after LSG) [10, 33, 34]. Although routine use often allows small leaks to go undetected giving a false sense of confidence, the decision to perform routine versus selective UGI contrast studies after bariatric surgery is left to the discretion of the surgeon. When CT scan and UGI contrast studies are used sequentially, up to one-third of patients with leaks will have both studies interpreted as normal. Therefore, the American Society for Metabolic and Bariatric Surgery (ASMBS) suggest operative re-exploration to be appropriate when postoperative leak is suspected clinically [35]. In chronic postoperative leaks presenting with signs and symptoms of left diaphragmatic erosion, plain abdominal and chest films followed by CT scan are performed and demonstrate the communicating tract, left pleural effusion and passive atelectasis of the left lower lobe with consolidation [28].

25.5 Management

The management of a leak is primarily dictated by the clinical presentation, the timing of presentation, and the location of the leak. Other influencing factors to consider include the size of the leak, extent of contamination, and whether the leak is a secondary consequence of other types of known complications, such as the presence of a distal obstruction. Based on the timing of the clinical presentation, postoperative leaks can be classified as acute (within 7 days), early (1–6 weeks), late (6–12 weeks), and chronic (> 12 weeks) [12, 13].

25.5.1 Non-Operative Management

Regardless of timing, conservative non-operative management can be considered for small, contained leaks without distal obstruction in hemodynamically stable patients. The goals of treatment are to control the local and systemic sepsis, control gastrointestinal secretions, and early nutrition. The patient should be kept nil per os (NPO) with enteric or parental nutritional support, and broad-spectrum IV antibiotics should be initiated [22, 29, 36–39]. Response to conservative management is measured clinically by assessing drain outputs and resolution of leukocytosis and fever. Additionally, studies have reported successful management of bariatric leaks using minimally invasive endoscopic techniques, such as placement of stents, clips, fibrin glue, internal drainage, and pyloric dilatation [36, 40].

Given their challenging nature, leaks may have difficulty spontaneously resolving and can collect into an abscess and chronic fistula. The persistence of injury by leaks and abscesses lead to chronic inflammation, impairing the adequacy of the gastrointestinal wound healing process, resulting in the activation of leukocytes, production of growth factors and cytokines, and increasing the occurrence of fistulas and fibrosis (adhesions subsequently leading to stenosis and distal obstructions) [41, 42]. If a distal obstruction is present it must be resolved. Most cases of distal obstructions are adequately treated with endoscopic balloon dilatation or bougie dilatation [43]. Endoscopic stenting has been described with some success; however, limitations exist.

Surgeons should maintain a low threshold for subsequent operative intervention in the face of clinical deterioration or unsuccessful non-operative management. However, before non-operative management is deemed unsuccessful, 12 weeks postoperatively should be allowed to give time to optimize the patient's nutrition and to control the local and systemic sepsis for the acute inflammation to go down for a less hostile surgical field.

25.5.2 Reoperative Management and Drainage

The choice of drainage modality is dictated by the hemodynamic status of the patient. If a patient is hemodynamically stable, less invasive, percutaneous drainage of intra-abdominal collections is performed. In the presence of hemodynamic compromise and uncontrolled sepsis, aggressive treatment with emergent operative re-exploration with extensive irrigation and drainage is mandatory to limit morbidity and mortality. Given the rapid progression to sepsis in the severely obese patient with comorbidities, when a leak is suspected clinically, even with negative or absence of imaging studies, emergent operative re-exploration is appropriate.

In an acute/early postoperative leak, the primary goal of re-exploration is to ensure extensive washout and drainage to manage the local abdominal sepsis. Never reconstruct in an acute situation with a hemodynamically unstable patient. In an emergency, always choose the smallest procedure. Secondary goals include confirmation of diagnosis and insertion of an enteral feeding tube (into the excluded stomach in RYGB; a JJ in LSG). Under these circumstances, primary repair can be attempted, although often may not be feasible due to extensive inflammatory changes and poor tissue integrity at the leak site. Nonetheless, the literature describes most effective outcomes of primary repair when performed within the first two days postoperatively, with significantly decreasing efficacy thereafter [24, 29, 37]. In most cases, extensive irrigation and control of the contamination is the only plausible intervention [22, 24, 25, 44].

Over time, persistent leaks become abscessed cavity that can evolve to fistula. The presence of a persistent leak, more than 4 weeks, despite conservative management should raise suspicion for secondary causes preventing healing, such as distal narrowing increasing intraluminal pressure (see Fig. 25.3) or the presence of a foreign body (e.g., drain). Less invasive non-operative management is preferred whenever possible, using proton-pump inhibitors (PPI) and cytoprotective agent [11]. However, if a patient is hemodynamically stable and nutrition is reasonable, reoperation for repair of a persistent leak can be performed not before 12 weeks postoperatively. Surgical options for repairing acute/early uncontained leaks include primary repair, serosal patching using the small intestine pulled up to the leak, wedge resection of the fundus to include the leaking region, and T-tube gastrostomy creating a controlled fistula directly into the defect [13, 22, 44, 45].

T-tube Gastrostomy Surgical Technique The T-tube converts a free draining fistulae to a controlled one. Uncover the leak site by careful blunt dissection of any omentum or tissue covering the defect. Once visible, irrigate and drain any intra-abdominal collections around the leak site. Using 2–0 sutures, narrow the gastric defect and insert a 14-French T-tube into the defect. Reinforce the T-tube using gastric sutures followed by a Graham patch [45].

Chronic, (usually gastric) non-healing fistulas despite adequate drainage and non-surgical management present more of a challenge. In this case, invasive surgical approaches are most effective. Before non-operative management is deemed

Fig. 25.3 Upper gastrointestinal contrast study demonstrating area of fixed narrowing between the proximal and distal stomach with contrast extravasation (*arrow*) following a LSG

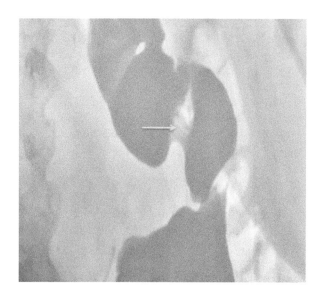

unsuccessful, 12 weeks should be allowed to give time to optimize the patient's nutrition and to control the local and systemic sepsis for the acute inflammation to go down for a less hostile surgical field. Surgical options for management of chronic, non-healing fistulas include suturing a Roux limb directly to the leak site creating a GJ anastomosis and proximal gastrectomy with Roux-en-Y esophagojejunostomy (PGEJ) reconstruction [13, 22, 44]. Advanced, chronic fistulas forming supradiaphragmatic communications into the pulmonary parenchyma or bronchus may require lobectomy [28].

Direct Jejunal-Gastric Fistula Anastomosis Reconstruction Surgical Technique The dissection begins at the pars flaccida, away from the area of most contamination. The dissection proceeds until the caudate lobe, vena cava and right crus of the diaphragm are identified. After incising the peritoneum overlying the medial edge of the right crus, the esophagus is identified. Retroesophageal dissection then allows for visualization of the left crus of the diaphragm. At this point the fistula tract is dissected in order to generously debride the sclerotic edges of the stomach defect to obtain healthy tissue. After transecting the jejunum 50 cm distal to the ligament of Trietz, the distal part of the jejunum is brought in an antecolic antegastric or retrocolic retrogastric fashion to the proximal stomach. Whichever route provides the least tension should be the one to be chosen. The anastomosis to the debrided fistula edge is then performed using a completely handsewn technique over an orogastric tube. The jejeuno-jejunostomy is then carried out 60–100 cm distally in a standard fashion, using a linear stapler or handsewn technique. In the presence of a sizable hiatal defect, this should be repaired posteriorly in a standard fashion [46].

PGEJ Reconstruction Surgical Technique The first part of the dissection is similar as described above through the pars flaccida. An orogastric tube aids in the identification of the esophagus. The hiatus is completely dissected and the distal esophagus mobilized. At this point the left gastric artery is divided using a vascular linear stapler. The fistulous tract is completely mobilized, starting from the most distal and less inflamed aspect of the sleeve. Esophageal stay sutures are placed at the 3 and 9 o'clock position, then transect the esophagus immediately proximal to the GEJ using a standard (3.5 mm) cartridge linear stapler. The distal sleeve is then transected distal to the fistulous tract using a thick cartridge (4.1 mm) linear stapler. When creating the esophagojejunostomy (EJ) widen the left crus of the diaphragm to allow the stapler to advance to the lower mediastinum. Transect the jejunum 50 cm distal to the ligament of Trietz, the Roux limb is then brought up to the esophagus in an antecolic antegastric fashion. The EJ anastomosis is fashioned using a standard (3.5 mm) cartridge linear stapler and the defect closed in two-layer handsewn technique (Fig. 25.4). Finally, 100 cm from the EJ, the JJ is fashioned using two firings of a vascular (2.5 mm) cartridge linear stapler and closing the enterotomy with more firings of a similar linear stapler [44].

Fig. 25.4 Laparoscopic creation of an esophagojejunostomy using a Roux limb during a laparoscopic proximal gastrectomy with Roux-en-Y esophagojejunostomy (PGEJ) reconstruction due to complication of a chronic non-healing fistula

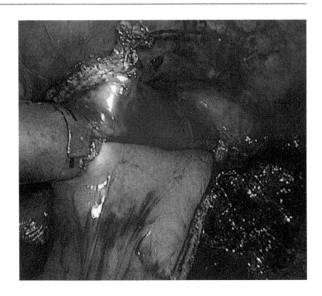

25.6   Management of Leaks of Less Common Bariatric Surgeries

Biliopancreatic Diversion with Duodenal Switch Biliopancreatic diversion with duodenal switch (BPD/DS) induces weight loss by utilizing restrictive, enterohormonal, and malabsorptive strategies, where a sleeve gastrectomy is created with the ileum anastomosed to the proximal duodenum, and the biliopancreatic limb then sutured to the distal ileum. BPD/DS is recognized as one of the most efficient bariatric surgeries, as it is associated with comorbidity remission and the greatest weight loss (60–70% at 5 year follow up). However, the associated morbidity and mortality rates are greater than LSG and RYGB [47]. At present, data on anastomotic leaks after BPD/DS surgery is limited.

One-Anastomosis Duodenal Switch Established as a bariatric procedure in 2018 by the International Federation for the Surgery of Obesity and Metabolic Disorders (IFSO), single anastomosis duodenoileal bypass with sleeve gastrectomy (SADI-S), also known as stomach intestinal pylorus-sparing surgery (SIPS) and one-anastomosis duodenal switch (OADS), emerged as a new bariatric operation that induces weight loss by utilizing restrictive, enterohormonal, and malabsorptive strategies. The configuration of this procedure resembles the BPD/DS except that the reconstruction is made with a loop duodenoileostomy with a single anastomosis [33, 48]. Described as a simplification of the BPD/DS, complications are fewer with SADI-S than with BPD/DS. In a single center retrospective study with 225 patients, the incidence of anastomotic leaks after SADI-S was 2.2%. Leak management was dictated by the patient's clinical presentation and timing [49]. At present, data on anastomotic leaks after SADI-S surgery is limited.

One-Anastomosis Gastric Bypass   One-anastomosis gastric bypass (OAGB), previously also known as the mini-gastric bypass (MGB), has emerged as a new bariatric operation that induces weight loss by utilizing restrictive, enterohormonal, and malabsorptive strategies. This procedure shares a divided gastric pouch, but more voluminous with the gastric bypass. To complete the intestinal bypass portion of the operation, OAGB utilizes a loop reconstruction with a single anastomosis between jejunum and gastric pouch. Anastomotic leaks occur in 0.1–1.9% of patients. This can most likely be attributed to the tension-free, densely vascular anastomosis to a narrow and thin-walled lesser curvature-based gastric pouch. Arterial hypertension and heavy smoking have been reported to be predictive factors for developing leaks after OAGB. If a leak is detected, management involves intra-abdominal washout and drainage with primary repair of the leak. However, in a leak that has become chronic with severely damaged gastric tissue, a PGEJ reconstruction is considered [50].

25.7   Conclusion

Despite an overall decrease in the incidence of anastomotic leaks over time, this dreaded complication remains a significant cause of morbidity and mortality after bariatric surgery [35]. While the causes for developing a leak are multifactorial, it is imperative that surgeons understand the distinct patient and technical factors of each bariatric surgery, to minimize the morbidity and mortality associated with the rapid progression from systemic inflammatory response to sepsis and shock. A high index of suspicion is critical to expedite recognition and early initiation of management. For patients who present hemodynamically stable, the surgeon's clinical suspicion can be confirmed with the assistance of laboratory studies, UGI contrast studies, and CT scan. Conservative management includes control of local and systemic sepsis, control of gastrointestinal secretions, and early nutritional support. Successful management has also been reported using minimally invasive endoscopic techniques. In the face of clinical deterioration or unsuccessful non-operative management, operative intervention involves re-exploration with extensive washout and drainage, with or without repair of the leak.

References

1. Hales CM, Carroll MD, Fryar CD, Ogden CL. Prevalence of obesity among adults and youth: United States, 2015–2016. NCHS data brief, no 288. Hyattsville, MD: National Center for Health Statistics. NCHS data brief, no 288 Hyattsville, MD Natl Cent Heal Stat [Internet]. 2017;2015–6. Available from: https://www.cdc.gov/nchs/products/databriefs/db288.htm
2. Jensen MD, Ryan DH, Apovian CM, Ard JD, Comuzzie AG, Donato KA, et al. A report of the American college of cardiology/American heart association task force on practice guidelines and the obesity society. Circulation. 2014;129:102–41.
3. Colquitt JL, Pickett K, Loveman E, Frampton GK. Surgery for weight loss in adults. Cochrane Database Syst Rev. 2014;8:CD003641.

4. Maciejewski ML, Arterburn DE, Van Scoyoc L, Smith VA, Yancy WS, Weidenbacher HJ, et al. Bariatric surgery and long-term durability of weight loss. JAMA Surg. 2016;151:1046–55.

5. Golomb I, David MB, Glass A, Kolitz T, Keidar A. Long-term metabolic effects of laparoscopic sleeve gastrectomy. JAMA Surg. 2015;150:1051–7.

6. DeMaria E, English WJ, Mattar SG, et al. State variation in obesity, bariatric surgery, and economic ranks: a tale of two americas. Surgery for Obesity and Related Diseases. 2018;14(11):S71.

7. Ballesta C, Berindoague R, Cabrera M, Palau M, Gonzales M. Management of anastomotic leaks after laparoscopic roux-en-Y gastric bypass. Obes Surg. 2008;18:623–30.

8. Aurora AR, Khaitan L, Saber AA. Sleeve gastrectomy and the risk of leak: a systematic analysis of 4,888 patients. Surg Endosc. 2012;26:1509–15.

9. Tiwari MM, Goede MR, Reynoso JF, Tsang AW, Oleynikov D, McBride CL. Differences in outcomes of laparoscopic gastric bypass. Surg Obes Relat Dis [Internet]. 2011;7:277–82. Elsevier, Available from: https://doi.org/10.1016/j.soard.2011.02.005

10. Gonzalez R, Sarr MG, Smith CD, Baghai M, Kendrick M, Szomstein S, et al. Diagnosis and contemporary Management of Anastomotic Leaks after gastric bypass for obesity. J Am Coll Surg. 2007;204:47–55.

11. Nguyen NT, Blackstone RP, Morton JM, Ponce J, Rosenthal RJ. The ASMBS textbook of bariatric surgery. 2nd ed. New York: Springer; 2020.

12. Noel P, Nedelcu M, Gagner M. Impact of the surgical experience on leak rate after laparoscopic sleeve gastrectomy. Obes Surg. 2016;26:1782–7.

13. Rosenthal RJ. International sleeve gastrectomy expert panel consensus statement: best practice guidelines based on experience of >12,000 cases. Surg Obes Relat Dis [Internet]. 2012;8:8–19. Elsevier, Available from: https://doi.org/10.1016/j.soard.2011.10.019

14. Chen B, Kiriakopoulos A, Tsakayannis D, Wachtel MS, Linos D, Frezza EE. Reinforcement does not necessarily reduce the rate of staple line leaks after sleeve gastrectomy. A review of the literature and clinical experiences. Obes Surg. 2009;19:166–72.

15. Baker RS, Foote J, Kemmeter P, Brady R, Vroegop T, Serveld M. The science of stapling and leaks. Obes Surg. 2004;14(10):1290–8.

16. Silecchia G, Iossa A. Complications of staple line and anastomoses following laparoscopic bariatric surgery. Ann Gastroenterol. 2018;31:56–64.

17. Dapri G, Bernard Cadière G, Himpens J. Reinforcing the staple line during laparoscopic sleeve gastrectomy: prospective randomized clinical study comparing three different techniques. Obes Surg. 2010;20:462–7.

18. Parikh M, Issa R, McCrillis A, Saunders JK, Ude-Welcome A, Gagner M. Surgical strategies that may decrease leak after laparoscopic sleeve gastrectomy: a systematic review and meta-analysis of 9991 cases. Ann Surg. 2013;257:231–7.

19. Berger ER, Clements ÃRH, Morton JM, Huffman KM, Wolfe BM, Nguyen NT, et al. The impact of different surgical techniques on outcomes in laparoscopic sleeve Gastrectomies. Ann Surg. 2016;264:473.

20. Cucchi SD, Pories WJ, MacDonald KG, Morgan EJ. Gastrogastric fistulas: a complication of divided gastric bypass surgery. Ann Surg. 1995;221:387–91.

21. Gagner M, Hutchinson C, Rosenthal R. Fifth international consensus conference: current status of sleeve gastrectomy. Surg Obes Relat Dis [Internet]. 2016;12:750–756. Elsevier, Available from: https://doi.org/10.1016/j.soard.2016.01.022

22. Sakran N, Goitein D, Raziel A, Keidar A, Beglaibter N, Grinbaum R, et al. Gastric leaks after sleeve gastrectomy: a multicenter experience with 2,834 patients. Surg Endosc. 2013;27:240–5.

23. Bellorin O, Abdemur A, Sucandy I, Szomstein S, Rosenthal RJ. Understanding the significance, reasons and patterns of abnormal vital signs after gastric bypass for morbid obesity. Obes Surg. 2011;21:707–13.

24. Burgos AM, Braghetto I, Csendes A, Maluenda F, Korn O, Yarmuch J, et al. Gastric leak after laparoscopic-sleeve gastrectomy for obesity. Obes Surg. 2009;19:1672–7.

25. Márquez MF, Ayza MF, Lozano RB, Del Mar Rico Morales M, García Díez JM, Poujoulet RB. Gastric leak after laparoscopic sleeve gastrectomy. Obes Surg. 2010;20:1306–11.

26. Hamilton EC, Sims TL, Hamilton TT, Mullican MA, Jones DB, Provost DA. Clinical predictors of leak after laparoscopic roux-en-Y gastric bypass for morbid obesity. Surg Endosc Other Interv Tech. 2003;17:679–84.
27. Garofalo F, Atlas H, Pescarus R. Laparoscopic treatment of gastrocolic fistula: a rare complication post-sleeve gastrectomy. Surg Obes Relat Dis [Internet]. 2016;12:1761–1763. Elsevier, Available from: https://doi.org/10.1016/j.soard.2016.08.023
28. Sakran N, Assalia A, Keidar A, Goitein D. Gastrobronchial fistula as a complication of bariatric surgery: a series of 6 cases. Obes Facts. 2012;5:538–45.
29. Csendes JA, Braghetto MI, LAM B, Palavecino BT, Iglesias FR, Torrijos CC. Conducta frente a fltraciones post gastrectomía vertical. Rev Chil Cir. 2013;65:315–20.
30. Warschkow R, Tarantino I, Folie P, Beutner U, Schmied BM, Bisang P, et al. C-reactive protein 2 days after laparoscopic gastric bypass surgery reliably indicates leaks and moderately predicts morbidity. J Gastrointest Surg. 2012;16:1128–35.
31. Maher JW, Bakhos W, Nahmias N, Wolfe LG, Meador JG, Baugh N, et al. Drain amylase levels are an adjunct in detection of gastrojejunostomy leaks after Roux-en-Y gastric bypass. J Am Coll Surg [Internet]. 2009;208:881–4. https://doi.org/10.1016/j.jamcollsurg.2008.12.022.
32. Gonzalez R, Nelson LG, Gallagher SF, Murr MM. Anastomotic leaks after laparoscopic gastric bypass. Obes Surg. 2004;14:1299–307.
33. Kim J. American Society for Metabolic and Bariatric Surgery statement on single-anastomosis duodenal switch. Surg Obes Relat Dis [Internet]. 2016;12:944–945. Elsevier, Available from: https://doi.org/10.1016/j.soard.2016.05.006
34. Doraiswamy A, Rasmussen JJ, Pierce J, Fuller W, Ali MR. The utility of routine postoperative upper GI series following laparoscopic gastric bypass. Surg Endosc Other Interv Tech. 2007;21:2159–62.
35. Kim J, Azagury D, Eisenberg D, Demaria E, Campos GM. ASMBS position statement on prevention, detection, and treatment of gastrointestinal leak after gastric bypass and sleeve gastrectomy, including the roles of imaging, surgical exploration, and nonoperative management. Surg Obes Relat Dis [Internet]. 2015;11:739–748. Elsevier, Available from: https://doi.org/10.1016/j.soard.2015.05.001
36. Casella G, Soricelli E, Rizzello M, Trentino P, Fiocca F, Fantini A, et al. Nonsurgical treatment of staple line leaks after laparoscopic sleeve gastrectomy. Obes Surg. 2009;19:821–6.
37. Csendes A, Braghetto I, León P, Burgos AM. Management of leaks after laparoscopic sleeve gastrectomy in patients with obesity. J Gastrointest Surg. 2010;14:1343–8.
38. Spyropoulos C, Argentou MI, Petsas T, Thomopoulos K, Kehagias I, Kalfarentzos F. Management of gastrointestinal leaks after surgery for clinically severe obesity. Surg Obes Relat Dis [Internet]. 2012;8:609–15. Elsevier, Available from: https://doi.org/10.1016/j.soard.2011.04.222
39. Tan JT, Kariyawasam S, Wijeratne T, Chandraratna HS. Diagnosis and management of gastric leaks after laparoscopic sleeve gastrectomy for morbid obesity. Obes Surg. 2010;20:403–9.
40. Mahadev S, Kumbhari V, Campos JM, Galvao Neto M, Khashab MA, Chavez YH, et al. Endoscopic septotomy: an effective approach for internal drainage of sleeve gastrectomy-associated collections. Endoscopy. 2017;49:504–8.
41. Thompson SK, Chang EY, Jobe BA. Clinical review: healing in gastrointestinal anastomoses, part I. Microsurgery. 2006;26:131–6.
42. Tabola R, Augoff K, Lewandowski A, Ziolkowski P, Szelachowski P, Grabowski K. Esophageal anastomosis how the granulation phase of wound healing improves the incidence of anastomotic leakage. Oncol Lett. 2016;12:2038–44.
43. Valli PV, Gubler C. Review article including treatment algorithm: endoscopic treatment of luminal complications after bariatric surgery. Clin Obes. 2017;7:115–22.
44. Thompson CE, Ahmad H, Lo Menzo E, Szomstein S, Rosenthal RJ. Outcomes of laparoscopic proximal gastrectomy with esophagojejunal reconstruction for chronic staple line disruption after laparoscopic sleeve gastrectomy. Surg Obes Relat Dis [Internet]. 2014;10:455–459. Elsevier, Available from: https://doi.org/10.1016/j.soard.2013.10.008

45. Court I, Wilson A, Benotti P, Szomstein S, Rosenthal RJ. T-tube gastrostomy as a novel approach for distal staple line disruption after sleeve gastrectomy for morbid obesity: case report and review of the literature. Obes Surg. 2010;20:519–22.
46. Van De Vrande S, Himpens J, El Mourad H, Debaerdemaeker R, Leman G. Management of chronic proximal fistulas after sleeve gastrectomy by laparoscopic roux-limb placement. Surg Obes Relat Dis [Internet]; 2013;9:856–861. Elsevier, Available from: https://doi.org/10.1016/j.soard.2013.01.003
47. Bariatric Surgery Procedures [Internet]. Am Soc Metab Bariatr Surg. [Cited 2019 Nov 21]. Available from: https://asmbs.org/patients/bariatric-surgery-procedures
48. Sánchez-Pernaute A, Herrera MAR, Pérez-Aguirre ME, Talavera P, Cabrerizo L, Matía P, et al. Single anastomosis duodeno-ileal bypass with sleeve gastrectomy (SADI-S). One to three-year follow-up. Obes Surg. 2010;20:1720–6.
49. Cottam A, Cottam D, Portenier D, Zaveri H, Surve A, Cottam S, et al. A matched cohort analysis of stomach intestinal pylorus saving (SIPS) surgery versus biliopancreatic diversion with duodenal switch with two-year follow-up. Obes Surg [Internet]. 2017;27:454–61. https://doi.org/10.1007/s11695-016-2341-7.
50. Solouki A, Kermansaravi M, Jazi AHD, Kabir A, Farsani TM, Pazouki A. One-anastomosis gastric bypass as an alternative procedure of choice in morbidly obese patients. J Res Med Sc [Internet]. 2018;23:84. Available from: http://www.jmsjournal.net/article.asp?issn=1735-1995;year=2018;volume=23;issue=1;spage=84;epage=84;aulast=Solouki

Gastric Sleeve Stricture, Twist or Kink, Now What?

26

Laurel L. Tangalakis and Jonathan A. Myers

26.1 Introduction

Laparoscopic sleeve gastrectomy (LSG) has gained popularity over recent years [1]. Although the risk profile of the sleeve gastrectomy is low, there are still multiple feared complications [2]. Specifically, gastric sleeve stenosis can occur in 0.1–3.9% of cases [3]. This complication can occur by two main mechanisms. First, from a mechanical obstruction or stricture, usually occurring more proximal and secondary to fibrosis. Second, is an axial deviation, or twist, of the sleeve, often present at the incisura angularis. This likely occurs as a result of progressive rotation of the staple line and scarring of the sleeve in a kinked fashion or from imbrications of the staple line and over-retraction of the greater curvature during stapling. Symptoms include regurgitation, dyspepsia, early satiety, abdominal pain, nausea, vomiting and rapid weight loss. Diagnosis includes endoscopic and fluoroscopic imaging [4]. Treatment options historically involved surgical revision, most commonly converting to a roux-en-y gastric bypass (RYGB). However, there are multiple endoscopic options that can be offered and have recently gained popularity.

Management of a stenosis following laparoscopic sleeve gastrectomy is an important topic given the high morbidity that can result from this complication. There are multiple case reports that suggest surgical revision should be the mainstay of treatment for gastric stenosis [5]. However, the use of endoscopy as treatment allows for a less invasive approach and avoids potential complications of revisional surgery. Endoscopic treatment is also not without risk and cost and length of therapy may add additional morbidity. There are a wide variety of studies that recommend algorithmic approaches to the treatment of gastric stenosis following LSG. The goal

L. L. Tangalakis · J. A. Myers (✉)
Department of Surgery, Rush University Medical Center, Chicago, IL, USA
e-mail: Jonathan_myers@rush.edu

© Springer Nature Switzerland AG 2021
J. Alverdy, Y. Vigneswaran (eds.), *Difficult Decisions in Bariatric Surgery*,
Difficult Decisions in Surgery: An Evidence-Based Approach,
https://doi.org/10.1007/978-3-030-55329-6_26

of this chapter is to address and grade the different treatment modalities available for stenosis following a gastric sleeve operation.

26.2 Search Strategy

A literature search of English language publications from 2014 to 2019 was used to identify published data of surgical revision versus endoscopic management of stenosis after a gastric sleeve operation. PubMed and Cochrane Evidence Based Medicine were used. Terms used in the search were ("2014" [Date—Publication]: "2019" [Date—Publication]) AND (sleeve gastrectomy) AND (stenosis or stricture or twist) AND (endoscopic management) AND (surgical revision). Articles were excluded that were over 10 years old and 11 articles were used. There were 10 retrospective chart review studies, and 1 case report. The data was classified using the GRADE system.

P (Patients)	I (Intervention)	C (Comparator)	O (Outcomes)
Patients with gastric sleeve stenosis after laparoscopic sleeve gastrectomy	Endoscopic balloon dilatation or stent placement	Surgical Revision	Symptom resolution, risks of therapy, treatment duration, cost

26.3 Results

26.3.1 Diagnosis of Sleeve Stenosis

Accurate diagnosis of gastric sleeve stenosis after laparoscopic sleeve gastrectomy is an important aspect of determining appropriate management. Multiple retrospective review studies that outline endoscopic treatment modalities for sleeve stenosis begin with review of proper diagnosis. Diagnosis is commonly made by x-ray with ingestion of radio-opaque contrast (barium swallow) or with esophagoduodenoscopy [4]. Some proposed algorithms also defined specific parameters for diagnosis. Rebibo et al. stated that for diagnosis of an organic gastric stenosis an upper endoscopy was mandated followed by a water-soluble contrast agent under radiologic guidance. This helped to define the site and length of the stenosis. For a functional gastric stenosis, an upper gastrointestinal endoscopy procedure was necessary as the swallow study was often normal. If a patient who presented with gastric stenosis symptoms had normal imaging, then esophageal manometry was essential to rule out a diagnosis of achalasia [6].

26.3.2 Management of Sleeve Stenosis

After a diagnosis is made, there are many proposed management options for gastric stenosis following LSG. There are multiple retrospective chart reviews that report varying rates and demographic data on patients who experience gastric stenosis.

These studies also review various treatment modalities, rates of success and need for revisional surgery (Table 26.1). There are a variety of balloon types and sizes used to treat this complication. Most commonly used are achalasia balloons and through the scope balloons (TTS). Some studies utilized one or the other, or a combination of both. Stent placement was used less often in these studies and was often a last resort prior to surgical revision.

26.3.3 Single Modality Management with Balloon Dilation

The most common management includes balloon dilation. Balloon dilation can be done with either through the scope balloons or achalasia balloons. Through the scope balloons range from 10 to 20 mm in size. They work by passing a wire through the scope and are endoscopically guided, so all dilation is performed under direct visualization. Achalasia balloons range from 30 to 40 mm in size. They are also passed over a wire, but with fluoroscopic guidance as opposed to endoscopic. Achalasia balloons were originally designed specifically for achalasia, but the use has become more widespread [7].

Some studies utilized through the scope balloon dilatation as opposed to achalasia balloon dilatation, or a combination of both. A retrospective study by Ellatif [8] reviewed 3634 patients undergoing LSG, with 2.3% of patients having either a gastric sleeve axial twist (45 patients) or a stricture (41 patients). Of the patients with an axial twist, they found that 27 patients were successfully managed by balloon dilation, and 16 patients by endoscopic stenting with an overall endoscopic success rate of 95.5%. Only balloons with size ranging from 15 to 18 mm (through the scope balloons) were used and 1.7 dilations were required. Two patients required three dilations and subsequently required revision. Both were found to be secondary to adhesions, and an adhesiolysis with gastropexy was performed on both patients.

A retrospective study by Deslauriers et al. also examined through the scope balloon dilation as a first attempt, with sequential therapy using 20 mm through the scope balloons followed by 30–40 mm achalasia balloons and stent placement in refractory cases. Revisional surgery was reserved for patients who did not have significant improvement in symptoms after endoscopic treatment. Twenty-seven patients underwent endoscopic treatment with a success rate of 56% (15/27 patients). Twenty percent of these patients had only moderate improvement in their symptoms and were considered partial responders. After three failed interventions, patients then underwent revisional surgery. There were 44% that were considered failures. All surgical revisions consisted of conversion to laparoscopic RYGB.

One study found that patients who had a dilation with a TTS balloon (20 mm) only had a 31% success rate compared to a 100% success rate in patients that had dilatation with an achalasia balloon (30 mm) [9]. Another retrospective study had a 69% success rate only using TTS balloons (10–18 mm) [10]. On the contrary, a study by Ogra et al. had a 100% success rate (26/26 patients) utilizing sequential therapy [3], starting with a TTS 20 mm balloon followed by a 30 and 35 mm achalasia balloon.

Table 26.1 Comparison of endoscopic treatment modalities and clinical outcomes

Authors	Publication year	% Successful cases treated endoscopically	Mean # of endoscopic treatments	Endoscopic modalities	Complications	% Failure (revisional surgery)
Shnell et al.	2014	44% (7/16)	N/A (1–3)	TTS 20 mm Achalasia balloon: 30 mm	None	56% (five RYGB, one re-sleeve, three lost to follow up)
Ogra et al.	2015	100% (26/26)	1.6 (1–4)	TTS <20 mm Achalasia balloon: 30 mm + 35 mm (15 psi)	4% (one stent migration)	N/A
Rebibo et al.	2016	88% (15/17)	2 (1–3)	Alchalasia balloon: 30 mm (20 psi), then 25–40 mm (20 psi), stent (2/17)	None	12% (RYGB)
Al Sabah et al.	2016	88% (23/36)	2.3 (N/A)	Achalasia balloon: 30–35–40 mm	None	12%
Nath et al.	2016	69% (23/33)	N/A	TTS (10–18 mm)	N/A	31%
Donatelli et al.	2017	60% (20/33)	1.5 (1–3)	Achalasia balloon: 30–35–40 mm (20 psi)	6% (one perforation; one bleeding)	40% (four RYGB, one total gastrectomy, seven unspecified revisional surgery)
Agnihotri et al.	2017	88.2% (15/17)	2 (1–4)	Achalasia balloon: 30–35 mm, stent	5.8% (mucosal tear)	11.8% (RYGB)
Manos et al.	2017	94.4% (17/18)	1.3 (1–4)	Achalasia balloon: 30–35 mm (25 psi), stent	None	6% (RYGB)
Ellatif et al.	2017	95.5% (43/45)	1.7	TTS (15–18 mm)	None	4.44% (Adhesiolysis and gastropexy)
Deslauriers et al.	2018	56% (15/27)	1.7 (1–5)	TTS 20 mm, 30–40 mm achalasia balloon, stent	3.7% (distal migration of stent)	44% (RYGB)

A case report by Farha et al. describes the use of gastric per oral endoscopy myotomy for treatment of organic gastric stenosis following LSG. The patient had failed endoscopic management and refused a conversion to a RYGB. The patient had marked improvement in symptoms and endoscopy at 5 weeks post procedure revealed improved stenosis. This procedure could be considered in the algorithm after other endoscopic treatments such as balloon dilatation and stent placement fail [11].

26.3.4 Sequential Algorithms Utilizing Balloons and Stent Placement

Multiple studies have attempted to create algorithmic approaches to treatment based on retrospective data, including retrospective studies by both Agnihortri et al., and Rebibo et al. These studies utilized stent placement as well as balloon dilation for the management of gastric sleeve stenosis.

The study by Agnihotri et al. created an algorithm based on the use of an achalasia balloon dilatation as a first line treatment modality. The algorithm recommends starting with achalasia 30 mm balloon dilation, followed by 35 mm dilation, and then repeating 3–4 times as needed. If this is unsuccessful, stent placement is then recommended. If patient is still symptomatic, surgical revision is considered last. The study found that out of the 17 patients initially treated with balloon dilatation, 3 went on to require stent placement and 2 patients underwent eventual surgical revision, with an 88.2% success rate.

The study by Rebibo et al. recommended a similar algorithm with minor deviations. Patients initially underwent serial balloon dilatations using progressively larger balloons (30–35–40 mm). However, they only recommended stent placement for early onset gastric stenosis, considered as occurring prior to post-operative day 7. After three failed dilatation attempts, surgical revision was then recommended. They examined 1210 patients who underwent laparoscopic sleeve gastrectomy. Seventeen (1.4%) were found to have gastric stenosis with 6 patients having a functional twist, and 11 patients having an organic cause for the stenosis. The rate of success of endoscopic management was 86.6%, with two patients requiring revisional surgery and one patient having a stent placed after an early diagnosis of gastric stenosis.

A study by Manos et al. [12] also had an algorithm that included stent placement. Ninety-four percent of patients were successful with endoscopic therapy. Stents were utilized in cases of complete stenosis (the endoscope was unable to be passed) or after patients had a failed attempt at balloon dilation.

There were also varying reports of achalasia balloons being used as a primary treatment modality with success rates ranging from 60 to 88% [13, 14].

26.3.5 Complications of Various Treatment Modalities

Overall the risk profile of endoscopic treatments was low. The complications are outline in Table 26.1. Complication rates ranged from 3.7 to 6% and including stent migration, perforation and bleeding, mucosal tear and distal migration of stents [2–4, 14]. The risk profile of revisional surgery as a treatment modality varies by the surgery and is fairly well established for the conversion to a Roux-en-Y gastric bypass.

26.4 Recommendations Based on Results

The overall quality of evidence relating to the topic of managing gastric sleeve stenosis is low. There are multiple retrospective reviews but there are no prospective or randomized control trials comparing various treatment modalities. Recommendations based on the data are listed in Table 26.2.

26.5 Personal View of the Data

The treatment of gastric stenosis after a sleeve gastrectomy can be complicated and time consuming. Meanwhile, surgical revision can offer a quick solution but may not be ideal for every patient. Endoscopic techniques such as balloon dilatations and stent placement may offer non-surgical treatment options. Although data is not strong to support this, it appears to be a reasonable treatment modality. It may be worthwhile to attempt endoscopic treatment prior to pursuing surgical revision, especially in patients who may not desire surgical revision. However endoscopic treatment in these patients may result in weight regain unlike revisional surgery to

Table 26.2 Evidence and recommendations regarding the treatment of gastric sleeve stenosis

Treatment modality	Grade of evidence	Recommendation	Strength of recommendation
Achalasia balloon dilatation	Moderate	Reasonable first line treatment for stenosis, up to three attempts	Weak
TTS balloon dilatation	Moderate	Reasonable balloon dilatation option to consider, up to three attempts	Weak
Stent placement	Low	Should be considered in early diagnosed gastric stenosis, in cases of complete stenosis or when balloon dilation has failed	Weak
Surgical Revision	Moderate	Surgical revision should be reserved for those cases that fail endoscopic management	Weak

RYGB and patients should be counseled of this risk with endoscopic treatments. Further prospective studies and randomized control trails comparing endoscopic techniques and surgical revision are essential to create algorithms based on high grade evidence.

References

1. English WJ, DeMaria EJ, Brethauer SA, Mattar SG, Rosenthal RJ, Morton JM. American Society for Metabolic and Bariatric Surgery estimation of metabolic and bariatric procedures performed in the United States in 2016. Surg Obes Relat Dis. 2018;14(3):259–63.
2. Deslauriers V, Beauchamp A, Garofalo F, et al. Endoscopic management of post-laparoscopic sleeve gastrectomy stenosis. Surg Endosc. 2018;32(2):601–9.
3. Ogra R, Kini GP. Evolving endoscopic management options for symptomatic stenosis post-laparoscopic sleeve gastrectomy for morbid obesity: experience at a large bariatric surgery unit in New Zealand. Obes Surg. 2015;25(2):242–8.
4. Agnihotri A, Barola S, Hill C, et al. An algorithmic approach to the management of gastric stenosis following laparoscopic sleeve gastrectomy. Obes Surg. 2017;27(10):2628–36.
5. Switzer NJ, Karmali S, Gill RS, Sherman V. Revisional bariatric surgery. Surg Clin North Am. 2016;96(4):827–42.
6. Rebibo L, Hakim S, Dhahri A, Yzet T, Delcenserie R, Regimbeau JM. Gastric stenosis after laparoscopic sleeve gastrectomy: diagnosis and management. Obes Surg. 2016;26(5):995–1001.
7. Siddiqui UD, Banerjee S, Barth B, et al. Tools for endoscopic stricture dilation. Gastrointest Endosc. 2013;78(3):391–404.
8. Abd Ellatif ME, Abbas A, El Nakeeb A, et al. Management options for twisted gastric tube after laparoscopic sleeve gastrectomy. Obes Surg. 2017;27(9):2404–9.
9. Shnell M, Fishman S, Eldar S, Goitein D, Santo E. Balloon dilatation for symptomatic gastric sleeve stricture. Gastrointest Endosc. 2014;79(3):521–4.
10. Nath A, Yewale S, Tran T, Brebbia JS, Shope TR, Koch TR. Dysphagia after vertical sleeve gastrectomy: evaluation of risk factors and assessment of endoscopic intervention. World J Gastroenterol. 2016;22(47):10371–9.
11. Farha J, Fayad L, Kadhim A, et al. Gastric per-oral endoscopic myotomy (G-POEM) for the treatment of gastric stenosis post-laparoscopic sleeve gastrectomy (LSG). Obes Surg. 2019;29(7):2350–4.
12. Manos T, Nedelcu M, Cotirlet A, Eddbali I, Gagner M, Noel P. How to treat stenosis after sleeve gastrectomy? Surg Obes Relat Dis. 2017;13(2):150–4.
13. Al Sabah S, Al Haddad E, Siddique I. Endoscopic management of post-laparoscopic sleeve gastrectomy stenosis. Surg Endosc. 2017;31(9):3559–63.
14. Donatelli G, Dumont JL, Pourcher G, et al. Pneumatic dilation for functional helix stenosis after sleeve gastrectomy: long-term follow-up (with videos). Surg Obes Relat Dis. 2017;13(6):943–50.

Hiatal Hernia Complicating Bariatric Surgery

Priya Rajdev, Phylicia Dupree, and Farah Husain

27.1 Introduction

As more people seek bariatric surgery for durable treatment of morbid obesity and its associated metabolic diseases, the decision of whether or not to concomitantly treat co-existing hiatal hernia (HH) has become increasingly relevant. The prevalence of symptomatic HH in the general population is thought to range between 16 and 22%. However, the problem is more significant in the morbidly obese population, with rates reported as high as 37% when diagnosed on preoperative barium swallow [1].

The distribution amongst the four types of HH in morbidly obese individuals is similar to the overall population, with type I "sliding" hernias being the most common (90–95%). Risk factors that predispose this population to widening and laxity of the hiatus as well as gastroesophageal sphincter incompetence are thought to be related to increased intraabdominal pressure [2, 3].

Generally, symptomatic sliding type I HH may be satisfactorily treated with medical therapy alone. Therefore, there is some uncertainty as to whether bariatric surgery alone and subsequent reduction in intraabdominal pressure with weight loss may improve reflux symptoms in morbidly obese patients with HH [4]. Conversely, recent short- and long-term data suggest that anatomic changes and increased intragastric pressure secondary to sleeve gastrectomy (SG) may either unmask or result in de novo reflux symptoms in obese patients with previously asymptomatic HH [5].

P. Rajdev · P. Dupree · F. Husain (✉)
Department of Surgery, Division of Bariatric Surgery, Oregon Health and Science University, Portland, OR, USA
e-mail: husain@ohsu.edu

© Springer Nature Switzerland AG 2021
J. Alverdy, Y. Vigneswaran (eds.), *Difficult Decisions in Bariatric Surgery*,
Difficult Decisions in Surgery: An Evidence-Based Approach,
https://doi.org/10.1007/978-3-030-55329-6_27

295

In the 2011 consensus guidelines on laparoscopic sleeve gastrectomy, 82% of expert surgeons surveyed agreed that the hiatus should be aggressively explored by routinely "dissecting the phrenoesophageal membrane and inspect[ing] the greater curvature side of the stomach for the presence of a hiatal hernia." Any hiatal defect should be repaired posteriorly [6]. However, subsequent data suggest varying symptom resolution or even worsening with the addition of routine hiatal exploration to SG.

The problem of hiatal hernia complicating bariatric surgery is sometimes approached from a slightly different angle when a morbidly obese patient is referred for treatment of symptomatic hiatal or paraesophageal hernia. Particularly for larger type III and IV HH or paraesophageal hernias, a second related question arises: since obesity is a risk factor for both occurrence and recurrence of HH, should morbidly obese patients undergoing HH repair undergo simultaneous bariatric surgery? Taken together, with the growing numbers of patients with BMI greater than 35 being referred for foregut surgery, as well as rising popularity of sleeve gastrectomy (SG) over Roux-en-y gastric bypass (RYGB), preoperative consideration of the patient's native anatomy and severity of reflux symptoms becomes an important part of the preoperative discussion and decision-making process.

27.2   Search Strategy

A literature search of English language publications from 2010 to 2020 was used to identify published data on hiatal hernia in the bariatric surgery population. Databases searched were PubMed, Cochrane Library, and Scopus Database. Terms used in the search were "hiatal hernia," "hiatal hernia repair," "obesity," "bariatric surgery," "sleeve gastrectomy," "gastric bypass," "bariatric surgical procedures," "crural repair," and "gastroesophageal reflux disease." Articles were excluded if they did not simultaneously address hiatal hernia and obesity surgery, Articles discussing laparoscopic gastric banding and simultaneous hiatal hernia repair were excluded and felt to be outside the scope of this chapter, given the declining popularity of this procedure. Articles reviewing perioperative reflux symptoms without addressing hiatal hernia repair were reviewed, but not included in the final analysis. Of note, many of the studies that will be discussed approached this challenging problem from the somewhat differing angles of (a) surgical treatment for obesity with incidental hiatal hernia versus (b) surgical treatment for symptomatic hiatal hernia in the setting of obesity. Both approaches were included if they specifically addressed concomitant surgery, as we felt based on clinical experience that the overlap in this patient population was too significant to exclude. In total, we included 23 articles.

P (Patients)	I (Intervention)	C (Comparator)	O (Outcomes)
Patients undergoing obesity surgery with hiatal hernia	Sleeve Gastrectomy with concomitant Hiatal hernia repair OR Roux-en-y gastric bypass with concomitant paraesophageal hernia repair	Sleeve gastrectomy without hiatal hernia repair OR Hiatal hernia repair without obesity surgery	Morbidity/mortality, postoperative reflux symptoms, hiatal hernia recurrence

27.3 Results

27.3.1 Clinical Relevance of Hiatal Hernias in Bariatric Surgery

As obesity continue to rise across the United States, the rate of hiatal hernias continues to increase. Che et al. identified the prevalence of HH to be 37% in a study of 181 morbidly obese patients with BMI of 43 g/m^2 [1]. Despite various pre-operative tests such as GERD questionnaires, pH monitoring, esophagogastroduodenoscopy (EGD), upper gastrointestinal series (UGI) or CT scans, hiatal hernias (HH) are commonly missed during the workup. One of the few studies that used preoperative pH monitoring to identify GERD was Ece et al. [7]. Their goal was to elucidate high risk patients with GERD by using GERD Health-Related Quality of Life questionnaire (GERD-HRQL), ambulatory pH monitoring and EGD. Based on the results of the GERD-HRQL questionnaire, this determined if the patient would undergo pH monitoring and 84% of these patients had a DeMeester score greater than 14.7%. These patients underwent HH repair. Post operatively, three patients had persistent GERD symptoms and 11% of patients had de novo GERD. There was no difference found in the excess weight loss between the two groups. Despite there being a small subset of de novo GERD patients, this study was able to elucidate that HH is feasible with SG as well as has no outcome in weight loss.

Author (year)	# of concomitant HHR (%)	Bariatric Procedure	Type of Repair	Preop known HH	BMI	Avg Follow-up (months)	Statistically significant difference in %EWL?	Difference in GERD Sx?	Preop GERD (%)	Study Type (quality of evidence)
Aridi [8]	76 (46%)	SG	Primary, posterior ± anterior	57.9%	42.7	12–24	No	No	61.8%	Retrospective cohort (low)
Boules [9]	83 (n/a)	SG (27%), RYGB (73%)	Anterior (45%), posterior (25%), mesh (8%)	39%	44.5 ± 7.9	12	No (matched controls)	Yes	Unknown	Retrospective matched control cohort (low)
Braghetto [10]	N/a, total n 20	SG	none	Not measured (all had normal LESP >12 mmHg)	38.3 ± 3.47	6	N/a	Not measured; 85% with incompetent postop LES	Excluded	Prospective case series (low)
Chaar [11]	99 (29%)	SG	Anterior (16%) posterior (13%) ± mesh	Not specified	42.6–43.5	1, 3, 6	Yes, at 6mo (0.02)	Unclear, preop not asked	Not assessed	Retrospective cohort (low)
Chaudhry [12]	14	RYGB		57%	42.0	24+	N/a	Yes, 785 improvement QoL	100%	Retrospective case series (low)
Csendes [13]	9/104	SG	Posterior ± anterior; no mesh	9/104	37.4 ± 5 in 9/104 group	1, 12–24, 126	N/a	No	100%	Prospective cohort (low)
Daes [14]	34/134 (25%)	SG	Anterior (82%), posterior	34 (25%)	36.5–39.3	1, 6, 12	Not specified	Yes (32/34 resolution)	48%	Prospective cohort (low)

Docimo [15]	23,408 (17.9%) of 130772 (MBSAQIP)	SG (21%), RYGB (10.8%)	Not specified	Not specified	45.7 ± 8.4	1	Not specified	Not specified	31.2% (~37% RYGB, 29% SG)	Retrospective cohort (low)
Ece [7]	59/402	SG	Posterior, +prolene mesh for >5 cm	28/402	43.4–44.6	12	No	Yes, reduction in DeMeester Score	92/402 met requirements for pH monitoring on preop GERD-HRQL; all SG-HHR pts had preop GERD score 38.6 ± 10.7	Retrospective cohort (low)
Hefler [16]	42379 (MBSAQIP propensity score matched)	SG (82.4%), RYGB (17.6%)	Anterior/posterior not specified; without (94%) or with (6%) mesh	Not specified	44.4 ± 6.7	1	Not specified	Not specified	36.1% in PEHR group vs. 30% in non-PEHR group	Retrospective cohort (low)
Kasotakis [17]	3	RYGB	Posterior	Yes	46	12	N/a	Yes	100%	Retrospective case series (low)
Kothari [4]	644	RYGB	Anterior/posterior not specified	6.2%	Not specified	1	Not specified	Not specified	Not specified	Retrospective cohort (low)

(continued)

(Continued)

Author (year)	# of concomitant HHR (%)	Bariatric Procedure	Type of Repair	Preop known HH	BMI	Avg Follow-up (months)	Statistically significant difference in %EWL?	Difference in GERD Sx?	Preop GERD (%)	Study Type (quality of evidence)
Lyon [18]	170	Extended SG	Anterior 57%, posterior 43%	Not specified	42 in posterior repair, 44 in anterior, 45 for no repair (p < 0.001)	14	Not specified	Yes, improved for severe sx regardless of repair; mildly worsened for mild preop GERD without hiatal management, improved with posterior closure	22% severe sx	Retrospective cohort (low)
Mahawar [19]	737	SG	Posterior (39%) or anterior (40%), with or without mesh	Not specified	44	Approx. 24–36	Not specified	Yes, gross improvement with hiatal closure	Not specified	Systematic Review (low)
Patel [20]	18	SG	Posterior	Yes	40.7 ± 8.0	20	Not applicable	67% sx resolution	Not specified, presumed yes	Retrospective cohort (low)
Pham [21]	23	SG	Posterior	4/23	41.9	6	Not specified	Not specified	Not specified	Retrospective cohort (low)
Rodriguez [22]	19	SG + PEH	Transverse	Yes	37.8 ± 4.1	13	Not applicable	Yes	100%	Retrospective cohort (low)

	n	Procedure	Repair		Age	Follow-up	Controls	Symptom improvement	Recurrence	Study type
Ruscio [23]	98	SG/HH (Group A) vs. SG/HH+mesh (Group B)	Posterior	Yes	Group A: 11 vs. Group B: 28	21	No	Yes improved	17 pts vs. 20 pts	Prospective cohort (low)
Samakar [24]	58	SG	Posterior	34.5%	44.2 ± 6.6	8	Not applicable	Yes	15.5%	Retrospective cohort (low)
Santonicola [25]	78	SG	Posterior	No	4.6	6	Not specified	No	38.4%	Retrospective cohort (low)
Snyder [26]	98	SG + HHR vs. SG	Posterior	Yes	44	1, 3, 6,9, 12	No	Yes GSRS score of 14 preop to 8.7	Not specified	Randomized control trial (high)
Soricelli [27]	97	SG + HHR	Posterior	11.1%	44 ± 3.5	18	Not specified	Yes (80.4%)	42%	Retrospective cohort (low)
Sutherland [28]	58	BAR(SG/ RYGB) + HHR vs. FP(fundo) + HHR	Posterior	Yes, 52%	44 ± 6	10	No matched controls	Yes	57 % in BAR group	Retrospective cohort (low)

HH are difficult to identify in patients pre-operatively and because of this, the operator should have a high index of suspicion. Soricelli and colleagues found that of the 97 patients found to have a HH, 56% were identified intra-operatively [27]. Intra-operatively, there are various measures used to identify a HH. Some authors described a method of identifying a fingerprint sign above the anterior esophagus at the hiatus while others explored every patient's hiatus by opening the phrenoesophageal ligament [7, 27]. There is no consensus on how to identify an intra-operative HH but more cases of HH are found at the time of surgery than pre-operatively. Once the abdomen is inspected and found to have a laxity or possible HH, the question becomes how to repair this find. These findings can be repaired anteriorly vs. posteriorly. Lyon et al. evaluated 262 patients undergoing SG and found 57% had GERD symptoms, 45% had a HH [18]. They performed anterior repair of the aperture for simple laxity and pre-operative GERD symptoms or performed a posterior repair for true hiatal hernia. They found that the patients who underwent anterior repair had worsening of post-operative GERD symptoms and the posterior group had significant improvement in frequency and severity of GERD symptoms. The decision then becomes to repair or not to repair. Also to repair and perform bariatric surgery separately. Snyder's RCT demonstrated that even when a patient is found to have a HH, solely performing the bariatric surgery can improve GERD symptoms.

Hefler used the Metabolic and Bariatric Surgery Accreditation and Quality Improvement Program (MBSAQIP) matched cohorts to compare outcomes of patients undergoing bariatric surgery compared to patients who underwent bariatric surgery with PEHR [16]. They demonstrated that the rate of PEH did not increase as BMI increased. The cohort undergoing PEHR had a higher percentage of patients undergoing SG + PEHR (82.6%) vs. SG alone (69.4%) ($p < 0.001$). When comparing the SG versus the RYGB, the rate of major complications was significantly higher in the RYGB group (3% vs. 7%, $p < 0.001$). This finding was not higher than previously published complication rates.

27.3.2 A Personal View of the Data

The data are variable and conflicting: some authors found that reflux was worsened after sleeve, while others found no difference if sleeve was performed with or without crural exploration and repair. One of the most compelling findings was the fact that patients who had more severe preoperative symptoms in the setting of hiatal hernia experienced the most relief with simultaneous cruroplasty at the time of bariatric surgery. Therefore, as with any patient, every preoperative bariatric patient should be approached thoughtfully with a thorough history and physical, including an assessment of their reflux symptoms. Our view is that this type of basic, methodical assessment can trigger further workup, including endoscopy and esophagram. Taken together, these studies and the patient's symptoms inform our preoperative discussion. At our institution, we currently offer sleeve gastrectomy and Roux-en-y gastric bypass. Our general approach to hiatal hernia is a posterior sutured cruroplasty with 0-gauge permanent braided suture. Bio-absorbable pledgets are used at the discretion of the surgeon. Bio-absorbable mesh is used only for hiatal defects greater than 5 cm.

Our current practice is broadly consistent with the trends suggested by the data. For patients with clinically significant reflux symptoms on medical therapy, we tend to favor RYGB, and recommend this to our patients. If patients have hiatal hernia, we offer concurrent repair at the time of bypass. We tend to agree with the general consensus that SG disrupts the crossing fibers near the angle of His, worsening or unmasking existing reflux symptoms. However, as implied by the majority of these studies, many patients still prefer SG for multiple reasons, including reduced morbidity related to anastomotic complications, internal hernia risk, and lower risk of malnutrition. Therefore, if the patient is adamant about undergoing SG, we have a thorough discussion regarding the risks and benefits of operation, including worsened GERD with change in angle of His, versus improvement with weight loss. In these patients, if hiatal hernia is seen on preoperative workup, we plan for exploration of the crus and repair. While we do not routinely explore the crus during SG, we do take down the left phrenoesophageal ligament in preparation for stapling, and assess for the presence of a hiatal hernia at that time.

There is clearly room for future work. More randomized control trials in the vein of Snyder should be undertaken. In an ideal world, preoperative workup and postoperative follow-up in future studies should include manometry, pH probe, upper endoscopy, and esophagram. Manometry and pH testing should be used to elucidate the clinical relevance of asymptomatic hiatal hernia recurrence in the SG population. One troubling effect of long-term acid exposure after SG is Barrett's esophagus; in our current practice, we do not routinely surveil patients postoperatively with endoscopy unless warranted by symptoms. A future study could follow SG patients with or without hiatal hernia repair at 6-, 12-, and 24-month intervals with pH probe and endoscopy to better understand how acid exposure at the gastroesophageal junction changes after disruption of the angle of His, with weight loss, and with or without gradual loosening of cruroplasty over time.

References

1. Che F, Nguyen B, Cohen A, Nguyen NT. Prevalence of hiatal hernia in the morbidly obese. Surg Obes Relat Dis. 2013;9(6):920–4. https://doi.org/10.1016/j.soard.2013.03.013.
2. Gordon C, Kang JY, Neild PJ, Maxwell JD. Review article: The role of the hiatus hernia in gastro-oesophageal reflux disease. Aliment Pharmacol Ther. 2004;20(7):719–32. https://doi.org/10.1111/j.1365-2036.2004.02149.x.
3. Lee YY, Mccoll KEL. Disruption of the gastroesophageal junction by central obesity and waist belt: Role of raised intra-abdominal pressure. Dis Esophagus. 2015;28(4):318–25. https://doi.org/10.1111/dote.12202.
4. Kothari V, Shaligram A, Reynoso J, Schmidt E, McBride CL, Oleynikov D. Impact on perioperative outcomes of concomitant hiatal hernia repair with laparoscopic gastric bypass. Obes Surg. 2012;22(10):1607–10. https://doi.org/10.1007/s11695-012-0714-0.
5. DuPree CE, Blair K, Steele SR, Martin MJ. Laparoscopic sleeve gastrectomy in patients with preexisting gastroesophageal reflux disease a national analysis. JAMA Surg. 2014;149(4):328–34. https://doi.org/10.1001/jamasurg.2013.4323.

6. Rosenthal RJ. International sleeve gastrectomy expert panel consensus statement: Best practice guidelines based on experience of >12,000 cases. Surg Obes Relat Dis. 2012;8(1):8–19. https://doi.org/10.1016/j.soard.2011.10.019.
7. Ece I, Yilmaz H, Acar F, Colak B, Yormaz S, Sahin M. A New Algorithm to Reduce the Incidence of Gastroesophageal Reflux Symptoms after Laparoscopic Sleeve Gastrectomy. Obes Surg. 2017;27(6):1460–5. https://doi.org/10.1007/s11695-016-2518-0.
8. Dakour Aridi H, Asali M, Fouani T, Alami RS, Safadi BY. Gastroesophageal Reflux Disease After Laparoscopic Sleeve Gastrectomy with Concomitant Hiatal Hernia Repair: an Unresolved Question. Obes Surg. 2017;27(11):2898–904. https://doi.org/10.1007/s11695-017-2702-x.
9. Boules M, Corcelles R, Guerron AD, et al. The incidence of hiatal hernia and technical feasibility of repair during bariatric surgery. Surgery (United States). 2015;158(4):911–8. https://doi.org/10.1016/j.surg.2015.06.036.
10. Braghetto I, Lanzarini E, Korn O, Valladares H, Molina JC, Henriquez A. Manometric changes of the lower esophageal sphincter after sleeve gastrectomy in obese patients. Obes Surg. 2010;20(3):357–62. https://doi.org/10.1007/s11695-009-0040-3.
11. El Chaar M, Ezeji G, Claros L, Miletics M, Stoltzfus J. Short-Term Results of Laparoscopic Sleeve Gastrectomy in Combination with Hiatal Hernia Repair: Experience in a Single Accredited Center. Obes Surg. 2016;26(1):68–76. https://doi.org/10.1007/s11695-015-1739-y.
12. Chaudhry UI, Marr BM, Osayi SN, et al. Laparoscopic Roux-en-Y gastric bypass for treatment of symptomatic paraesophageal hernia in the morbidly obese: Medium-term results. Surg Obes Relat Dis. 2014;10(6):1063–7. https://doi.org/10.1016/j.soard.2014.02.004.
13. Csendes A, Orellana O, Martínez G, Burgos AM, Figueroa M, Lanzarini E. Clinical, Endoscopic, and Histologic Findings at the Distal Esophagus and Stomach Before and Late (10.5 Years) After Laparoscopic Sleeve Gastrectomy: Results of a Prospective Study with 93% Follow-Up. Obes Surg. 2019;29(12):3809–17. https://doi.org/10.1007/s11695-019-04054-5.
14. Daes J, Jimenez ME, Said N, Daza JC, Dennis R. Laparoscopic sleeve gastrectomy: Symptoms of gastroesophageal reflux can be reduced by changes in surgical technique. Obes Surg. 2012;22(12):1874–9. https://doi.org/10.1007/s11695-012-0746-5.
15. Docimo S, Rahmana U, Bates A, Talamini M, Pryor A, Spaniolas K. Concomitant Hiatal Hernia Repair Is more Common in Laparoscopic Sleeve Gastrectomy than During Laparoscopic Roux-en-Y Gastric Bypass: an Analysis of 130,772 Cases. Obes Surg. 2019;29(2):744–6. https://doi.org/10.1007/s11695-018-3594-0.
16. Hefler J, Dang J, Mocanu V, Switzer N, Birch DW, Karmali S. Concurrent bariatric surgery and paraesophageal hernia repair: an analysis of the Metabolic and Bariatric Surgery Association Quality Improvement Program (MBSAQIP) database. Surg Obes Relat Dis. 2019;15(10):1746–54. https://doi.org/10.1016/j.soard.2019.08.025.
17. Kasotakis G, Mittal SK, Sudan R. Combined treatment of Symptomatic Massive Paraesophageal Hernia in the Morbidly Obese. J Soc Laparoendosc Surg. 2011;15(2):188–92. https://doi.org/10.4293/108680811X13022985132164.
18. Lyon A, Gibson SC, De-Loyde K, Martin D. Gastroesophageal reflux in laparoscopic sleeve gastrectomy: Hiatal findings and their management influence outcome. Surg Obes Relat Dis. 2015;11(3):530–7. https://doi.org/10.1016/j.soard.2014.08.010.
19. Mahawar KK, Carr WRJ, Jennings N, Balupuri S, Small PK. Simultaneous Sleeve Gastrectomy and Hiatus Hernia Repair: a Systematic Review. Obes Surg. 2015;25(1):159–66. https://doi.org/10.1007/s11695-014-1470-0.
20. Patel AD, Lin E, Lytle NW, et al. Combining laparoscopic giant paraesophageal hernia repair with sleeve gastrectomy in obese patients. Surg Endosc. 2015;29(5):1115–22. https://doi.org/10.1007/s00464-014-3771-8.
21. Pham DV, Protyniak B, Binenbaum SJ, Squillaro A, Borao FJ. Simultaneous laparoscopic paraesophageal hernia repair and sleeve gastrectomy in the morbidly obese. Surg Obes Relat Dis. 2014;10(2):257–61. https://doi.org/10.1016/j.soard.2013.08.003.
22. Rodriguez JH, Kroh M, El-Hayek K, Timratana P, Chand B. Combined paraesophageal hernia repair and partial longitudinal gastrectomy in obese patients with symptomatic paraesophageal hernias. Surg Endosc. 2012;26(12):3382–90. https://doi.org/10.1007/s00464-012-2347-8.

23. Ruscio S, Abdelgawad M, Badiali D, et al. Simple versus reinforced cruroplasty in patients submitted to concomitant laparoscopic sleeve gastrectomy: prospective evaluation in a bariatric center of excellence. Surg Endosc. 2016;30(6):2374–81. https://doi.org/10.1007/s00464-015-4487-0.
24. Samakar K, McKenzie TJ, Tavakkoli A, Vernon AH, Robinson MK, Shikora SA. The Effect of Laparoscopic Sleeve Gastrectomy with Concomitant Hiatal Hernia Repair on Gastroesophageal Reflux Disease in the Morbidly Obese. Obes Surg. 2016;26(1):61–6. https://doi.org/10.1007/s11695-015-1737-0.
25. Santonicola A, Angrisani L, Cutolo P, Formisano G, Iovino P. The effect of laparoscopic sleeve gastrectomy with or without hiatal hernia repair on gastroesophageal reflux disease in obese patients. Surg Obes Relat Dis. 2014;10(2):250–5. https://doi.org/10.1016/j.soard.2013.09.006.
26. Snyder B, Wilson E, Wilson T, Mehta S, Bajwa K, Klein C. A randomized trial comparing reflux symptoms in sleeve gastrectomy patients with or without hiatal hernia repair. Surg Obes Relat Dis. 2016;12(9):1681–8. https://doi.org/10.1016/j.soard.2016.09.004.
27. Soricelli E, Iossa A, Casella G, Abbatini F, Calì B, Basso N. Sleeve gastrectomy and crural repair in obese patients with gastroesophageal reflux disease and/or hiatal hernia. Surg Obes Relat Dis. 2013;9(3):356–61. https://doi.org/10.1016/j.soard.2012.06.003.
28. Sutherland V, Kuwada T, Gersin K, Simms C, Stefanidis D. Impact of bariatric surgery on hiatal hernia repair outcomes. Am Surg. 2016;82(8):743–7.

Management of GERD in Duodenal Switch

28

Michelle Campbell and Mustafa Hussain

28.1 Introduction

Morbid obesity is a major risk factor in the development of gastroesophageal reflux disease (GERD). Not surprisingly, the rise of the worldwide obesity epidemic has seen a concurrent rise of GERD prevalence with estimates among obese patients ranging from 37 to 72% [1, 2]. Biliopancreatic diversion with duodenal switch (BPD-DS), or simply duodenal switch (DS), has been shown to be the most powerful tool for durable weight loss currently available, achieving target total body weight loss of ~35–45% [3, 4]. Today DS remains the least commonly performed of four bariatric surgeries currently approved by the American Society of Metabolic and Bariatric Surgery (ASMBS), representing only 2% [4]. The low rate of adaptation of this procedure since its development by Scopinaro in the 1970s [5] is likely multifactorial, including increased technical difficulty and greater risk of serious macro and micronutrient deficiencies related to malabsorption in comparison to the more commonly performed vertical sleeve gastrectomy (VSG) and Roux-en-Y gastric bypass (RYGB). It has also been associated with worsening or de novo development of GERD symptoms as high as 43.8% in one 10-year follow up series [6].

28.2 Search Strategy

A literature review of the PubMed database (title and abstract) was conducted using the search term 'duodenal switch' AND 'gastroesophageal reflux disease'. The results pertaining to management of GERD in the post-operative period following

M. Campbell · M. Hussain (✉)
Minimally Invasive Gastrointestinal and Bariatric Surgery, University of Chicago Medical Center, Chicago, IL, USA
e-mail: mhussain@surgery.bsd.uchicago.edu

© Springer Nature Switzerland AG 2021
J. Alverdy, Y. Vigneswaran (eds.), *Difficult Decisions in Bariatric Surgery*,
Difficult Decisions in Surgery: An Evidence-Based Approach,
https://doi.org/10.1007/978-3-030-55329-6_28

duodenal switch were limited. Therefore, an additional search was conducted using the search term 'sleeve gastrectomy' AND 'gastroesophageal reflux disease'. The search results were reviewed for publications pertaining to management of GERD in the post-operative setting. Additional search terms utilized to further narrow the results for focused review included 'hiatal hernia', 'intractable GERD', 'GERD management', and 'revisional surgery'. The search was largely limited to studies written in the English language; no publication date filter was utilized.

28.3 Results

28.3.1 Current Evidence

The difficult question arises what to do for those patients who develop worsening or de novo GERD symptoms following DS. There is little to no evidence regarding management of GERD after DS at the time of this publication. Prior to being a stand-alone surgical procedure, vertical sleeve gastrectomy was described by Hess in 1988 as a component in the modified approach to the original biliopancreatic diversion described by Scopinaro which involved distal partial gastrectomy [7]. Therefore, the modern DS shares significant similarity to the VSG. Because the DS utilizes a larger sleeve diameter, it is inherently less at risk for development of reflux given decreased intragastric pressure. This may contribute to the relative lack of incidence and literature on the subject of GERD after reflux. Despite this difference, management strategies for GERD in the DS patient are able to be extrapolated from the SG population with reasonable utility.

28.3.2 Extrapolation from Vertical Sleeve Gastrectomy Literature

The relationship between VSG and the development of new or worsening GERD is related to several structural factors including removal of the gastric fundus, disruption of the sling muscle fibers at the gastroesophageal junction (GEJ), reduced gastric volume, and decreased antral pump action proximal to an intact pylorus resulting in increased pressure in the proximal sleeve [8]. However, there has been little consensus in the literature regarding the true effect of SG on GERD [9]. A systematic review of the existing literature in 2016 showed a pooled incidence of new-onset GERD symptoms in 20% of patients following VSG, as well as a slight propensity for SG to worsen existing GERD prevalence [2]. The management strategies summarized below have been recommended for management of GERD in VSG populations and are similarly advised for management of GERD in DS populations.

28.3.2.1 Pre-operative Screening

Recent updated clinical practice guidelines advised that all patients planning bariatric surgery undergo pre-operative screening with detailed questioning for existing GERD symptoms. If present, these should be evaluated with imaging studies, upper

GI series, or endoscopy [4]. Endoscopic detection of hiatal hernia has a reported sensitivity of 78% while clinical detection has a sensitivity of only 55% [10] leading some experts to advise that pre-operative endoscopy should be considered routinely prior to all VSG [4]. This recommendation may similarly be applied to patients considering DS.

28.3.2.2 Concomitant Hiatal Hernia Repair

The prevalence of hiatal hernias in morbidly obese patients is estimated to be around 40% [11]. The presence of a hiatal hernia has a role in both initiation and promotion of GERD symptoms and should therefore ideally be repaired at the time of the index weight loss operation. There is growing literature and consensus amongst experts that concomitant repair of hiatal laxity or hiatal hernia results in improved GERD symptoms and increased patient satisfaction post-operatively [12, 13]. An international panel of experts saw 83% consensus amongst panelists advising an aggressive approach to identification and repair of intraoperatively identified hiatal hernia [14]. A similar approach is recommended for both VSG and DS.

28.3.2.3 Subsequent Hiatal Hernia Repair

For those patients who develop de novo or worsening GERD symptoms post-operatively following DS, an initial approach with optimized medical management beginning with proton pump inhibitors should be undertaken. If medical management is unsuccessful in achieving adequate relief, diagnostic evaluation is recommended for the presence of hiatal hernia. If confirmed, consider re-operation for subsequent hiatal hernia repair. While traditional fundoplication is not an option following VSG or DS, hiatoplasty with or without mesh has been shown to be safe and effective in alleviating GERD symptoms after previous sleeve gastrectomy [15, 16]. Resection of dilated or retained neo-fundus that may be within the hernia may aid in resolution of symptoms and prevent hernia recurrence.

28.3.2.4 Rescue Conversion

An established re-operative intervention in sleeve gastrectomy patients with intractable GERD is rescue conversion to RYGB [17, 18]. However, extrapolation of this recommendation to the DS population should be considered a last resort given the increased technical difficulty and risk associated with revisional surgery from DS to RYGB.

28.3.2.5 Novel Approaches

There is some new literature on the use of magnetic sphincter augmentation as another tool for managing reflux after bariatric surgery. The device has been used in patients undergoing all types of bariatric surgery, including VSG, RYGB, and DS. Post-operatively patients were shown to have decreased use of acid-reducing medication and increased GERD-specific quality of life scores [19]. While early results are promising, this approach has not yet been widely investigated or adapted.

28.4   Conclusions and Recommendations

Biliopancreatic diversion with duodenal switch is our preferred intervention for patients with a BMI greater than 50 kg/m^2. As compared to Roux-en-Y gastric bypass, DS has superior outcomes for weight loss, and resolution of all co-morbid conditions with the exception of GERD [20]. Therefore, when we encounter patients with BMI > 50kg/m^2 who have GERD, we weigh the risks of ongoing or worsening GERD with the benefits of superior weight loss and resolution of metabolic conditions afforded by DS. Our pre-operative assessment includes pH testing, esophageal manometry, upper GI contrast study and EGD. Patients with pathologic reflux, esophageal dysmotility or reflux induced changes to esophageal mucosa (esophagitis, stricture, Barrett's) are designates to undergo Roux-en-Y gastric bypass. Patients with hiatal hernia that may contribute to reflux, but without esophageal mucosal changes, may undergo RYGB or DS with concomitant hiatal hernia repair. Severely obese patients with significant metabolic conditions and without esophageal mucosal changed may benefit more from duodenal switch.

Patients who have undergone DS and subsequently develop worsening reflux, our first step is to counsel them on diet and behavior modifications that may contribute to their symptoms along with PPI therapy. Patients with refractory symptoms often have a hiatal hernia that can be addressed surgically. Many times, these hernias are associated with a dilated neo-fundus that needs resection or "re-sleeve" along with hiatal hernia repair. This serves to reduce acid producing gastric mucosa and eliminates a "lead-point" for gastric herniation. We have not needed to convert a duodenal switch to a Roux-en-Y gastric bypass to date, nor have we employed the use of magnetic sphincter augmentation. Prior to doing so, we would recommend pH and manometry testing to confirm pathologic reflux.

28.5   Personal View of Data

Clearly there is need for more research and publication in this particular area. The lack of literature may be due to selection of patients with significant preoperative GERD to have procedures other than DS, the overall low numbers of DS performed or perhaps the lower incidence of post-operative GERD in patients with a larger capacity/lower pressure sleeve. Another issue not examined is the contribution of bile reflux to pathologic GERD. The diversion of biliopancreatic secretions away from the stomach and esophagus in DS, may also lead to a reduced incidence of symptomatic GERD resulting in lower reports. Nevertheless, when encountering DS patients with significant GERD, extrapolating from the VSG experience can be instructive and therapeutic.

28.6   Recommendations

1. Thorough pre-operative screening for symptoms of GERD ± diagnostic studies such as endoscopy, contrast upper GI radiography, manometry, and pH monitoring.

2. Adequate intra-operative dissection of the hiatus for identification of existing laxity or hiatal hernia with low threshold for simultaneous repair during the index weight loss operation.
3. Subsequent hiatal hernia repair for those patients who develop de novo or worsening GERD symptoms post-operatively and fail optimal medical management.
4. Rescue conversion to Roux-en-Y gastric bypass should be considered a last resort given technical difficulty.

References

1. Hampel H, Abraham NS, El-Serag HB. Meta-analysis: obesity and the risk for gastroesophageal reflux disease and its complications. Ann Intern Med. 2005;143(3):199–211. https://doi.org/10.7326/0003-4819-143-3-200508020-00006.
2. Oor JE, Roks DJ, Ünlü Ç, Hazebroek EJ. Laparoscopic sleeve gastrectomy and gastroesophageal reflux disease: a systematic review and meta-analysis. Am J Surg. 2016;211(1):250–67. https://doi.org/10.1016/j.amjsurg.2015.05.031.
3. Hess DS, Hess DW, Oakley RS. The biliopancreatic diversion with the duodenal switch: results beyond 10 years. Obes Surg. 2005;15(3):408–16. https://doi.org/10.1381/0960892053576695.
4. Mechanick JI, Apovian C, Brethauer S, Garvey WT, Joffe AM, Kim J, et al. Clinical practice guidelines for the perioperative nutrition, metabolic, and nonsurgical support of patients undergoing bariatric procedures—2019 update: cosponsored by American association of clinical endocrinologists/American college of endocrinology, the obesity society, American society for metabolic & bariatric surgery, obesity medicine association, and American society of anesthesiologists—executive summary. Endocr Pract. 2019;25(12):1346–59. https://doi.org/10.4158/GL-2019-0406.
5. Scopinaro N, Gianetta E, Pandolfo N, Anfossi A, Berretti B, Bachi V. Bilio-pancreatic bypass: proposal and preliminary experimental study of a new type of operation for the functional surgical treatment of obesity. Minerva Chir. 1976;31(10):560–6.
6. Bolckmans R, Himpens J. Long-term (>10 yrs) outcome of the laparoscopic biliopancreatic diversion with duodenal switch. Ann Surg. 2016;264(6):1029–37. https://doi.org/10.1097/SLA.0000000000001622.
7. Hess DS, Hess DW. Biliopancreatic diversion with a duodenal switch. Obes Surg. 1998;8(3):267–82. https://doi.org/10.1381/096089298765554476.
8. Del Genio G, Tolone S, Limongelli P, Brusciano L, D'Alessandro A, Docimo G, et al. Sleeve gastrectomy and development of "de novo" gastroesophageal reflux. Obes Surg. 2014;24:71–7.
9. Chiu S, Birch DW, Shi X, Sharma AM, Karmali S. Effect of sleeve gastrectomy on gastroesophageal reflux disease: a systematic review. Surg Obes Relat Dis. 2011;7(4):510–5. https://doi.org/10.1016/j.soard.2010.09.011.
10. Mohammed R, Fei P, Phu J, Asai M, Antanavicius G. Efficiency of preoperative esophagogastroduodenoscopy in identifying operable hiatal hernia for bariatric surgery patients. Surg Obes Relat Dis. 2017;13(2):287–90. https://doi.org/10.1016/j.soard.2016.08.015.
11. Che F, Nguyen B, Cohen A, Nguyen NT. Prevalence of hiatal hernia in the morbidly obese. Surg Obes Relat Dis. 2013;9(6):920–4. https://doi.org/10.1016/j.soard.2013.03.013.
12. El Chaar M, Ezeji G, Claros L, Miletics M, Stoltzfus J. Short-term results of laparoscopic sleeve gastrectomy in combination with hiatal hernia repair: experience in a single accredited center. Obes Surg. 2016;26:68–76. https://doi.org/10.1007/s11695-015-1739-y.
13. Lyon A, Gibson SC, De-loyde K, Martin D. Gastroesophageal reflux in laparoscopic sleeve gastrectomy: hiatal findings and their management influence outcome. Surg Obes Relat Dis. 2015;11(3):530–7. https://doi.org/10.1016/j.soard.2014.08.010.

14. Rosenthal RJ, International Sleeve Gastrectomy Expert Panel, Diaz AA, Arvidsson D, Baker RS, Basso N, et al. International sleeve gastrectomy expert panel consensus statement: best practice guidelines based on experience of >12,000 cases. Surg Obes Relat Dis. 2012;8(1):8–19. https://doi.org/10.1016/j.soard.2011.10.019.
15. Macedo FIB, Mowzoon M, Mittal VK, Sabir M. Outcomes of laparoscopic hiatal hernia repair in nine bariatric patients with prior sleeve gastrectomy. Obes Surg. 2017;27(10):2768–72. https://doi.org/10.1007/s11695-017-2880-6.
16. Soong TC, Almalki OM, Lee WJ, Ser KH, Chen JC, Wu CC, Chen SC. Revision of sleeve gastrectomy with hiatal repair with gastropexy for gastroesophageal reflux disease. Obes Surg. 2019 Aug;29(8):2381–6. https://doi.org/10.1007/s11695-019-03853-0.
17. Langer FB, Bohdjalian A, Shakeri-Leidenmühler S, Schoppmann SF, Zacherl J, Prager G. Conversion from sleeve gastrectomy to Roux-en-Y gastric bypass—indications and outcome. Obes Surg. 2010;20(7):835–40. https://doi.org/10.1007/s11695-010-0125-z.
18. Abdemur A, Han SM, Lo Menzo E, Szomstein S, Rosenthal R. Reasons and outcomes of conversion of laparoscopic sleeve gastrectomy to Roux-en-Y gastric bypass for nonresponders. Surg Obes Relat Dis. 2016;12(1):113–8. https://doi.org/10.1016/j.soard.2015.04.005.
19. Broderick RC, Smith CD, Cheverie JN, Omelanczuk P, Lee AM, Dominguez-Profeta R, Cubas R, Jacobsen GR, Sandler BJ, Fuchs KH, Horgan S. Magnetic sphincter augmentation: a viable rescue therapy for symptomatic reflux following bariatric surgery. Surg Endosc. 2019;34(7):3211–5. https://doi.org/10.1007/s00464-019-07096-z.
20. Prachand VN, Ward M, Alverdy JC. Duodenal switch provides superior resolution of metabolic comorbidities independent of weight loss in the super-obese (BMI > or = 50 kg/m2) compared with gastric bypass. J Gastrointest Surg. 2010;14(2):211–20.

Endoscopic Management of the Dilated Gastrojejunal Anastomosis

Ye Eun Kwak and Christopher G. Chapman

29.1 Introduction

Roux-en-Y gastric bypass (RYGB) is a very effective weight loss surgery that can achieve significant and sustained weight loss [1, 2]. In the United States, over a million RYGB have been performed in the past decade, and it is currently the second most commonly performed bariatric surgery for obesity [3]. On average, excess weight loss (EWL) after RYGB is 60–70% [1, 4] and resolution or improvement of obesity related comorbidities such as diabetes, dyslipidemia, hypertension and sleep apnea have been reported in 75–94% of cases [4].

Weight regain, defined as gaining more than 15% of maximum weight loss is common in all bariatric surgeries [5]. In RYGB, twenty to fifty percent of patients experience significant weight regain in 5 to 10 years after surgery [6, 7] and weight regain can occur as early as 1 year after RYGB [8]. Most RYGB patients regain more than 30% of lost weight and over a quarter of RYGB patients regain almost all of their lost weight [8]. Weight regain is suspected to be caused by combination of multiple factors including genetic susceptibility, hormonal/metabolic changes, environmental/nutritional/psychosocial aspects and modifiable anatomic changes such as dilated gastrojejunal stoma, dilated pouch and/or gastro-gastric fistula formation. This chapter will review the endoscopic interventions for revision of a dilated gastrojejunal stoma for weight regain.

Y. E. Kwak
Section of Gastroenterology, Hepatology and Nutrition, Department of Medicine, University of Chicago Medicine, Chicago, IL, USA

C. G. Chapman (✉)
Center for Endoscopic Research and Therapeutics (CERT), University of Chicago Medicine, Chicago, IL, USA
e-mail: christopher.chapman@uchospitals.edu

© Springer Nature Switzerland AG 2021
J. Alverdy, Y. Vigneswaran (eds.), *Difficult Decisions in Bariatric Surgery*,
Difficult Decisions in Surgery: An Evidence-Based Approach,
https://doi.org/10.1007/978-3-030-55329-6_29

29.2   Search Strategy

PubMed database were used in the majority of search and Google Scholar database were searched if no study was found in PubMed related to each subject. References of included articles were searched to identify additional studies. Two independent reviewers (YEK and CC) manually reviewed all articles to ensure the qualification of the study in each endoscopic procedure criteria. Search keyword used included, but not limited to: bariatric endoscopy, StomaphyX, incisionless operating platform, transoral outlet reduction, endoscopic suturing, gastrojejunal stoma and Roux-en-Y gastric bypass revision.

29.3   Clinical Relevance of a Dilated Gastrojejunal Stoma

Although controversial, studies have demonstrated that a dilated gastrojejunal stoma after RYGB is a strong independent risk factor associated with weight regain and the diameter of the gastrojejunal stoma demonstrates a positive linear correlation with the amount of weight regain [9]. One study showed each 10 mm increase in the stoma diameter resulted in 8% increase in the percent of maximal weight lost that was regained in 5 years after RYGB [9]. Stoma size ≥15 mm is defined as dilated and endoscopic or surgical revision should be considered in those patients [10].

Certain surgical revision techniques including gastrojejunal outlet reduction surgery for weight regain after initial RYGB have shown to be effective in additional weight loss. One study showed laparoscopic RYGB revision resulted in 54% of additional percentage of EWL at 4 years after revision surgery [11]. However, various surgical revision procedures have major complication rates ranging from 20 to 50% and mortality rates up to 2% [11–16]. To overcome morbidity and mortality from surgical revision, minimally invasive endoscopic revision procedures have been proposed. Multiple endoscopic modalities using various tissue plication techniques and sclerotherapy have been investigated to achieve reduction of dilated gastrojejunal stoma and/or gastric pouch size.

29.4   Endoscopic Plication Techniques

29.4.1 StomaphyX

The StomaphyX™ (EndoGastricSolutions, Inc., Redmond, WA, USA) is a transoral plication device that creates tissue approximation and ligation using polypropylene SerosaFuse™ fasteners (Fig. 29.1a). In this procedure, a vacuum suctions gastric tissue into the device creating a large tissue fold. A stylet is advanced through the tissue and polypropylene H-fasteners are deployed across the base of the created fold [17]. The procedure creates a series of 3–4 rows of 4–6 plications

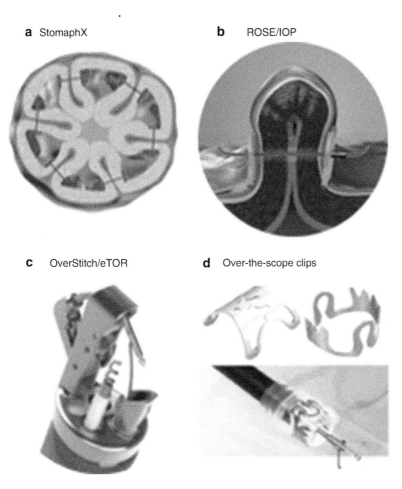

Fig. 29.1 Plication devices and techniques. (**a**) StomaphX, (**b**) ROSE/IOP, (**c**) OverStitch/eTOR and (**d**) Over-the-scope clips

circumferentially from the most distal end of the pouch to the stoma, with a goal of reducing ≥75% of gastric pouch volume and ≥ 50% of stoma diameter.

Four retrospective case series evaluating StomaphX for RYGB revision for weight regain have been reported in the literature [18–21]. The first report in 2009 consisted of 39 patients with >10% weight regain from the nadir and > 2 years from the RYGB [18]. After 6 months (n = 14), the mean weight loss was 8.7 kg (17.0% EBWL), and at 1 year (n = 6) was 10.0 kg (19.5% EBWL). A second series with 64 patients, the mean weight loss was similar, with 7.6 kg lost at a mean follow-up of nearly 6 months [19]. However, subsequent retrospective case series started raising concerns about the durability of the revisional weight loss. In 2011, Ong'uti et al. reported 29 patients undergoing Stomaphyx revision had a median weight loss of

47% of regained weight at 6 months, but this declined to 20% at 1 year [21]. A similar concern for durability of weight loss was reported by Goyal et al. reviewing 59 post-RYGB patients who underwent revision of gastric pouch using StomaphyX from 2007 to 2008 [20]. At 6 months, EBWL was $11.5 \pm 17.9\%$ (n = 10), however in a cohort of 53 patients with 24–48 months of follow-up, the average weight loss declined to 1.7 ± 9.7 kg, and EBWL was $4.3 \pm 29.8\%$. Further, endoscopy performed in 12 patients at average 18 months follow-up showed no sustained reduction in pouch and stoma size (Table 29.1).

A prospective, single-center, randomized, single-blinded study for RYGB revision was initiated in 2009 [22]. However, due to the preliminary results indicating a failure to achieve the primary efficacy end point ($\geq$15% excessive BMI loss and BMI <35) in at least 50% of StomaphyX-treated patients, enrollment was closed prematurely. 45 patients treated with StomaphyX and 29 patients in the sham treatment group completed 1 year of post-randomization follow up. 22.2% of the StomaphyX patients achieved the primary endpoint compared to 3.4% in sham procedure group (p < 0.1). In the StomaphyX cohort there was a gastric perforation causally related to the device which required laparoscopic exploration and repair surgery. The failure to reach the primary study endpoint resulted in early termination of the study and the device is no longer available for RYGB revision.

29.4.2 ROSE Procedure/Incisionless Operating Platform

Restorative Obesity Surgery Endolumenal (ROSE) procedure is an endoscopic revision technique using the Incisionless Operating Platform™ (USGI Medical, Inc., San Clemente, CA, USA). The device creates full thickness gastric tissue plications and decreases the size of gastric pouch or gastrojejunal stoma (Fig. 29.1b).

Four prospective studies and one retrospective case series evaluating ROSE procedure in RYGB patients were reported in the literature. The first prospective pilot study involving 5 patients who regained a mean of 14.7 kg with dilated pouch and GJA noted on endoscopy showed technical success in 100% of patients with mean weight loss of 7.8 kg at months without major complications [23]. Subsequently, Mullady et al. performed prospective case series study with 20 patients who had a mean of 13 kg weight regain with dilated pouch and GJA [24]. Procedure success rate was 85% with average reduction in stoma diameter of 16 mm and pouch length of 2.5 cm, and of those successful cases, mean weight loss 8.8 kg at 3 months.

This prompted a prospective multicenter registry study published in 2010 involving 116 patients who had regained significant weight $\geq$ 2 years after RYGB after achieving $\geq$50% EWL [25]. Technical success rate was 96%, with average stoma diameter reduction of 50% and pouch length reduction of 44%. At 6 months, an average of 32% of weight regain after RYGB had been lost, with average EWL of 18%. Follow up EGD at 12 months showed durable tissue folds and anchors. A follow up data from this study showed safety and durability of ROSE procedure, with 14.5% EWL at 12 months without serious adverse events. This study highlighted that aggressive reduction of stoma dilation to less than 10 mm was associated with

Table 29.1 Summary of literature

Study	Study type	No	Procedure	Selection criteria	M:F	Mean age (years)	Mean pre-revision weight (kg)	Mean pre-revision BMI (kg/M²)	Mean time since initial surgery (months)
Mikami et al. [18]	Retro case series	39	StomaphyX	>2 years post-op >10% of nadir weight	3:36	47.8 (29–64)	108 (65.9–172.2)	39.8 (22.7–63.2)	
Leitman et al. [19]	Pro case series	64	StomaphyX	Inadequate weight loss, dumping syndrome (42), GERD (15)		48		39.5	60
Goyal et al. [20]	Retro case series	55	StomaphyX		1:53	49.6 (30–68)	96.6	36.1	68.4 (12–156)
Ong'Uti et al. [21]	Retro case series	27	StomaphyX	> 2 years post-op	2:25	49 (44–54)	103 (88.5–115)	37 (32–40)	72 (60–96)
Eid et al. [22]	Pros RCT	90	StomaphyX	> 2 years post-op initial weight loss ≥60% of excess BMI. BMI ≤35 followed by regaining ≥20% of pre-RYGB excess weight	1:1.2	51 (43–56)		29.2	6.4 (5.0–7.5)
Ryou et al. [23]	Pros case series	5	ROSE	WR, satiety, dilated pouch/GJA	0:5	48 (41–55)	100.4	36.3	
Mullady et al. [24]	Pros case series	20	ROSE	WR/ no weight loss, satiety	1:19	48 (36–62)		36.7 (28.4–48.8)	63 (24–117)
Horgan et al. [25]	Pros case series	116	ROSE	> 2 yrs. postop, >50% EWL after RYGB	15:101	45.6 ± 8.7	110.8 ± 20.5	39.9 ± 6.7	

(continued)

Table 29.1 (continued)

Study	No	Procedure	Selection criteria	M:F	Mean age (years)	Mean pre-revision weight (kg)	Mean pre-revision BMI (kg/M²)	Mean time since initial surgery (months)
Thompson, Jacobsen et al. [26]	116	ROSE	> 2 yrs. after RYGB	15:101	46 ± 9	110.5 ± 20.5	39.9 ± 6.7	
Gallo et al. [27]	27	ROSE	> 50% EWL, significant weight gain 2 years post-op	2:25	49.2 ± 9.6 (26–68)	106.2 ± 21.2	40.6 (30–67)	142.8 ± 51.6
Thompson, Chand et al. [28]	50	eTOR	BMI 30–60 at >6 months post-op, inadequate WL > 50% EWL/ WR > 5% EWL, GJA > 2 cm	3:47	47.6 ± 9.46	101.5 ± 16.4	37.6 ± 4.9	58
Jirapinyo et al. [29]	25	eTOR	WR, GJA > 15 mm	7:18	48 (34–69)		43	
Kumar and Thompson [29]	150	eTOR	GJA > 15 mm	27:123	51.2 ± 0.8	110.7 ± 2.2	40.1 ± 0.7	103.2 ± 3.6
Vargas et al. [32]	130	eTOR	WR	16:114	47.12 ± 8.55		36.8 ± 6.84	100.8 ± 57.4

Jirapinyo et al. [33]	Pros case series	331	eTOR	Adequate weight loss (loss of <50% excess weight loss after bariatric surgery) or weight regain (gaining of 15% of maximal weight initially lost)	1:6	50 ± 11	110.0 ± 26.3	40.1 ± 9.1	111.6 ± 56.4
Heylen et al. [34]	Pros case series	46	OTSC-clip	> 10% WG 2 yrs. post-op, reappearing comorbidities, volume/ frequency of meals	19:75			32.8	
Dayyeh et al. [35]	Pros case series	231	Sclerotherapy (sodium morrhuate)	Weight regain	1:9	47 ± 10			68.4
Jirapinyo et al. [31]	Pros case series	43	Sclerotherapy (sodium morrhuate)	> 1 yr. postop >20% of nadir weight	3:31	47 ± 9			72 ± 60
Moon et al. [36]	Retro case series	558	APC	> 18 months post-op, regain of >10% of nadir weight, satiety, size of GJ stoma >15 mm	103:455	40.9 ± 9.5	94.5 ± 18.6	34.0 ± 5.7	90

(continued)

Table 29.1 (continued)

Study	Study type	No	Procedure	Selection criteria	M:F	Mean age (years)	Mean pre-revision weight (kg)	Mean pre-revision BMI (kg/M^2)	Mean time since initial surgery (months)
Baretta et al. [38]	Pros case series	30	APC	> 18 months post-op, regain of >10% of nadir weight, stoma diameter > 15 mm	4:26	42.83 (22–59)	121.77 ± 22.50	45.63 ± 7.63	
de Quadros et al. [37]	RCT	42	APC		13:29	39.5 ± 9.96	101 ± 25.2	36.1 ± 7.45	
Abidi et al. [39]	Case report	1	Modified ESD	Weight regain, dilated GJA	Female	34			
de Moura et al. [40]	Case report	1	Modified ESD	Weight regain	Female	55			
Abrams et al. [41]	Single arm, unblinded, multicenterstudy	25	RFA	Achieved >40% excess body weight loss and then regained >25% of lost weight	4:21	45.4	110.9	40.2	109

	Mean post-surgical weight or BMI				% Excess weight loss <3mo					
Study	3 mo	6 mo	1 year	3 years	<3 mo	3 mo	6 mo	12 mo	24 mo	≥36 mo
Mikami et al. [18]	101.3 kg	99.3 kg	98 kg		7.4 at 2 weeks, 10.6 at 1mo, 13.1 at 2mo	13.1	17	19.5		
Leitman et al. [19]							Mean weight loss 7.3 kg (0–31)			

Goyal et al. [20]	92.9 (1 mo)	92.8	94.9		7.3 ± 7.1 at 1 week 11.6 ± 12.1 at 1mo		11.5 (17.9)		4.3 ± 29.8
Ong'Uti et al. [21]	101.3 BMI 33(29–36) at 0 month	94.5	93.9 (81.6 ± 102)		24 at 2 weeks	33	47	20	
Eid et al. [22]	7.9 (1mo) 11.3 (3mo)	10.1	9.9 (9mo) 7.8 (12mo)						
Ryou et al. [23]	92.6 BMI 33.4				4.2 kg weight loss at 1mo	7.8 kg			
Mullady et al. [24]					5.8 kg weight loss at 1mo	8.8 kg			
Horgan et al. [25]							21.5 ± 15.3		
Thompson, Jacobsen et al. [26]			104.6					14.5 ± 3.1	
Gallo et al. [27]	BMI 39.2 ± 7		BMI 39.9 ± 10.1	BMI 37.7 ± 6.3	8.9	9.3	8	6.7	− 10.7 at 36 mo − 13.5 at 48 mo −5.8 at 60 mo −4.5 at 72 mo

(continued)

Table 29.1 (continued)

| Study | Mean post-surgical weight or BMI | | | | % Excess weight loss <3mo | | | | | |
	3 mo	6 mo	1 year	3 years	<3 mo	3 mo	6 mo	12 mo	24 mo	≥36 mo
Thompson, Chand et al. [28]							15.9			
Jirapinyo et al. [29]						Mean 11.5	Mean 11.7	Mean 10.8		
Kumar and Thompson [29]	101.1 BMI 36.6	100.1 BMI 36.3	100.2 BMI 36.3	90.7 at 2 year BMI 36.8 at 2 year 91.5 at 3 year BMI 36.7 at 3 year		25.0 ± 1.9	28.8 ± 2.7	24.9 ± 2.6	20.0 ± 6.4	19.2 ± 4.6
Vargas et al. [32]							9.31 ± 6.7	20.2 ± 10	8 ± 8.8 (18–24 mo)	
Jirapinyo et al. [33]			Lost 9.4 ± 12.3 kg	Lost 8.7 ± 13.8 kg				% total weight loss 8.5 ± 8.5%		% total weight loss 6.9 ± 10.1% at 36 mo 8.8 ± 12.5% at 60 mo
Heylen et al. [34]	BMI 29.7		BMI 27.4							
Dayyeh et al. [35]		Mean weight loss 4.5 kg								

Jirapinyo et al. [31]		Mean % total body weight loss 2.7 ± 5.5%		Mean % total body weight loss 6.1 ± 6.8 (9 months)
Moon et al. [36]	83.29 (4 months)		Mean weight loss 6.5	Mean weight loss 7.7
Baretta et al. [38]	78.87 BMI 31.14 ± 5.81			Mean weight loss 8.3
de Quadros et al. [37]	93.1		%total weight loss 15.6%	
Abidi et al. [39]		19 kg weight loss		
de Moura et al. [40]			9 kg weight loss 12.5%total body weight loss	6.3 kg weight loss 8.6%TBWL
Abrams et al. [41]		11.4% at 3.5mo	10.0% at 7.5 mo	18.40%

(continued)

Table 29.1 (continued)

Study	Avg stoma diameter at the end of procedure (mm)	Definition of successful endoscopy	Success number (rate %)	Recurrence rate	Post-procedure complication
Mikami et al. [18]					Minor: Sore throat (87.1), epigastric pain (76.9)
Leitman et al. [19]				21% weight regain	
Goyal et al. [20]	12.8	1. Ability to reduce pouch and stoma size 2. Weight loss	35 (63.6)	2 (3.6)–progressed to further procedure	N/A
Ong'Uti et al. [21]	20 (20–30)			3 (4.7%)	
Eid et al. [22]		Reduction in pre-RYGB excess weight by ≥15% excess BMI loss and BMI < 35 at 12 months after the procedure	22.2% with StomaphyX vs 3.4% sham (p < 0.01)		One patient major gastric perforation
Ryou et al. [23]		1. Ability to reduce pouch and stoma size 2. Weight loss	5 (100)		N/A
Mullady et al. [24]		1. Ability to reduce pouch and stoma size 2. Weight loss	17 (85)		Minor: Abdominal bloating, mild sore throats
Horgan et al. [25]	11.5	1. Ability to reduce pouch and stoma size 2. Weight loss	112 (97)		Mild: Pharyhgitis, nausea, vomiting, abdominal pain moderate: Superficial distal esophagus tear (3)
Thompson, Jacobsen et al. [26]	11.5	1. Ability to reduce pouch and stoma size 2. Weight loss	112 (97)		

Study					
Gallo et al. [27]	8 ± 4				n/a
Thompson, Chand et al. [28]		Ability to reduce the GJ to <10 mm	89.60%		
Jirapinyo et al. [29]	6 (3–10)	Ability to reduce the GJ to <12 mm	25 (100)		
Kumar and Thompson [29]	9.0 ± 0.2				Pain 6 (4.0), bleeding 5 (3.3), nausea 3 (2.0)
Vargas et al. [32]		Ability to reduce the GJ to <10 mm		11 (8)—Repeat EGD performed	Nausea 18 (14), pain 23 (18), Oesophageal tear requiring endoscopic clipping 1 (< 1), balloon dilation of narrowed GJA after TORe 5 (4)
Jirapinyo et al. [33]					No severe adverse events
Heylen et al. [34]					Mild: Sore throat moderate: 5(10.9) dysphagia (repeat OGD), 2 persistent dysphagia had endoscopic dilatation)
Dayyeh et al. [35]					Moderate: Bleeding, transient elevation of diastolic BP, ulcer, abdominal pain
Jirapinyo et al. [31]	21 ± 6	Ability to reduce the GJ to <12 mm			Pain 1, heartburn 1, hypertensive urgency 1, bleeding 1

(continued)

Table 29.1 (continued)

Study	Avg stoma diameter at the end of procedure (mm)	Definition of successful endoscopy	Success number (rate %)	Recurrence rate	Post-procedure complication
Moon et al. [36]	14.0 ± 6.3				Stenosis 9, GJ ulcer 3, vomiting 3, GJ leakage 2, melena 1
Baretta et al. [38]	8.40 ± 1.85				Severe stenosis (stoma diameter < 3 mm) 2, ulcers at stoma 10
de Quadros et al. [37]	14.8 at 6 mo				N/A
Abidi et al. [39]					
de Moura et al. [40]	12 at 12 mo				
Abrams et al. [41]			92.30%		Minor mucosal tears with self-limited bleeding occurred in 38 of 65 cases(58.5%). Gastric ulcer bleeding (1), severe dehydration (1)

Table was adapted and revised from Goh et al. [43]

more than double EWL compare to the one who did not (24% vs 10% EWL, p = 0.03) [26].

However, a retrospective study following up 27 patients after ROSE procedure showed that statistically significant sustained weight loss was achieved only until 12 months, and among those who had follow up data, EWL were − 10.7%, −13.5%, −5.8% and − 4.5% at 36, 48, 60, and 72 months respectively. Of note, only 15% patient followed up after 2 years and authors attributed the loss of sustained weight loss to lack of follow up and possible anatomical failure [27]. Currently, the ROSE procedure with the IOP is not routinely performed in the United States.

29.4.3 Endoscopic Transoral Outlet Reduction (eTOR)

The endoscopic transoral outlet reduction, or eTOR, procedure has emerged as the most widely used technique across the US and internationally. The standard eTOR procedure utilizes ablation of gastric mucosa adjacent to the stoma followed by full thickness sutures to reduce the gastrojejunal anastomosis size (Fig. 29.2a–d). The

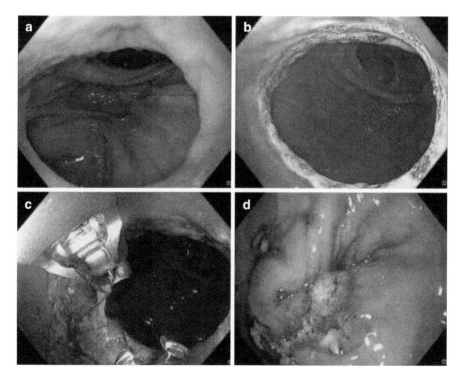

Fig. 29.2 Endoscopic Transoral outlet reduction (eTOR) procedure. (**a**) Dilated gastrojejunal stoma. (**b**) Argon plasma coagulation treatment of the dialted gastrojejunal stoma. (**c**) Endoscopic transoral outlet reduction (eTOR) using the Overstitch endoscopic suturing device in a modified figure 8 suturing pattern. (**d**) Completed eTOR procedure

eTOR procedure is currently performed using the OverStitch™ platform (Apollo Endosurgery, Austin, TX, USA) (Fig. 29.1c) and is an effective, durable and safe weight regain intervention after RYGB.

Thompson et al. performed a multicenter randomized sham control trial to evaluate the efficacy of the eTOR using superficial suction-based device in 77 patients who had weight regain or inadequate weight loss after RYGB and GJ diameter > 2 cm [28]. This study proved the concept of eTOR could be effective in weight loss with greater mean percentage weight loss from baseline (3.5% in eTOR compared to 0.4% in control group, p = 0.021). The small scale of weight loss was attributed to superficial suction-based device, hence subsequent studies using OverStitch™ platform (Apollo Endosurgery, Austin, TX, USA) which allows a full thickness suturing had been performed. In a retrospective case series of 25 patients who underwent TORe for dilated GJA and weight regain, technical success was achieved in all patients with a mean reduction in GJA diameter to 6 mm (77.3% reduction) with sustained weight loss mean of 11.5 kg, 11.7 kg and 10.8 kg at 3, 6, and 12 months respectively, without major complications [29]. A prospective case series was published in 2016 proving durability of weight loss and safety with TORe at 3 years (EWL 24.9% at 1 year, 20.0% at 2 years and 19.2% at 3 years) [30]. This study highlights a low number needed to treat for arrest of weight regain with 1.0 at 6 months, 1.1 at 1 year, 1.2 at 2 and 3 years. The number needed to treat to maintain weight loss of ≥5 kg from TORe was also low (1.2 at 6 months, 1.5 at 1 year, 1.9 at 2 years and 2.0 at 3 years). In a prospective study comparing endoscopic suturing and sclerotherapy, endoscopic suturing resulted in greater reduction in outlet size (reduction of the outlet diameter by 15.0 mm in suture and 2.6 mm in sclerotherapy group), which was the only predictor of weight loss (p < 0.01). In the endoscopic suturing group, patients had significant improvement in eating behavior and weight loss than sclerotherapy [31]. A large, multicenter meta-analysis of TORe procedure using full thickness suturing device from 2013 to 2016 involving 130 patients showed average weight loss of 9.3 kg, 7.8 kg and 8 kg at 6, 12 and 18 months, respectively [32]. Overall 14% of patient had nausea, 18% had pain and 8% required a repeat EGD, however, no serious adverse events were reported.

Most recently, a five-year follow-up retrospective review of prospectively collected data on 331 RYGB patients who underwent TORe showed 8.5%, 6.9% and 8.8% total weight loss at 1, 3, and 5 years, with no severe adverse events [33]. The mean BMI was 40 kg/ m^2 and mean pre-TORe GJA size was 23 mm which was decreased to 8.4 mm after TORe. The amount of weight loss at 1 year was a predictor of percentage of total weight loss at 5 years (β = .43, p = 0.01). Interestingly, follow up rates were 83.3% at 1 year, 81.8% at 3 years and 82.9% at 5 years and 39.3% patients had additional weight loss therapy with either pharmacotherapy or procedure, with 3.6% getting repeat TORe. An additional endoscopic weight loss procedure was associated with higher percentage of total weight loss at 5 years (p = 0.01).

29.4.4 Over-the-Scope Clips

The Over-the-scope clip (OTSC®, Ovesco Endoscopy GmbH, Tübingen, Germany) is a biocompatible jaw shaped clip made of Nitinol which is loaded on a transparent applicator cap to be mounted on the tip of the scope (Fig. 29.1d). The OTS clips are larger in size (11–12 mm) and can capture more tissue than standard through-the-scope clips. There is a single prospective case series conducted that used a large OTSCs to decrease the size of dilated gastrojejunal anastomosis outlet in 46 patients with post-RYGB weight regain. This study showed two clips placed at the opposite sites of dilated gastrojejunostomy could successfully reduce the outlet by more than 80%. In this series, the mean BMI at one year decreased from 32.8 to 27.4 after OTSC clip revision procedure [34]. However, due to lack of larger prospective trial using OTSC clip for weight regain revision, it has not been adopted as a mainstream procedure.

29.5 Endoscopic Ablation and Resection Techniques

29.5.1 Sclerotherapy

Ablation therapies decrease the size of the dilated gastrojejunal stoma by forming scar tissue resulting in delayed gastric emptying and increased restriction. Gastrojejunal anastomosis reduction was first reported using sclerotherapy with submucosal needle injection of sodium morrhuate. In multiple case series and retrospective studies, sclerotherapy was effective in achieving mean weight loss of 11.7 lbs. at 12 months follow up, and 2 or 3 sclerotherapy sessions showed higher rates of weight regain stabilization than a single session (90 vs 60% at 12 months, p = 0.003) [35]. However, in a prospective study directly comparing endoscopic suturing and sclerotherapy in reducing gastrojejunal anastomosis size, an endoscopic suturing resulted in greater reduction in outlet size and improvement in weight loss than sclerotherapy [31]. Moreover, due to safety concerns in using sclerotherapy (2.4% bleeding rate with 67% of bleeding requiring clipping and transient diastolic blood pressure elevation [35]) as well as lack of availability of sclerotherapy in many centers, the sclerotherapy is no longer used [10].

29.5.2 Argon Plasma Coagulation

Similar to the sclerotherapy but with less safety concern, argon plasma coagulation (APC) has been increasingly adopted for the treatment of dilated gastrojejunal stomas. APC is a noncontact electrocoagulation method using ionized argon gas that results in tissue devitalization and ablation. When treating weight regain in post-RYGB patients, the gastrojejunal anastomosis is ablated 360 degrees around the circumference of the outlet with 1 cm width to induce tissue scar formation. APC settings vary based on duration of activation, power setting and probe distance. Commonly used settings are pulsed or forced APC, flow of 0.7–2.0 L/min, effect 2 and 50 Watts resulting in a light char on the mucosa with no impact to submucosa. However, recent data indicate that a higher dose (70–80 Watts) with increased depth of penetration to the submucosa may result in increased scar tissue formation and enhanced weight loss [36, 37].

In the largest series published to date, a retrospective chart review was performed for 558 patients at eight bariatric centers in the USA (1) and Brazil (7) who underwent APC procedure for post-RYGB weight regain between 2009 and 2017 [36]. 81.5% of the patients were female with a mean age of 40.9 years, and the mean BMI at the time of APC was 34.0 kg/m2 (with 25.1% having a BMI less than 30 kg/m2). Using an APC setting of Pulse, flow 2 L, 70 Watts, many patients underwent multiple treatments with the median number of interventions in these patients being two sessions. Mean size of the gastrojejunostomy before APC intervention was 24.4 mm, and this decreased to a mean size of 14.0 mm after the intervention. The mean weight loss was 6.5, 7.7, and 8.3 kg at 6, 12, and 24 months, respectively. The % TWL was 6.7, 8.3, and 11.0 at 6, 12, and 24 months, respectively. Among 333 patients at four centers for whom information on complications was provided, there were nine cases of stenosis, three cases of gastrojejunal ulcers, three cases of vomiting, two cases of gastrojejunal leakage, and one case of melena.

In a prospective study looking at the efficacy of APC (2 L/min, 90 W) as a weight regain intervention in 30 post-RYGB patients, three, 8-weeks apart consecutive sessions of APC have shown to decrease the stoma size by 66.9% with mean weight loss of 15.5 kg of the 19.6 kg of regained weight after RYGB. The effect of APC was maintained at 8 weeks after the final session, both endoscopically and weight loss wise, with only complication being stenosed aperture of less than 3 mm in 2 patients [38].

Most recently in 2020, a parallel, randomized controlled study was published comparing APC to exclusive multidisciplinary management after weight regain [37]. 42 patients were divided into two groups: APC at 1 L/min, 80 W every 8 weeks (n = 22) and control (n = 20). After 14 months of follow-up with a crossover at 6 months, significant improvement in satiety and greater weight loss were found in the APC group and after crossover. Mean pre-APC weight was 101 ± 25.2 kg, mean weight regain was 19.4 kg from the minimum weight achieved after the initial surgical procedure, and mean BMI was 36.1 ± 7.45. The average anastomosis diameter was 21 mm, with a pouch size of 5.05 cm. APC was associated with significant weight loss (9.73 kg vs. + 1.38 kg) at 6 months, a reduction in the anastomosis diameter, early satiation, and increased quality of life. In the control group, no change in weight occurred, however after crossing over to receive APC, these patients demonstrated 9.8 kg weight loss (10.7%TWL). Patients in the APC arm were followed up for 1 year with no reported APC-related complications, such as ulcers or strictures. Based on the above published findings, endoscopic APC appears to be a safe and effective tool for the treatment of weight regain following RYGB surgery in select patients, enabling the avoidance of revisional surgeries.

29.6 Endoscopic Mucosal Resection/Endoscopic Submucosal Resection

Endoscopic submucosal dissection (ESD) or endoscopic mucosal resection have been reported to be safe and effective methods for endoscopic malignant and pre-malignant tissue removal. A common side effect of the tissue resection methods is scar formation suggesting that tissue resection at the post-RYGB gastrojejunal anastomosis may result in scar-induced aperture decrease. Data for this indication currently remains limited to anectdotal case reports. In two case reports, modified ESD was performed to incise the mucosa surrounding the gastrojejunal anastomosis in order to directly expose the submucosa and muscularis propria for suturing. After injecting methylene blue and epinephrine in saline solution into the submucosa, circumferential incision approximately 5 mm away from the gastrojejunal anastomosis using needle knife followed by the extension of the incision using insulated tip knife was performed. APC and purse-string endoscopic suturing to reduce the size of the aperture were then performed resulting in 42 lbs. of weight loss in 3 months in one case [39] and 14 lbs. of weight loss at 1 year in another case [40].

29.7 Radiofrequency Ablation

Another resurfacing technique using radiofrequency ablation (RFA) by causing subepithelial scarring and fibrosis to reduce compliance of the stomach has shown to be effective in a pilot study. Among patients who regained >25% of lost weight after RYGB, RFA was applied to the gastrojejunal anastomosis as well as the entire surface area of the remnant gastric pouch, with repeat sessions at 4 and 8 months if the patients did not meet the weight loss target. This study showed mean EWL of 18.4% at 12 months with a significant trend for continued weight loss over the 12 months period. Among 25 study subjects, two patients developed significant GI bleeding requiring hospitalization, including one patient on dual anti-platelet agents [41]. Further clinical studies are needed to investigate durability and selection criteria for RFA as a weight regain revision procedure.

29.8 Cryotherapy

Cryoballoon ablation therapy that is typically used for treatment of Barrett's esophagus has been used experimentally to induce stricture formation to achieve outlet and pouch reduction. In a pilot study, among 22 patients who had weight regain after RYGB with dilated pouch for 3–6 cm or dilated outlet of 20–30 mm, cryoballoon therapy was performed to ablate 75% of the pouch surface area and/or the entire outlet circumference. This study showed over 90% of technical success, with significant reduction in outlet size at 8 weeks but no reduction in pouch size. Significant correlation of weight loss (%TBWL was 8.1 +/− 12.8 at 8 weeks) with reduction in outlet size was observed, however not with reduction in pouch size as observed in other weight regain revision procedures. However, major side effects included upper gastrointestinal bleeding requiring transfusion, intractable emesis and gastric stenosis requiring endoscopic intervention [42]. Further data including safety, long-term success are required before this technique could be recommended.

29.9 Conclusion

Bariatric surgery remains the most effective procedure for the treatment of morbid obesity and obesity associated co-morbidities. However, in a large proportion of patients, weight regain can occur resulting in recurrence of co-morbidities and decreased quality of life. Patients who develop weight regain after RYGB should be evaluated for dilation of the gastrojejunal anastomosis. Transoral outlet reduction (eTOR) is a safe and effective treatment of weight regain after RYGB and should be offered as a part of a multidisciplinary management strategy. Endoscopic revision procedures for weight regain will continue to have a role in patients who are poor surgical candidates, as an early intervention to halt weight regain, as a bridge to revision surgery, or as a primary alternative to the revision surgery.

29.10 A Personal View of the Data

Weight regain after RYGB is multi-factorial in etiology and there remains controversy whether or not a dilated stoma or pouch is causative factor. Regardless, surgical options for revision of RYGB require increased operating time and are associated with increased patient morbidity. Given the limitations with surgery, several intraluminal endoscopic approaches have emerged in effort to provide alternative minimally-invasive options for RYGB revision. Of the trialed endoscopic approaches, endoscopic transoral outlet reduction of the gastrojejunal anastomosis has the most evidence (including Level 1 evidence) supporting routine use in clinical practice. In particular endoscopic transoral outlet reduction using the Overstitch device has long-term data supporting safe, durable weight loss over a 5-year period. APC alone appears to be an emerging second line endoscopic option, and is currently the procedure I perform if not a candidate for eTOR. At the current time, the alternative endoscopic RYGB revision approaches discussed should be considered experimental or investigational.

However, in my personal experience, success with endoscopic transoral outlet reduction requires a multidisciplinary approach with frequent follow-up, appropriate patient selection, and setting realistic expectations and goals. The eTOR procedure will not routinely result in similar total weight loss or rate of weight loss as the primary RYGB, and the majority of patients will not achieve their post-surgical nadir. However, if weight regain is addressed early, even aborting the weight regain trend should be considered a success with likely subsequent clinical benefit.

Additionally, instituting this procedure into practice, providers will encounter patients that have limited or no response with the eTOR. This is likely due to the fact weight regain is multi-factorial with significant post-surgical changes to patient's metabolism, hormones, behaviors and psychologic factors all playing a role beyond restriction or dilation of the pouch/stoma. However, the balance of safety and efficacy, ability to be repeated without difficulty and relative technical ease for adoption all make eTOR an attractive first-line option for post-RGYB weight regain. In addition to working to identifying novel solutions to this common clinical problem, professional societies need to work together to develop a procedure coding with appropriate reimbursement to increase the availability of eTOR.

References

1. Nguyen NT, Slone JA, Nguyen XM, et al. A prospective randomized trial of laparoscopic gastric bypass versus laparoscopic adjustable gastric banding for the treatment of morbid obesity: outcomes, quality of life, and costs. Ann Surg. 2009;250(4):631–41.
2. Angrisani L, Lorenzo M, Borrelli V. Laparoscopic adjustable gastric banding versus roux-en-Y gastric bypass: 5-year results of a prospective randomized trial. Surg Obes Relat Dis. 2007;3(2):127–32.
3. Ponce J, DeMaria EJ, Nguyen NT, et al. American Society for Metabolic and Bariatric Surgery estimation of bariatric surgery procedures in 2015 and surgeon workforce in the United States. Surg Obes Relat Dis. 2016;12(9):1637–9.
4. Farrell TM, Haggerty SP, Overby DW, et al. Clinical application of laparoscopic bariatric surgery: an evidence-based review. Surg Endosc. 2009;23(5):930–49.
5. King WC, Hinerman AS, Belle SH, et al. Comparison of the performance of common measures of weight regain after bariatric surgery for association with clinical outcomes. JAMA. 2018;320(15):1560–9.
6. Christou NV, Lo D, Maclean LD. Weight gain after short- and long-limb gastric bypass in patients followed for longer than 10 years. Ann Surg. 2006;244(5):734–40.
7. Magro DO, Geloneze B, Delfini R, et al. Long-term weight regain after gastric bypass: a 5-year prospective study. Obes Surg. 2008;18(6):648–51.
8. Sjöström L, Lindroos AK, Peltonen M, et al. Lifestyle, diabetes, and cardiovascular risk factors 10 years after bariatric surgery. N Engl J Med. 2004;351(26):2683–93.
9. Abu Dayyeh BK, Lautz DB, Thompson CC. Gastrojejunal stoma diameter predicts weight regain after roux-en-Y gastric bypass. Clin Gastroenterol Hepatol. 2011;9(3):228–33.
10. Storm AC, Thompson CC. Endoscopic treatments following bariatric surgery. Gastrointest Endosc Clin N Am. 2017;27(2):233–44.
11. Himpens J, Coromina L, Verbrugghe A, Cadière GB. Outcomes of revisional procedures for insufficient weight loss or weight regain after roux-en-Y gastric bypass. Obes Surg. 2012;22(11):1746–54.
12. Behrns KE, Smith CD, Kelly KA, Sarr MG. Reoperative bariatric surgery. Lessons learned to improve patient selection and results. Ann Surg. 1993;218(5):646–53.
13. Coakley BA, Deveney CW, Spight DH, et al. Revisional bariatric surgery for failed restrictive procedures. Surg Obes Relat Dis. 2008;4(5):581–6.
14. Linner JH, Drew RL. Reoperative surgery-indications, efficacy, and long-term follow-up. Am J Clin Nutr. 1992;55(2 Suppl):606S–10S.
15. Iannelli A, Schneck AS, Hébuterne X, Gugenheim J. Gastric pouch resizing for roux-en-Y gastric bypass failure in patients with a dilated pouch. Surg Obes Relat Dis. 2013;9(2):260–7.
16. Schwartz RW, Strodel WE, Simpson WS, Griffen WO Jr. Gastric bypass revision: lessons learned from 920 cases. Surgery. 1988;104(4):806–12.

17. Overcash WT. Natural orifice surgery (NOS) using StomaphyX™ for repair of gastric leaks after bariatric revisions. Obes Surg. 2008;18(7):882–5.
18. Mikami D, Needleman B, Narula V, et al. Natural orifice surgery: initial US experience utilizing the StomaphyX device to reduce gastric pouches after roux-en-Y gastric bypass. Surg Endosc. 2010;24(1):223–8.
19. Leitman IM, Virk CS, Avgerinos DV, et al. Early results of trans-oral endoscopic plication and revision of the gastric pouch and stoma following roux-en-Y gastric bypass surgery. JSLS. 2010;14(2):217–20.
20. Goyal V, Holover S, Garber S. Gastric pouch reduction using StomaphyX in post roux-en-Y gastric bypass patients does not result in sustained weight loss: a retrospective analysis. Surg Endosc. 2013;27(9):3417–20.
21. Ong'uti SK, Ortega G, Onwugbufor MT, et al. Effective weight loss management with endoscopic gastric plication using StomaphyX device: is it achievable? Surg Obes Relat Dis. 2013;9(1):113–7.
22. Eid GM, McCloskey CA, Eagleton JK, et al. StomaphyX vs a sham procedure for revisional surgery to reduce regained weight in roux-en-Y gastric bypass patients: a randomized clinical trial. JAMA Surg. 2014;149(4):372–9.
23. Ryou M, Mullady DK, Lautz DB, Thompson CC. Pilot study evaluating technical feasibility and early outcomes of second-generation endosurgical platform for treatment of weight regain after gastric bypass surgery. Surg Obes Relat Dis. 2009;5(4):450–4.
24. Mullady DK, Lautz DB, Thompson CC. Treatment of weight regain after gastric bypass surgery when using a new endoscopic platform: initial experience and early outcomes (with video). Gastrointest Endosc. 2009;70(3):440–4.
25. Horgan S, Jacobsen G, Weiss GD, et al. Incisionless revision of post-roux-en-Y bypass stomal and pouch dilation: multicenter registry results. Surg Obes Relat Dis. 2010;6(3):290–5.
26. Thompson CC, Jacobsen GR, Schroder GL, Horgan S. Stoma size critical to 12-month outcomes in endoscopic suturing for gastric bypass repair. Surg Obes Relat Dis. 2012;8(3):282–7.
27. Gallo AS, DuCoin CG, Berducci MA, et al. Endoscopic revision of gastric bypass: holy grail or epic fail? Surg Endosc. 2016;30(9):3922–7.
28. Thompson CC, Chand B, Chen YK, et al. Endoscopic suturing for transoral outlet reduction increases weight loss after roux-en-Y gastric bypass surgery. Gastroenterology. 2013;145(1):129–37.
29. Jirapinyo P, Slattery J, Ryan MB, et al. Evaluation of an endoscopic suturing device for transoral outlet reduction in patients with weight regain following roux-en-Y gastric bypass. Endoscopy. 2013;45(7):532–6.
30. Kumar N, Thompson CC. Transoral outlet reduction for weight regain after gastric bypass: long-term follow-up. Gastrointest Endosc. 2016;83(4):776–9.
31. Jirapinyo P, Dayyeh BKA, Thompson CC. Gastrojejunal anastomotic reduction for weight regain in roux-en-y gastric bypass patients: physiological, behavioral, and anatomical effects of endoscopic suturing and sclerotherapy. Surg Obes Relat Dis. 2016;12(10):1810–6.
32. Vargas EJ, Bazerbachi F, Rizk M, et al. Transoral outlet reduction with full thickness endoscopic suturing for weight regain after gastric bypass: a large multicenter international experience and meta-analysis. Surg Endosc. 2018;32(1):252–9.
33. Jirapinyo P, Kumar N, Alsamman MA, Thompson CC. Five-year outcomes of transoral outlet reduction for the treatment of weight regain after roux-en-Y gastric bypass. Gastrointest Endosc. 2019;91(5):1067–73. https://doi.org/10.1016/j.gie.2019.11.044.
34. Heylen AM, Jacobs A, Lybeer M, Prosst RL. The OTSC®-clip in revisional endoscopy against weight gain after bariatric gastric bypass surgery. Obes Surg. 2011;21(10):1629–33.
35. Abu Dayyeh BK, Jirapinyo P, Weitzner Z, Barker C, Flicker MS, Lautz DB, Thompson CC. Endoscopic sclerotherapy for the treatment of weight regain after roux-en-Y gastric bypass: outcomes, complications, and predictors of response in 575 procedures. Gastrointest Endosc. 2012;76(2):275–82.

36. Moon RC, Teixeira AF, Neto MG, et al. Efficacy of utilizing argon plasma coagulation for weight regain in roux-en-Y gastric bypass patients: a multi-center study. Obes Surg. 2018;28(9):2737–44.
37. De Quadros LG, Neto MG, Marchesini JC, et al. Endoscopic argon plasma coagulation vs multidisciplinary evaluation in the management of weight regain after gastric bypass surgery: a randomized controlled trial with SHAM group. Obes Surg. 2020;30:3260–2. https://doi.org/10.1007/s11695-020-04414-6.
38. Baretta GA, Alhinho HC, Matias JE, et al. Argon plasma coagulation of gastrojejunal anastomosis for weight regain after gastric bypass. Obes Surg. 2015;25(1):72–9.
39. Abidi WM, Aihara H, Thompson CC. Modified endoscopic submucosal dissection techniques before endoscopic revision of a gastric bypass. Gastrointest Endosc. 2016;83(6):1281–2.
40. de Moura DTH, Jirapinyo P, Thompson CC. Modified-ESD plus APC and suturing for treatment of weight regain after gastric bypass. Obes Surg. 2019;29(6):2001–2.
41. Abrams JA, Komanduri S, Shaheen NJ, et al. Radiofrequency ablation for the treatment of weight regain after roux-en-Y gastric bypass surgery. Gastrointest Endosc. 2018;87(1):275–9.
42. Fayad L, Simsek C, Raad M, et al. Cryoballoon ablation for gastric pouch and/or outlet reduction in patients with weight regain post Roux-en-Y gastric bypass. Gastrointest Endosc. 2019;89(6):sAB275–6.
43. Goh YM, James NE, Goh EL, Khanna A. The use of endoluminal techniques in the revision of primary bariatric surgery procedures: a systematic review. Surg Endosc. 2020;34:2410–28. https://doi.org/10.1007/s00464-020-07468-w.

Suboptimal Weight Loss and Weight Regain: Is it Prime Time for Pharmacotherapy?

30

Silvana Pannain

30.1 Introduction

Bariatric surgery is undoubtfully the most effective weight loss intervention in severe obesity and leads to significant improvement of obesity associated health conditions, health-related quality of life and reduction in overall mortality and morbidity [1, 2].

However the variability in weight loss outcome and the longer-term durability of weight loss and control of comorbidity after bariatric procedures are a new concern.

In this chapter we will briefly review the prevalence and possible etiology of suboptimal weight loss (SWL) and weight regain (WR) as complications of bariatric surgery. We will then discuss the evaluation and treatment of these conditions, with a more specific focus on the possible role of weight loss medications as a rescue therapy in patients who experience these complications.

30.2 Search Strategy

A literature search was conducted between November 2019 and January 2020 and aimed to find published clinical trials and systematic reviews. The databases searched was PubMed (January 1921 to January 2020). The key terms used were suboptimal weight loss, weight regain, bariatric surgery, anti-obesity medication, obesity pharmacotherapy, re-operative bariatric surgery, re-operative intervention, conversional procedures, endoscopic procedures.

Laparoscopic Roux-en-Y gastric bypass (RYGB) and vertical sleeve gastrectomy (SG) are the two most common weight reduction surgeries in the world,

S. Pannain (✉)
Department of Medicine, University of Chicago, Chicago, IL, USA
e-mail: spannain@medicine.bsd.uchicago.edu

© Springer Nature Switzerland AG 2021   339
J. Alverdy, Y. Vigneswaran (eds.), *Difficult Decisions in Bariatric Surgery*,
Difficult Decisions in Surgery: An Evidence-Based Approach,
https://doi.org/10.1007/978-3-030-55329-6_30

therefore most attention was given in this chapter to these two procedures. Additionally, seen that the SG has been available in the US only since 2010, a larger number of the studies available and discussed here are in RYGB patients.

30.3   Suboptimal Weight Loss after Bariatric Surgery

There is consensus that some patients experience SWL after bariatric surgery [3]. SWL is often defined as never achieving more than 50% excess weight loss (EWL) [4]. Depending on the report, 5–20% of patients do not lose weight successfully, despite perceived optimal surgical technique and regular follow-up [5–7]. Interestingly a retrospective review of 375 post RYGB, showed that an early prediction of insufficient weight loss can be made at 6 months: patients who lost <30% of their initial excess weight were unlikely to loose ≥50% at 24 months [8]. A large retrospective review on approximately 1450 patients who underwent either RYGB (n=918) or SG (n=538) showed that weight loss at 3–6 months was an independent predictor of maximal % weight loss in both SG and RYGB patients [9], ultimately suggesting that early identification and treatment of suboptimal weight loss post bariatric surgery may not be unreasonable when utilizing lifestyle and medical interventions as an initial approach.

30.4   Weight Regain after Bariatric Surgery

There is also growing recognition that post bariatric surgery patients may experience WR which can be associated with diminished health benefits, including recurrence of type 2 diabetes and other comorbidities, which had seen an initial remission [10, 11].

So far there isn't an univocal definition of WR after bariatric surgery. With lack of uniform reporting the prevalence of this condition cannot be conclusively estimated. A systematic review identified nine heterogeneous studies which reported weight regain of 5.7% at 2 years all the way to 75.6% at 6 years [4]. But the majority of the studies were small, in different populations, and the methodology of definition and report was different. There has been a handful of larger longitudinal studies looking at the long term weight loss outcomes after bariatric surgery [2, 3, 12], which show consistently that patients generally regain 5 to 10% of their TWL within the first decade. In a study of 55 patients post SG, Lauti et al. demonstrated the importance of using standardized definitions of weight regain and found that when in their cohort they selected 3 best definitions of weight regain, 40 to 64% of patients regained some weight at 5 years after SG [13]. Across the board the studies show that the susceptibility to weight regain increases as time from surgery increases. However, while some weight regain needs to be expected after bariatric surgery, and patients accept it, there is a subgroup of patient who may regain a significant amount of weight and that is associated with decreased quality of life and possibly recurrence of comorbidities as well as emotional impact and dissatisfaction from the procedure [3, 14]. In a large study which included 1406 RYGB patients, weight regain quantified as percentage of maximum weight lost correlated best with most clinical outcomes. Utilizing this definition, at 5 years 67.3% of post RYGB patients had regained ≥20% of maximum weight loss [15]. In this study instead the rate of weight regain was largest during the first year after reaching nadir weight and decreased over time, but continued throughout the 5 year follow-up.

Additionally the finding from this study in RYGB [15] combined with the data of Jirapinyo et al. [16] as well as those reported by Lauti et al. in SG [13] suggest a dose-response relationship between weight regain and some bariatric surgery outcomes such as diabetes, hypertension, and physical health–related quality of life, highlighting the importance of effectively intervene to limit or correct the weight regain.

A 5 years prospective weight loss study suggests that super obesity [Body Mass Index (BMI) >50 kg/m^2] puts patients at higher risk of SWL and WR after gastric bypass [17]. In 782 patients post gastric bypass weight loss was completed by 24 months and WR become significant at 48 months. Some WR was observed in approximately 50% of the patients (46% within 24 months and 63.6% within 48 months) who had received gastric bypass. Patients with WR experienced a mean gain of 8.8 kg within 60 months, which represented a 8% increase from the lowest weight after surgery. Again, WR was higher in the patients with super obesity (BMI >50 kg/m^2) with a BMI increase from 34.2 kg/m^2 at 18 months after surgery to 39.4 kg/m^2 at 60 months. SWL was defined as excess weight loss less than 50%, and was highest in the group with super obesity at all times studied, reaching 18.8% at 48 months after surgery.

30.5 Evaluation of Suboptimal Weight Loss and Weight Regain after Weight Loss Surgery

The recommended approach is to perform a multidisciplinary evaluation to determine the potential causes of the poor weight loss response. It should include a nutritional evaluation, a behavioral assessment and an evaluation of the anatomy when indicated. Lifestyle and behavioral modification should be optimized before considering other therapy or revisional endoscopic or surgical procedure. Iatrogenic weight gain due to obesogenic medications should be excluded as it will be discussed in more detail in the coming section.

Nevertheless, even with the most diligent evaluation, the cause of SWL and WR is not always identified and often life style and behavioral interventions alone do not improve the outcome.

30.6 Etiology of SWL and WR Post Bariatric Surgery

Besides cases where obvious anatomic abnormalities exist which may explain a suboptimal weight loss outcome, such as pouch or stoma dilation and gastro-gastric fistula in RYGB or dilated sleeve in SG [18], the mechanisms of SWL and WR after bariatric surgery remains poorly understood, and are likely to be distinct at least in part, and to involve physiologic processes as well as behavioral and psychological factors. In general, the choice of weight loss surgery is still often empirical, therefore individual factors such as the anatomy of the gastrointestinal tract in relationship to the hormonal function and the CNS response to peripheral hunger and satiety signals are all factors which could affect behavior and determine individual responses to the different weight loss bariatric surgery procedures and ultimately explain both SWL and WR. At this stage there isn't a valid approach to study the unique physiology of each patient after surgery but factors such as the limb length are regarded as important in determining the post-bariatric surgery physiology [19].

A publication studying 49 patients with SWL or WR after 1 year post RYGB compared with 38 matched controls with acceptable weight loss, indicated that lower levels of physical activity, disordered eating behavior and lower quality of life were associated with the unsuccessful weigh loss outcome [20]. While association does not imply causation, it is conceivable that those behaviors may have contributed, at least in part, to the poorer weight loss outcome. In fact, previous studies have shown the importance of physical activity in weight maintenance and prevention of weight regain after RYGB [21–23].

A systematic review of 115 selected articles published between 1998 and 2010 found that the predictors of weight loss outcomes post bariatric surgery (RYGB or laparoscopic adjustable gastric banding (LAGB)) are quite heterogenous across the studies but factors such as the preoperative mandatory weight loss, the initial BMI, the presence of super obesity, eating disorders/maladaptive eating habits and psychiatric disorders/substance abuse may be more often implicated [6]. Similarly, a recent review by Sarwer et al. discusses that the presence of impulsivity, which is an element of overeating, disinhibited eating, substance abuse and mood regulation, is a predictor of weight loss outcomes of bariatric surgery [24]. A prospective observational study in 2365 patients undergoing RYGB found that higher baseline BMI, preoperative use of any diabetes medications, non-use of buproprion medications, no history of smoking, age > 50 years and the presence of fibrosis at liver biopsy were associated with lower % EBWL at 36 months [25]. In a multivariate analysis of 310 RYGB patients with a mean presurgical BMI of 52 kg/m^2 followed up to 12 months, only the presence of diabetes (odds ratio [OR], 3.09; 95% confidence interval [CI], 1.35–7.09 [P =.007]) and larger pouch size (OR, 2.77; 95% CI, 1.81–4.22 [P < .001]) were independently associated with poor weight loss (defined in this study as ≤ 40% excess weight loss) [26]. Similarly, a previous review published in 2012, which included only RYGB and gastric banding (GB) (as SG was only approved in 2010) identified nutritional non-compliance, hormonal/metabolic imbalance, mental health, physical inactivity and anatomical/surgical factors as possible mechanisms [10]. Specifically, the hormonal factors refer to a blunting of the changes in the appetite regulating hormone levels which have been called to explain in part the satiety, the decreased food intake and consequently the weight loss after bariatric procedures [27–29].

A review of the studies looking at possible causes of post SG weight regain pointed to initial sleeve size, sleeve dilatation, increased ghrelin levels, inadequate follow-up support and maladaptive lifestyle behaviors as proposed mechanisms [4]. Finally, prescription of one or more medication from a list of 32 obesogenic medications has shown to lead to decreased weight loss at one year in a group of 150 patient versus 173 patients who were not prescribed such medications [30], suggesting that scrutiny of the patients' medication list should be included in the evaluation of insufficient weight loss and weight regain post bariatric surgery.

In general, several classes of medications are known to be associated with weight gain, including steroids, contraceptives, and other hormonal agents as well as some antidiabetic, antihypertensive, antidepressant, antipsychotic, anti-epileptic, and antihistamine agents [31]. Therefore, it is necessary to make a careful review of a patient's medications to identify those which may be limit weight loss and possibly contribute to weight regain. Consideration of alternatives which are weight-neutral and weight-loss promoting [31] should be part of an initial intervention (together with diet and exercise counseling) when assisting patients with an unsatisfactory response to weight loss surgery. Finally, post-bariatric surgery hypoglycemia may represent a rare risk factor for weight regain [32].

In conclusion the patients who present with insufficient weight loss, continued co-morbidities or weight regain present a challenge to the surgeons which may warrant re-assessment and additional therapy. Re-operative interventions and more recently pharmacotherapy are potential treatments.

30.7   Re-Operative Bariatric Surgery and Procedures

Beyond life style interventions, re-operative interventions (correction of an anatomical abnormality or conversation to a different procedure) have been the traditional treatment approach to SWL and WR after bariatric surgery.

In 2014 a task force reviewed the data on re-operative bariatric surgery [18]. They included 175 articles in a systematic review and analysis. The analysis of re-operative surgery for unsuccessful bariatric surgery highlights that the majority of studies available so far are single center retrospective reviews, and/or the outcomes are inconsistently reported in the literature and vary based on the population studied. Conversely one large study reports the outcomes of 449,753 bariatric operations from a large data base, the Bariatric Outcomes Longitudinal Database (BOLD) [33]: a rate of reoperation of 6.3% was observed and the overall complication rate was low. The general sense is that the outcome after re-operative interventions (correction of an anatomical abnormality or conversation to a different procedure) are favorable and demonstrate additional weight loss, but the risk is higher than the initial bariatric surgery [33]. Therefore the decision to proceed for an invasive reintervention needs to be carefully weighted, especially in cases in which an anatomical abnormality suitable for a correction procedure is not identified or the surgical risk of a conversion is high or finally the patient's preference is for a non-invasive approach.

30.8   Adjuvant Medical Therapy

In this chapter we suggest that weight loss medications should be considered as a rescue therapy in patients with SWL or significant WR after bariatric surgery. Currently there aren't weight loss medications approved for use post bariatric surgery but weight loss medications could be a currently underutilized strategy in SWL and WR.

Additionally, even when patients have attained the expected weight loss with a bariatric surgery procedure, they are likely to have residual obesity and therefore in principle they still meet eligibility criteria for weight loss medications. Weight loss medication are in fact indicated for a BMI ≥ 27 kg/m^2 with at least one comorbid condition, including diabetes mellitus (DM), medication-controlled hypertension (blood pressures consistently <140/80), hypercholesterolemia, and/or obstructive sleep apnea; or a BMI ≥ 30 kg/m^2 without co-morbidities [31, 34].

Table 30.1 reviews the currently approved weight loss medications, their efficacy, safety and dosing [31, 34].

For the most part in the current obesity medicine practice the choice of weight loss medications is still empirical and often driven by the efficacy (tested in non-post bariatric surgery patients), coverage, cost, patients preferences (injectable versus oral) and potential dual benefit, meaning potential amelioration of coexisting conditions, such as diabetes, migraines, depression, addiction, tobacco abuse [36].

At this stage there is a limited number of studies looking at the efficacy of weight loss medications after weight loss surgery. These studies are summarized in Table 30.2.

One important limitation of these studies is that for the most part these are retrospective chart reviews [39–43] or not strictly controlled prospective studies [37, 38]. Additionally, some studies utilize the older and less effective off label drugs which have approved indications outside weight loss such as for depression, migraines, seizure and mood stabilization [38–40]. Of note in most of the studies the medications were given on a background of diet and exercise intervention: this is worth underscoring as generally in obesity a larger weight loss can be achieved when more than on approach is utilized simultaneously, as it is the case when pharmacotherapy is added to lifestyle modifications and more so to intensive behavioral therapy [44]. Therefore, even with the limited evidence available, we recommend that diet and exercise counseling and, when possible, behavioral therapy are adopted as the background to any intervention in SWL and WR after bariatric surgery.

The largest study of pharmacotherapy after bariatric surgery is retrospective and enrolled 319 patients (RYGB = 258; sleeve gastrectomy = 61) treated in two medical centers [40]. More than one medication was trialed in the course of the treatment and the average number of medication trialed was two. More than half of the patients in treatment with a weight loss medication post-surgery lost $\geq 5\%$ of their weight, 30.1% lost $\geq 10\%$ and 16% of patients lost $\geq 15\%$. The authors describe even one case where the weight loss with pharmacotherapy lead to a BMI decrease from 36 to 26 kg/m^2, surpassing the nadir weight loss of BMI of 33 kg/m^2 achieved with surgery alone.

Table 30.1 Drugs currently approved for weight loss: efficacy, safety and dosing. Data reported are from the RCT in overweight and obese patients without history of bariatric surgery [31, 34, 35]. These drugs have not been evaluated in post-bariatric surgery

Agent	Mechanism of action	Weight loss (% from baseline) in completers vs. placebo	Dosing	Most common side effects
Phentermine	Sympathomimetic; suppresses appetite, possibly increases resting energy expenditure.	7.38% vs 2.28% (15 mg)	8 mg TID orally before meals, 15 mg QD or BID, 30 mg QD	Headache, dry mouth, insomnia, dizziness, irritability, constipation.
Orlistat 120 TID (or OTC Alli 60 TID)	Pancreatic lipase inhibitor, decreases the absorption of 30% of dietary fat.	8.8% vs 5.8%	120 (or 60) mg orally TID before meals	Loose stools, flatulence, fecal urgency, oily stool, fecal incontinence small but significant decreases in fat-soluble vitamins.
Phentermine/ Topiramate ER 7.5/46 mg	Sympathomimetic; possible modulation of gamma-aminobutyric acid receptors, inhibition of carbonic anhydrase, and glutamate antagonism, suppresses appetite.	9.6% vs 1.2%	Orally qAM: 3.75/23 mg for 14 days then 7.5/46 mg	Paresthesias, dizziness, dysgeusia, insomnia, constipation, dry mouth.
Phentermine/ Topiramate ER 15/92 mg	See above.	12.4% vs 1.2%	At 12 weeks on 7.5/46 qAM, option to titrate to 11.25/69 for 2 weeks, then 15/92 mg	Paresthesias, dizziness, dysgeusia, insomnia, constipation, dry mouth.
Lorcarserin 20 mg	5HT-2C receptor agonist, suppresses appetite.	7.9% vs 4.0%	10 mg BID orally or 20 mg QD, no titration needed	Headache, dizziness, fatigue, nausea, dry mouth, constipation. **Withdrawn from the market on February 13 2020 because of potential increased cancer risk.**

(continued)

Table 30.1 (continued)

Agent	Mechanism of action	Weight loss (% from baseline) in completers vs. placebo	Dosing	Most common side effects
Naltrexone ER/bupropion ER 32/360	Dopamine/ noradrenaline reuptake inhibitor; opioid receptor antagonist, suppresses appetite	8.1% vs 1.8%	Orally Wk 1–1 table (8/90 mg) in am Wk 2–1 in am and 1 in pm Wk 3–2 in am and 1 in pm Wk 4–2 in am and 2 in pm, titrate slower if side effects	Nausea, vomiting, constipation, headache, dizziness, insomnia, dry mouth.
Liraglutide 3 mg	GLP-1 receptor agonist Suppresses appetite Decreases gastric emptying Has additional independent effects on insulin and glucagon secretion	9.2% vs 3.5%	Inject SQ Wk 1–0.6 daily, increase weekly by 0.6 until 3 mg daily, titrate slower if side effects	Nausea, vomiting, diarrhea, constipation, dyspepsia, abdominal pain.

Abbreviations/symbols: *TID* 3 times per day; *QD* once per day; *BID* 2 times per day, typically before breakfast and before dinner; *OTC* over the counter; *Wk* week; *qAM* once per day in the morning

In this study the most frequent medications prescribed for weight loss were topiramate, phentermine, metformin, buproprion and zonisamide. All except for phentermine are off label for the treatment of obesity. The mean added weight loss was 7.6% (17.8 lbs) of total postsurgical weight. When looking at predictors for weight loss with medication use after weight loss surgery, the authors had some interesting findings. The type of surgery (RYGB over SG) regardless of the postoperative BMI, as well as female gender, history of psychiatric conditions fared better while the presence of one comorbidity or of obstructive sleep apnea were associated with less weight loss [40].

Interestingly, those patients prescribed the medication at weight plateau rather than after some weight regain, experienced the larger percent weight loss from preoperative weigh. While the difference was not statistically significant it suggests that early intervention at weight loss plateau, rather than waiting for weight regain, may lead to a better response.

In a subgroup analysis of 37 young adults from the same data set, predominantly female, of which 75.7% had a RYGB, 54.1% of patients experienced ≥5% weight

Table 30.2 Studies utilizing obesity drugs after bariatric surgery

Author	Sample size	Study design	Surgery	Medication	Summary of findings	Side effects
Zoss et al. [37]	N = 38 Gender non reported	Prospective randomized, unblinded, non-placebo controlled 8 ± 6 months after laparoscopic SAGB 8 months	SAGB	Orlistat 120 before each meal	Weight loss 8 ± 2 kg (p < 0.01) vs 3 ± 2 kg (NS) (p < 0.02 between groups)	Increased gas-bloating and increased stool frequency (to a maximum of double frequency).
		Group A = 19 dietary counseling				
		Group B = 19 orlistat + dietary counseling				
Zilberstein et al. 2004 [38]	N = 16 2 ♂, 14 ♀ 10/16 patients diagnosed with binge eating disorder or episodes	Prospective, non-controlled 3 months	SAGB	Topiramate 25 mg (2 pts at 12.5 mg, 2 pts at 50 mg, 2 pts discontinued)	Additional mean EWL 14.8% (from 20.9% to 34.1%)	2 patients discontinued due to drug side effects; the nature of the side effects is not reported
Pajecki et al. 2012 [39]	N = 15 4 ♂, 11 ♀ <50% EWL ≥ 2 years (mean 5.6 years) or regained 15% of lowest weight	Retrospective 12.5 ± 4.7 weeks (range 8 to 28 weeks)	4 GB, 9 RYGB,1 DS, 1 longitudinal gastrectomy.	Liraglutide 1.2 to 1.8 mg daily (53.3% received 1.8 mg)	Mean weight loss −7.5 ± 4.3 kg (range 2 to 18 kg)	40% experienced nausea (3 pts post GB and 3 pts post RYGB). No discontinuation of the drug due to side effects

(continued)

Table 30.2 (continued)

Author	Sample size	Study design	Surgery	Medication	Summary of findings	Side effects
Cody Stanford et al. 2017 [40]	N = 319 72 ♂, 247 ♀	Retrospective 3 and 12 months	258 RYGB, 61 SG 78.5% had medications prescribed at weight regain, 21.5% at plateau	Topiramate Phentermine Metformin Buproprion Zonisamide	At 12 months mean added weight loss 7.6% (17.8 lbs) ≥5% TWL = 56%, ≥10% TWL = 30.1%, ≥15% TWL = 16% Predictors of better response: Topiramate; RYGB (vs sleeve gastrectomy); Female gender; Psychiatric co-morbidity; Higher preoperative BMI;	Not reported
Schwartz et al. 2016 [41]	N = 65 11 ♂, 47 ♀	Retrospective 90 days	51 RYGB 14 LAGB	Phentermine Phentermine–topiramate ER	Data at 90 days available for 30 pts Phentermine group (N = 24): mean weight loss 6.3 kg (12.8% EWL) Phentermine–Topiramate ER group (N = 6): mean weight loss 3.8 kg (12.9% EWL)	No patients required cessation of medical therapy due to hypertension, cardiac arrhythmias, or insomnia. One patient stopped phentermine due to headaches and one patient due to nausea.

Hanipah et al. 2018 [42]	N = 209 ♂ 14 ♀195	Retrospective 12 months	126 RYGB, 52 SG, 21 LAGB, 4 gastric plication, 6 revisional bariatric surgery	Phentermine N = 156 Phentermine-topiramate ER N = 25 Lorcaserin N = 18 Naltrexone SR/buproprion SR N = 10	5% TWL: 37% of pts >10% TWL: 19% of pts Mean % weight loss 2.2% Predictors of weight loss: Type of procedure: (4.6% in LAGB pts, 2.8% in RYGB pts, 0.3% in SG pts); BMI at the start of pharmacotherapy	Not reported
Wharton et al. 2019 [43]	N = 117 ♀ 87.2%	Retrospective chart review 7.6 ± 7.1 months	50 GB, 53 RYGB, 14 SG	Liraglutide 3 mg	Weight loss 6.3 ± 7.7 kg, $p < 0.05$	Nausea 29.1%

Abbreviations/symbols: *SAGB* Swedish adjustable gastric band; *GB* Gastric banding *LAGB* laparoscopic adjustable gastric banding; *RYGB* Roux-en-Y gastric bypass; *DS:* duodenal switch; *pt:* patient; *pts:* patients; *EWL* excess weight loss; *TWL* total weight loss
♂: male; ♀: female

loss, 34.5% and 22% experienced ≥10% and ≥15% weight loss, respectively [45]. The RYGB group achieved larger weight loss on the medication (compared with the SG group) with the difference near statistical significant (P=.051).

Since 2012 we have 4 new medications approved for weight loss, phentermine-topiramate ER, lorcaserine, naltrexone SR/buproprion SR, liraglutide 3 mg [31, 34] (Table 30.1). The efficacy of the newer approved medication options is generally 6%–13% baseline-weight loss, but weight losses of 15% and even 20% of baseline weight are not uncommonly observed with these drugs. Of note, most of the medications utilized in the studies post bariatric surgery, with the exception of two studies, are old obesity drugs or do not have a label for weight loss and are indeed less effective than the newer medications specifically designed for weight loss. Therefore it is conceivable but not yet demonstrated that the newer FDA approved weight loss medication will fare better also in post bariatric surgery patients.

30.9   Conclusions

The small set of uncontrolled data from the studies listed in Table 30.2 suggest that the addition of a medication may give an additional weight loss benefit in patients post bariatric surgery. Additionally, while conclusions cannot be derived, there are limited data suggesting that the optimal time to initiate post-bariatric surgery pharmacotherapy is at weight loss plateau [40], rather than after weight regain.

Given the low risk profile of the medications compared to revisional therapy, we suggest that a trial of pharmacotherapy in weight loss failure after bariatric surgery is warranted in appropriate cases. Larger studies and randomized controlled trials are necessary to determine the optimal medications and the timing of adjuvant medical therapy. At this time the data is insufficient to provide evidence based recommendations and a proven practical guidance on how medical therapy should be utilized as adjuvant to bariatric surgery. Therefore, based on the current knowledge, we suggest that when prescribing pharmacotherapy in post bariatric surgery we adopt the practice utilized in non-bariatric surgery patients. In general pharmacotherapy should be recommended on a background of behavioral counseling focusing on diet, physical activity, and lifestyle modifications, which also in post bariatric surgery should be regarded as the cornerstones of weight management [31, 34]. The efficacy and safety of a prescribed weight loss medication should be assessed monthly for the first three months and every three months thereafter and the medication should be discontinued if at anytime it is determined to be poorly effective or does not meet acceptable tolerability or safety. In that case a different medications with a different mechanism of action or an alternative treatment approach should be considered. A weight loss medication, when effective, should be prescribed long term to promote weight loss maintenance. A practical guideline on the use of medications in suboptimal weight loss outcome after weight loss surgery has been published in the last couple of years but is based on uncontrolled data and mostly on the practical experience of two US medical centers [46].

30.10 A Personal View of the Data

In conclusion, weight regain and even suboptimal weight loss after bariatric surgery are not infrequent and are likely multifactorial. The usefulness of adding obesity medications for SWL or WR after bariatric surgery appears promising and deserves further investigation with larger randomized trials, including controlled studies looking at the best time to add the pharmacotherapy and the most effective medication or combination of medications.

The experience available so far from small, non-randomized studies or retrospective chart reviews cannot support an evidence based standard of care but does suggest that pharmacotherapy after bariatric surgery is safe and that patients who are prescribed a weight loss medication after bariatric surgery are likely to experienced additional weight loss. Therefore pharmacotherapy could be attempted as adjuvant to bariatric surgery in combination with lifestyle modifications to counteract suboptimal weight loss, weight recidivism and to enhance weight maintenance.

Recommendations
- In SWL and/or WR after bariatric surgery a systematic approach including a nutritional evaluation, a behavioral assessment and an evaluation of the anatomy is essential. With the lack of an obvious anatomic abnormality, lifestyle and behavioral modification should be optimized before considering revisional endoscopic or surgical procedure.
- Limited data suggest that anti-obesity medications as adjuvant therapy give an additional weight loss benefit to patients post bariatric surgery. The optimal time to initiate post-bariatric surgery pharmacotherapy may be at weight loss plateau rather than after weight regain. Similarly to what non infrequently we see in patients without history of weight loss surgery, often more than one weight loss medication need to be trialed in each individual patient before finding the effective one.

References

1. Gloy VL, Briel M, Bhatt DL, Kashyap SR, Schauer PR, Mingrone G, Bucher HC, Nordmann AJ. Bariatric surgery versus non-surgical treatment for obesity: a systematic review and meta-analysis of randomised controlled trials. BMJ. 2013;347:f5934. Epub 2013/10/24; PubMed PMID: 24149519; PMCID: PMC3806364. https://doi.org/10.1136/bmj.f5934.
2. Sjostrom L. Review of the key results from the Swedish obese subjects (SOS) trial - a prospective controlled intervention study of bariatric surgery. J Intern Med. 2013;273(3):219–34. Epub 2012/11/21; PubMed PMID: 23163728. https://doi.org/10.1111/joim.12012.
3. Courcoulas AP, King WC, Belle SH, Berk P, Flum DR, Garcia L, Gourash W, Horlick M, Mitchell JE, Pomp A, Pories WJ, Purnell JQ, Singh A, Spaniolas K, Thirlby R, Wolfe BM, Yanovski SZ. Seven-year weight trajectories and health outcomes in the longitudinal assessment of bariatric surgery (LABS) study. JAMA Surg. 2018;153(5):427–34. . Epub 2017/12/08.; PubMed PMID: 29214306; PMCID: PMC6584318. https://doi.org/10.1001/jamasurg.2017.5025.

 4. Lauti M, Kularatna M, Hill AG, MacCormick AD. Weight regain following sleeve gastrec-
    tomy-a systematic review. Obes Surg. 2016;26(6):1326–34. Epub 2016/04/07; PubMed
    PMID: 27048439. https://doi.org/10.1007/s11695-016-2152-x.
 5. de Raaff CA, Coblijn UK, de Vries N, Heymans MW, van den Berg BT, van Tets WF, van
    Wagensveld BA. Predictive factors for insufficient weight loss after bariatric surgery: does
    obstructive sleep apnea influence weight loss? Obes Surg. 2016;26(5):1048–56. Epub
    2015/07/30; PubMed PMID: 26220241. https://doi.org/10.1007/s11695-015-1830-4.
 6. Livhits M, Mercado C, Yermilov I, Parikh JA, Dutson E, Mehran A, Ko CY, Gibbons
    MM. Preoperative predictors of weight loss following bariatric surgery: systematic review.
    Obes Surg. 2012;22(1):70–89. Epub 2011/08/13; PubMed PMID: 21833817. https://doi.
    org/10.1007/s11695-011-0472-4.
 7. Perugini RA, Mason R, Czerniach DR, Novitsky YW, Baker S, Litwin DE, Kelly JJ. Predictors
    of complication and suboptimal weight loss after laparoscopic roux-en-Y gastric bypass: a
    series of 188 patients. Arch Surg. 2003;138(5):541–5; discussion 5-6. Epub 2003/05/14;
    PubMed PMID: 12742960. https://doi.org/10.1001/archsurg.138.5.541.
 8. Ritz P, Caiazzo R, Becouarn G, Arnalsteen L, Andrieu S, Topart P, Pattou F. Early prediction
    of failure to lose weight after obesity surgery. Surg Obes Relat Dis. 2013;9(1):118–21. Epub
    2012/01/10; . PubMed PMID: 22222302. https://doi.org/10.1016/j.soard.2011.10.022.
 9. Manning S, Pucci A, Carter NC, Elkalaawy M, Querci G, Magno S, Tamberi A, Finer N,
    Fiennes AG, Hashemi M, Jenkinson AD, Anselmino M, Santini F, Adamo M, Batterham
    RL. Early postoperative weight loss predicts maximal weight loss after sleeve gastrectomy
    and roux-en-Y gastric bypass. Surg Endosc. 2015;29(6):1484–91. Epub 2014/09/23; PubMed
    PMID: 25239175; PMCID: PMC4422859. https://doi.org/10.1007/s00464-014-3829-7.
10. Karmali S, Brar B, Shi X, Sharma AM, de Gara C, Birch DW. Weight recidivism post-bariatric
    surgery: a systematic review. Obes Surg. 2013;23(11):1922–33. Epub 2013/09/03;. PubMed
    PMID: 23996349. https://doi.org/10.1007/s11695-013-1070-4.
11. Laurino Neto RM, Herbella FA, Tauil RM, Silva FS, de Lima SE Jr. Comorbidities remission
    after roux-en-Y gastric bypass for morbid obesity is sustained in a long-term follow-up and
    correlates with weight regain. Obes Surg. 2012;22(10):1580–5. Epub 2012/08/22; PubMed
    PMID: 22907795. https://doi.org/10.1007/s11695-012-0731-z.
12. Adams TD, Davidson LE, Litwin SE, Kim J, Kolotkin RL, Nanjee MN, Gutierrez JM, Frogley
    SJ, Ibele AR, Brinton EA, Hopkins PN, McKinlay R, Simper SC, Hunt SC. Weight and meta-
    bolic outcomes 12 years after gastric bypass. N Engl J Med. 2017;377(12):1143–55. Epub
    2017/09/21; PubMed PMID: 28930514; PMCID: PMC5737957. https://doi.org/10.1056/
    NEJMoa1700459.
13. Lauti M, Lemanu D, Zeng ISL, Su'a B, Hill AG, MacCormick AD. Definition determines
    weight regain outcomes after sleeve gastrectomy. Surg Obes Relat Dis. 2017;13(7):1123–9.
    Epub 2017/04/26; . PubMed PMID: 28438493. https://doi.org/10.1016/j.soard.2017.02.029.
14. Jones L, Cleator J, Yorke J. Maintaining weight loss after bariatric surgery: when the spectator
    role is no longer enough. Clin Obes. 2016;6(4):249–58. Epub 2016/06/09; PubMed PMID:
    27273813. https://doi.org/10.1111/cob.12152.
15. King WC, Hinerman AS, Belle SH, Wahed AS, Courcoulas AP. Comparison of the perfor-
    mance of common measures of weight regain after bariatric surgery for association with clini-
    cal outcomes. JAMA. 2018;320(15):1560–9. Epub 2018/10/17; PubMed PMID: 30326125;
    PMCID: PMC6233795. https://doi.org/10.1001/jama.2018.14433.
16. Jirapinyo P, Abu Dayyeh BK, Thompson CC. Weight regain after roux-en-Y gastric bypass
    has a large negative impact on the bariatric quality of life index. BMJ Open Gastroenterol.
    2017;4(1):e000153. Epub 2017/09/26; PubMed PMID: 28944069; PMCID: PMC5596836.
    https://doi.org/10.1136/bmjgast-2017-000153.
17. Magro DO, Geloneze B, Delfini R, Pareja BC, Callejas F, Pareja JC. Long-term weight
    regain after gastric bypass: a 5-year prospective study. Obes Surg. 2008;18(6):648–51. Epub
    2008/04/09; . PubMed PMID: 18392907. https://doi.org/10.1007/s11695-007-9265-1.
18. Brethauer SA, Kothari S, Sudan R, Williams B, English WJ, Brengman M, Kurian M, Hutter
    M, Stegemann L, Kallies K, Nguyen NT, Ponce J, Morton JM. Systematic review on reop-
    erative bariatric surgery: American Society for Metabolic and Bariatric Surgery Revision

Task Force. Surg Obes Relat Dis. 2014;10(5):952–72. Epub 2014/04/30; PubMed PMID: 24776071. https://doi.org/10.1016/j.soard.2014.02.014.

19. Zorrilla-Nunez LF, Campbell A, Giambartolomei G, Lo Menzo E, Szomstein S, Rosenthal RJ. The importance of the biliopancreatic limb length in gastric bypass: a systematic review. Surg Obes Relat Dis. 2019;15(1):43–9. Epub 2018/12/07; PubMed PMID: 30501957. https://doi.org/10.1016/j.soard.2018.10.013.

20. Amundsen T, Strommen M, Martins C. Suboptimal weight loss and weight regain after gastric bypass surgery-postoperative status of energy intake, eating behavior, physical activity, and psychometrics. Obes Surg. 2017;27(5):1316–23. . Epub 2016/12/04; PubMed PMID: 27914028; PMCID: PMC5403843. https://doi.org/10.1007/s11695-016-2475-7.

21. Freire RH, Borges MC, Alvarez-Leite JI, Toulson Davisson Correia MI. Food quality, physical activity, and nutritional follow-up as determinant of weight regain after roux-en-Y gastric bypass. Nutrition. 2012;28(1):53–8. Epub 2011/09/03; PubMed PMID: 21885246. https://doi.org/10.1016/j.nut.2011.01.011.

22. Faria SL, de Oliveira KE, Lins RD, Faria OP. Nutritional management of weight regain after bariatric surgery. Obes Surg. 2010;20(2):135–9. Epub 2008/06/26; PubMed PMID: 18575942. https://doi.org/10.1007/s11695-008-9610-z.

23. Welch G, Wesolowski C, Piepul B, Kuhn J, Romanelli J, Garb J. Physical activity predicts weight loss following gastric bypass surgery: findings from a support group survey. Obes Surg. 2008;18(5):517–24. Epub 2008/03/28; PubMed PMID: 18365295. https://doi.org/10.1007/s11695-007-9269-x.

24. Sarwer DB, Allison KC, Wadden TA, Ashare R, Spitzer JC, McCuen-Wurst C, LaGrotte C, Williams NN, Edwards M, Tewksbury C, Wu J. Psychopathology, disordered eating, and impulsivity as predictors of outcomes of bariatric surgery. Surg Obes Relat Dis. 2019;15(4):650–5. Epub 2019/03/13; PubMed PMID: 30858009; PMCID: PMC6538470. https://doi.org/10.1016/j.soard.2019.01.029.

25. Still CD, Wood GC, Chu X, Manney C, Strodel W, Petrick A, Gabrielsen J, Mirshahi T, Argyropoulos G, Seiler J, Yung M, Benotti P, Gerhard GS. Clinical factors associated with weight loss outcomes after Roux-en-Y gastric bypass surgery. Obesity (Silver Spring). 2014;22(3):888–94. Epub 2013/06/28; PubMed PMID: 23804287; PMCID: PMC3819407. https://doi.org/10.1002/oby.20529.

26. Campos GM, Rabl C, Mulligan K, Posselt A, Rogers SJ, Westphalen AC, Lin F, Vittinghoff E. Factors associated with weight loss after gastric bypass. Arch Surg. 2008;143(9):877–83.; discussion 84; Epub 2008/09/17; PubMed PMID: 18794426; PMCID: PMC2747804. https://doi.org/10.1001/archsurg.143.9.877.

27. Laferrere B. Bariatric surgery and obesity: influence on the incretins. Int J Obes Suppl. 2016;6(Suppl 1):S32–S6. Epub 2017/07/08; PubMed PMID: 28685028; PMCID: PMC5485883. https://doi.org/10.1038/ijosup.2016.8.

28. Dimitriadis GK, Randeva MS, Miras AD. Potential Hormone Mechanisms of Bariatric Surgery. Curr Obes Rep. 2017;6(3):253–65. Epub 2017/08/07; PubMed PMID: 28780756; PMCID: PMC5585994. https://doi.org/10.1007/s13679-017-0276-5.

29. Meek CL, Lewis HB, Reimann F, Gribble FM, Park AJ. The effect of bariatric surgery on gastrointestinal and pancreatic peptide hormones. Peptides. 2016;77:28–37. Epub 2015/09/08; . PubMed PMID: 26344355. https://doi.org/10.1016/j.peptides.2015.08.013.

30. Leggett CB, Desalermos A, Brown SD, Lee E, Proudfoot JA, Horgan S, Gupta S, Grunvald E, Ho SB, Zarrinpar A. The effects of provider-prescribed obesogenic drugs on post-laparoscopic sleeve gastrectomy outcomes: a retrospective cohort study. Int J Obes (Lond). 2019;43(6):1154–63. Epub 2018/09/23; PubMed PMID: 30242239; PMCID: PMC6428627. https://doi.org/10.1038/s41366-018-0207-x.

31. Apovian CM, Aronne LJ, Bessesen DH, McDonnell ME, Murad MH, Pagotto U, Ryan DH, Still CD, Endocrine S. Pharmacological management of obesity: an endocrine society clinical practice guideline. J Clin Endocrinol Metab. 2015;100(2):342–62. Epub 2015/01/16; PubMed PMID: 25590212. https://doi.org/10.1210/jc.2014-3415.

32. Varma S, Clark JM, Schweitzer M, Magnuson T, Brown TT, Lee CJ. Weight regain in patients with symptoms of post-bariatric surgery hypoglycemia. Surg Obes Relat Dis.

2017;13(10):1728–34. Epub 2017/08/29; PubMed PMID: 28844575; PMCID: PMC5657438. https://doi.org/10.1016/j.soard.2017.06.004.

33. Sudan R, Nguyen NT, Hutter MM, Brethauer SA, Ponce J, Morton JM. Morbidity, mortality, and weight loss outcomes after reoperative bariatric surgery in the USA. J Gastrointest Surg. 2015;19(1):171–178; discussion 8-9. Epub 2014/09/05; PubMed PMID: 25186073. doi: https://doi.org/10.1007/s11605-014-2639-5

34. Igel LI, Kumar RB, Saunders KH, Aronne LJ. Practical use of pharmacotherapy for obesity. Gastroenterology. 2017;152(7):1765–79. Epub 2017/02/14; . PubMed PMID: 28192104. https://doi.org/10.1053/j.gastro.2016.12.049.

35. Saunders KH, Shukla AP, Igel LI, Kumar RB, Aronne LJ. Pharmacotherapy for obesity. Endocrinol Metab Clin N Am. 2016;45(3):521–38. Epub 2016/08/16; PubMed PMID: 27519128. https://doi.org/10.1016/j.ecl.2016.04.005.

36. Saunders KH, Umashanker D, Igel LI, Kumar RB, Aronne LJ. Obesity pharmacotherapy. Med Clin N Am. 2018;102(1):135–48. Epub 2017/11/21; PubMed PMID: 29156182. https://doi.org/10.1016/j.mcna.2017.08.010.

37. Zoss I, Piec G, Horber FF. Impact of or list at therapy on weight reduction in morbidly obese patients after implantation of the Swedish adjustable gastric band. Obes Surg. 2002;12(1):113–7. Epub 2002/03/01; PubMed PMID: 11868286. https://doi.org/10.1381/096089202321144685.

38. Zilberstein B, Pajecki D, Garcia de Brito AC, Gallafrio ST, Eshkenazy R, Andrade CG. Topiramate after adjustable gastric banding in patients with binge eating and difficulty losing weight. Obes Surg. 2004;14(6):802–5. Epub 2004/08/21; PubMed PMID: 15318986. https://doi.org/10.1381/0960892041590926.

39. Pajecki D, Halpern A, Cercato C, Mancini M, de Cleva R, Santo MA. Short-term use of liraglutide in the management of patients with weight regain after bariatric surgery. Rev Col Bras Cir. 2013;40(3):191–5. Epub 2013/08/06; PubMed PMID: 23912365. https://doi.org/10.1590/s0100-69912013000300005.

40. Stanford FC, Alfaris N, Gomez G, Ricks ET, Shukla AP, Corey KE, Pratt JS, Pomp A, Rubino F, Aronne LJ. The utility of weight loss medications after bariatric surgery for weight regain or inadequate weight loss: A multi-center study. Surg Obes Relat Dis. 2017;13(3):491–500. Epub 2016/12/18; PubMed PMID: 27986587; PMCID: PMC6114136. https://doi.org/10.1016/j.soard.2016.10.018.

41. Schwartz J, Chaudhry UI, Suzo A, Durkin N, Wehr AM, Foreman KS, Tychonievich K, Mikami DJ, Needleman BJ, Noria SF. Pharmacotherapy in conjunction with a diet and exercise program for the treatment of weight recidivism or weight loss plateau post-bariatric surgery: a retrospective review. Obes Surg. 2016;26(2):452–8. Epub 2015/11/30; PubMed PMID: 26615406. https://doi.org/10.1007/s11695-015-1979-x.

42. Nor Hanipah Z, Nasr EC, Bucak E, Schauer PR, Aminian A, Brethauer SA, Cetin D. Efficacy of adjuvant weight loss medication after bariatric surgery. Surg Obes Relat Dis. 2018;14(1):93–8. Epub 2017/12/31; PubMed PMID: 29287757. https://doi.org/10.1016/j.soard.2017.10.002.

43. Wharton S, Kuk JL, Luszczynski M, Kamran E, Christensen RAG. Liraglutide 3.0 mg for the management of insufficient weight loss or excessive weight regain post-bariatric surgery. Clin Obes. 2019;9(4):e12323. Epub 2019/06/12; PubMed PMID: 31183988; PMCID: PMC6771702. https://doi.org/10.1111/cob.12323.

44. Phelan S, Wadden TA. Combining behavioral and pharmacological treatments for obesity. Obes Res. 2002;10(6):560–74. Epub 2002/06/11; PubMed PMID: 12055334. https://doi.org/10.1038/oby.2002.77.

45. Toth AT, Gomez G, Shukla AP, Pratt JS, Cena H, Biino G, Aronne LJ, Stanford FC. Weight loss medications in young adults after bariatric surgery for weight regain or inadequate weight loss: A multi-center study. Children (Basel). 2018;5(9) Epub 2018/08/31; PubMed PMID: 30158481; PMCID: PMC6162731 https://doi.org/10.3390/children5090116.

46. Stanford FC. Controversial issues: A practical guide to the use of weight loss medications after bariatric surgery for weight regain or inadequate weight loss. Surg Obes Relat Dis. 2019;15(1):128–32. Epub 2018/12/12; PubMed PMID: 30527889; PMCID: PMC6441616. https://doi.org/10.1016/j.soard.2018.10.020.

Does Resizing the Gastric Pouch Aid in Weight Loss?

31

Michael S. McCormack and Michael B. Ujiki

31.1 Introduction

Despite the rise in popularity of restrictive bariatric surgical procedures such as the sleeve gastrectomy in the US [1] the Roux-En-Y Gastric Bypass (RYGB) still maintains a more sustainable long-term weight loss outcome and larger reduction in co-morbid metabolic conditions [2]. After undergoing a RYGB, patients can expect initial weight-loss followed by a minor amount of weight regain after reaching their weight nadir. Up to a quarter of patients have been reported to regain even further weight often accompanied by return of metabolic co-morbidities [3]. This is thought to be attributed to a complex inter-play of various social, psychological, physiological, and anatomical factors [3, 4]. In this chapter we will explore if a specific anatomical factor, namely pouch size, has any effect on the weight loss awarded the RYGB or the weight regain plaguing up to a quarter of patients in the published literature.

31.2 Search Strategy

We conducted an online literature search using PubMed, Google Scholar, and Cochrane Clinical Trials databases. We limited our search to articles published in the English language between January first, 2000 until January first, 2020. The search terms and key-words were derived from our PICO table and included 'Roux-En-Y' or 'stomach' or 'gastric' and 'pouch' and 'size' or 'revised' or 'revision' and 'weight' or 'body mass' and 'loss' or 'regain'. We also included studies referenced

M. S. McCormack · M. B. Ujiki (✉)
NorthShore University HealthSystem, Evanston, Illinois, USA
e-mail: mujiki@northshore.org

© Springer Nature Switzerland AG 2021
J. Alverdy, Y. Vigneswaran (eds.), *Difficult Decisions in Bariatric Surgery*,
Difficult Decisions in Surgery: An Evidence-Based Approach,
https://doi.org/10.1007/978-3-030-55329-6_31

by the studies we selected from the search if they were relevant. We excluded case reports, animal studies, and articles pertaining to other bariatric procedures where a gastric pouch is not created (sleeve gastrectomy, gastroplasties, etc.). We also excluded studies with restrictive bands placed around the gastrum since this approach primarily targets restricting the size of the gastrojejunal stoma rather than the volume of the gastric pouch. Finally, we also excluded articles in which stoma reduction was the primary focus of the operation.

31.3   Results

We included a total of 20 studies examining the effect of gastric pouch size to either weight loss, recidivism, or response to revisional surgery following initial bariatric surgery. This includes 2 randomized controlled trials, 2 systematic reviews, and 3 prospective cohort studies. The remainder of studies were retrospective in design.

Table 31.1 demonstrates the 10 studies which did not find a correlation between a smaller pouch size and better weight loss outcome. One of the 10 studies had a contradictory outcome: a randomized controlled trial showed increased weight loss with a larger sized (elongated) pouch. Additionally, this table includes 2 prospective cohort studies, 4 retrospective comparative studies, 2 retrospective cohort studies, and 1 retrospective database review. N ranged from 14–14,168 with a median of 74.5. Subjects were on average 79.6% female (62.5–100%) with an average age of 44.43 years (41.6–51 years) and average original BMI of 47.3 kg/m^2 (42–54.6 kg/m^2). The studies followed the subjects for an average of 24.6 months (12–48 months). The method used to measure the size of the gastric pouch varied with the upper gastrointestinal contrast study being the most common method (4/10), while 3D-CT (2/10) and calculated staple length (2/10) tied for the second most common method, and endoscopy (1/10) or intraoperative direct measurement (1/10) accounted for the remaining methods used. The size of a small pouch was defined differently depending on the methodology used but when measured in volume varied from >10 mL to <49 mL. Complication rates were underreported with only 4/10 studies revealing an average total complication rate of 9.93% (7–17%). In this table, a randomized controlled trial evaluating a longer and larger pouch versus a smaller and shorter pouch demonstrated an increase in weight loss by 36 months in the larger pouch group (BMI $\triangle$ −2 kg/m^2, EWL% $\triangle$ 11% p = 0.023), however, this was not seen until the 36-month follow-up and the authors attribute this difference to a decrease in weight regain in the larger pouch group [6]. Three studies in this table, including a large Scandinavian database review (n = 14,168), demonstrated an initial (<12-month post-revision) weight loss after resizing the gastric pouch however, beyond 2 years, the weight loss was negated or non-significant [9, 10, 15]. One of these studies included concurrent revision of the GJ-stoma size [10]. The same Scandinavian database review also demonstrated an increase in the relative risk of developing a marginal ulcer by 14% per every 10 mm of linear stapler used (CI 9–20%, p = 0.05) [9]. Madan et al. [13] also explored if fundus size correlated to weight loss outcome,

Table 31.1 Studies with no association between smaller pouch size and better weight loss outcome

Author/design	Subjects	Pouch size	Revision/method	Weight △/complications	Findings	Comments
Boerboom et al. [6] Year: 2019 Design: Single-site RCT Follow up: 36 months Level of evidence: I	N = 132 Mean age: 47 ± 9 Female(%): 52.5% Original BMI: 44 ± 5 kg/m²	Method: Intraoperative Large pouch: 4×60 mm staplers Small pouch: 3×60mm staplers	Small pouch vs elongated & larger pouch size RCT.	EWL% △: −11% BMI △: 2 kg/m² Complications: 17%	Elongated pouch statistically significant more weight loss at 3 years.	No difference seen first 2 years, no weight regain seen in extended pouch group by third year accounting for difference in weight loss.
Edholm et al. [9] Year: 2015 Design: Retrospective database Follow up: 12 months Level of evidence: III	N = 14,168 Mean age: 41.6 ± 11.1 Female(%): 76 Original BMI: 42 ± 5 kg/m²	Method: Length of staplers Staple length: 145 ± 28 mm	Intraoperative staple length used as surrogate for pouch size. Correlated to weight loss and marginal ulcer risk.	EWL% △: N/A BMI △: N/A Complications: N/A	Initial correlation between staple length used and weight loss, but by 12 months no correlation remained.	Multivariate analysis at 12 months for staple length and EBMIL% -0.05 (p = 0.29). Staple length correlated with higher risk for marginal ulcer.
Hamdi et al. [10] Year: 2014 Design: Retrospective cohort Follow up: 24 months Level of evidence: III	N = 25 Mean age: 42 Female (%): 100% Original BMI: 54.6 kg/m²	Method: Endoscopy Large pouch: >5 cm in depth Small pouch: Pouch redone, 4 cm from angle of his	GJ anastomosis resected, new GJ anastomosis and pouch created <5 cm in any dimension.	EWL% △: 2.9% BMI △: 3.2 kg/m² Complications 8%	Initial weight loss at 3–12 month post revision, however at 24 months weight regain higher than prerevision.	Only 5 patients followed up at 24 months.

(continued)

Table 31.1 (continued)

Author/design	Subjects	Pouch size	Revision/method	Weight Δ/complications	Findings	Comments
Madan et al. [13] Year: 2007 Design: Retrospective comparative	N = 59 Mean age: N/A Female(%): 85%	Method: UGI Method: UGI 1. Smaller than average 2. Average	Radiographic/anatomical volume of pouch correlated to EWL	EWL% smallest pouch: 70%	No statistically significant difference in EWL% between different pouch size groups.	Attempted to subjectively determine volume of fundus and weight loss.
	Original BMI: 48.5 ± 6 kg/m²	3. Larger than average 4. ×3 times larger than average		EWL% largest pouch: 64% p = 0.59		No significant correlation found.
Follow up: 19.4 months Level of evidence: III				Complications: N/A		
Robert et al. [20] Year: 2005 Design: Prospective cohort	N = 39 Mean age: 46 Female(%): 61.5%	Method: 3D-CT Large pouch size: 47 cc	Ascertain weight loss at 12 months post RYGB comparative to pouch size.	EWL% Δ: N/A BMI Δ: N/A	No correlation between pouch volume and EWL% at 3, 6, 9, 12 or 24 months.	Original BMI correlated to initial pouch volume (r = 0.4, p = 0.01)
Follow up: 12 months Level of evidence: II	Original BMI: 43.4 kg/m²	Small pouch size: 43 cc		Complications: N/A		
Nishie et al. [15] Year: 2007 Design: Prospective cohort	N = 82 Mean age: 41.7 Female(%): 75.8%	Method: UGI Average pouch size: 30.1cm²	Correlation between area of pouch to EWL% following pouch revision.	EWL% Δ: 2.9% BMI Δ: 3.2 kg/m²	Initial weight loss at 3–12 month post revision, however at 24 months weight regain higher than prerevision.	Pouch volume estimated by calculating 2D measurements.
Follow up: 24 months Level of evidence: II	Original BMI: 47.4 kg/m²			Complications 8%		

OConnor et al. [16]	N = 231	Method: Intraoperative	Increments of pouch size compared for correlation to differences in weight loss at 12 months.	EWL% △: None	No correlation between EWL% and pouch size found for pouches 10-20 cc in size out to 12 months.	Size of pouch was subjective to operators interpretation. Largest pouch 20 cc is small compared to literature.
Year: 2007	Mean age: 45	Pouch size: 10-20 cc		BMI △: None		
Design: Retrospective cohort	Female (%): 90%	Stratified in		Complications: N/A		
Follow up: 12 months	Original BMI: 48 kg/m²	2.5 cc				
Level of evidence: III		increments.				
Parikh et al. [17]	N = 14	Method: UGI	14 patients with weight regain had their pouch size revised and weight loss measured over >1 year.	EWL% △: 12.8%	No statistically significant difference in weight at 12 months after revision of pouch.	Underpowered, a third of patients also had roux limb lengthening.
Year: 2010	Mean age: 43	Large pouch size: >120 cc		BMI △: −2.7 kg/m²		
Design: Retrospective comparative	Female (%): N/A	Small pouch size: 20-25 cc		p = 0.16		
Follow up: 12.2 months	Original BMI: 46.8 kg/m²			Complications: N/A		
Level of evidence: III						
Riccioppo et al. [19]	N = 67	Method: 3D-CT	Compared outcomes including weight loss and	Nadir EWL% △: −5.5%	More weight loss at nadir but slightly more weight regain in larger pouch group however neither statistically significant.	Smaller pouch lead to faster pouch emptying. Longer emptying time associated with more weight regain (regained EWL% 29.8% vs 11.7% p = 0.036)
Year: 2017	Mean age: 51	Large pouch size: >40 cc	Regain for two groups based on their pouch volume.	p = 0.41 Wt regain		
Design: Retrospective comparative	Female(%): 91%	Small pouch size: <40 cc		EWL%: 1.1%		
Follow up: 47 months	Original BMI: 51.4 kg/m²	Method: 3D-CT		p = 0.195		
Level of evidence: III				Complications:N/A		

(continued)

Table 31.1 (continued)

Author/design	Subjects	Pouch size	Revision/method	Weight Δ/ complications	Findings	Comments
Topart et al. [22]	N = 132	Method: UGI 2–4 years postop	Compared patients with large vs small pouch and EWL%.	>50 mL EWL%: 68 ± 3.6%	No significant weight loss difference based on pouch size, even when including pouches >100 mL.	Post op UGI performed 2–4 yrs. after RYGB, unknown if pouch dilated over time.
Year: 2011	Mean age: 42.6	Large pouch size: >50 mL		<49 mL EWL%: 66 ± 3.6%		
Design: Retrospective comparative	Female(%): 85%	Small pouch size:<49 mL		Complications: N/A		
Follow up: 48 months	Original BMI: 47 kg/m^2					
Level of evidence: III						

however no such correlation was discovered. Robert et al. [20] demonstrated that pre-operative BMI correlated to pouch volume following index-RYGB (r = 0.4, p = 0.01), suggesting that patients with larger BMI at onset of intervention end up with a larger pouch post-operatively. O'Connor et al. [16] demonstrated in a non-randomized format that there was no difference in weight loss at 10 months between small (<20 cc) and really small (<10 cc) pouches suggesting that if a size of at least <20 cc can be reached, there is no additional weight loss benefit in reducing the size of the gastric pouch.

P (Patients)	I (Intervention)	C (Comparator)	O (Outcomes)
Patients undergoing/gone RYGB	Adjusting size of gastric pouch	No pouch size revision/large size pouch	Weight loss

Table 31.2 depicts 10 studies which did find a correlation between the size of the pouch and weight loss outcome; specifically, larger pouches conferred poorer weight loss outcome. This includes 1 randomized controlled trial, 2 systematic reviews, 1 prospective cohort study, 3 retrospective comparative studies, 2 retrospective cohort studies, and 1 retrospective case-control study. Study populations ranged from 20 to 16,055 with a median of 261. Subjects were on average 78.9% female (43–90%) with an average age of 44.1 years (38.3–48 years) and average original BMI of 47.3 kg/m^2 (33.7–52 kg/m^2). The studies followed the subjects for an average of 26.2 months (12–49 months). The most common modality of measuring the gastric pouch size was the upper gastrointestinal contrast study (6/10); however, in half of these studies (3/6), an additional modality or 2 were used. This included endoscopy (3/6) and 3D-CT (1/6). Endoscopy was the second most common (4/10) modality used to measure pouch size but was only used as a single modality in 1 study. Intraoperative estimation of size was used the least (1/10). The 2 systematic reviews included studies using multiple varying methods of measuring pouch size. The size of the small pouch was in most studies defined in volume and ranged from >10 mL to <59 mL. Complication rates again were poorly reported with only 3 out of 10 studies depicting an average complication rate of 24.2% (15.6–30%). In this Table, 3 studies [5, 7, 12] demonstrated significant weight loss following revision of the size of the gastric pouch; however, in 2 of the 3 studies the size of the gastrojejunal stoma was revised as well [5, 7]. Borbely et al. [7] also demonstrated quite a significant perioperative morbidity (27%) with revisional bariatric surgery for pouch reduction. Roberts et al. [21] demonstrated with 320 subjects that pouch size was inversely related to weight loss (r = −0.302 p < 0.02) in the short term (12 month follow-up) with 320 subjects; however, he also demonstrated a positive correlation (r = 0.19 P < 0.01) between preoperative BMI and pouch size. Similarly, Campos et al. [8] demonstrated with 361 subjects that pouch size was inversely related to weight loss (r = −0.25 p < 0.01) in the short term (12 month follow-up), and Henegan et al. [11] demonstrated with 380 subjects that pouch size also was inversely related to weight loss (r = 0.127 p = 0.02) with a longer follow up of 49 months. Interestingly,

Table 31.2 Studies which demonstrate an association between smaller pouch size and greater weight loss

Author/design	Subjects	Pouch size	Revision/method	Weight △/ complications	Findings	Comments
Al-bader et al. [5]	N = 32	Method: UGI, endoscopy	Patients with weight regain after RYGB with a dilated gastric pouch underwent revision of pouch and stoma.	EWL% △: 29%	Pouch and stoma revision for weight regain with significant weight loss (+29% EWL) at 14 ± 6 months.	Stapled across and narrowed GJ-anastomosis as well. Less than 2-year follow-up.
Year: 2015	Mean age: 38.3	Large pouch size: >30 cc		BMI △: −5.5 kg/m²		
Design: Retrospective comparative	Female (%): 84%	Small pouch size: 20-25 cc		Complications: 15.6%		
Follow up: 14 ± 6 months	Original BMI: 50.7 kg/m²					
Level of evidence: III						
Borbely et al. [7]	N = 26	Method: UGI, endoscopy	Pouch and stoma revision for weight regain >30% EWL from nadir.	EWL% △: N/A	Significant weight reduction at 48 months with BMI 32.9 vs 39.1 prior to revision.	Stapled across and narrowed GJ-anastomosis as well.
Year: 2016	Mean age: 46.5	Large pouch size: N/A		BMI △: −6.2 kg/m²		Higher than average morbidity.
Design: Prospective cohort	Female(%): 85%	Small pouch size: N/A		Complications: 27%		
Follow up: 48 months (24–60)	Original BMI: 48.9 kg/m²					
Level of evidence: III						

Campos et al. [8] Year: 2008 Design: Retrospective cohort Follow up: 12 months Level of evidence: III	N = 361 Mean age: 45 Female (%): 86.1% Original BMI: 52 kg/m²	Method: UGI Large pouch size: 39 cc Small pouch size: 25 cc	Gastric pouch compared between two groups of EWL% >40% vs <40% at 12 months.	EWL% △: 31.7% BMI △: −7.8 kg/m² Complications N/A	Size of pouch inversely related to weight loss with a Pearson correlation of −0.25 (p < 0.01).	Only 12-month follow up for 85.9% of patients. 2 risk factors related to poor weight loss absent in the patients omited.
Henegan et al. [11] Year: 2012 Design: Retrospective comparative Follow up: 49 months Level of evidence: III	N = 380 Mean age: 48 Female (%): 86.3% Original BMI: 52 ± 10 kg/m²	Method: Endoscopy Large pouch size: 26 cc Small pouch size: 21.8 cc	Patients requiring EGD post-RYGB for GI symptoms were compared to patients with weight regain post-RYGB.	EWL% △: 43.4% BMI △: −12.9 kg/m² Complications: N/A	Pouch volume inversely related to EWL with Pearson correlation −0.127 (p = 0.02).	Multivariate analysis of weight regain after RYGB did not show pouch volume as statistically significant (OR 1.7 (0.4–6.2 p = 0.455). BMI and duration from RYGB did however.

(continued)

Table 31.2 (continued)

Author/design	Subjects	Pouch size	Revision/method	Weight Δ/complications	Findings	Comments
Iannelli et al. [12]	N = 20	Method: UGI, endoscopy, 3D-CT	Patient with weight loss failure And enlarged pouch underwent pouch revision and followed for 18 months.	EWL% Δ: 32.3%	Significant weight loss following revision of pouch size, GJ-anastomosis left intact.	Less weight loss at 18 months if pouch enlarges over time after index RYGB vs large pouch present right after index RYGB.
Year: 2013	Mean age: 44	Pouch size criteria varied based on modality.		BMI Δ: −4.4 kg/m²		
Design: Retrospective cohort	Female(%): 90%					
Follow up: 18 months				Complications: 30%		
Level of evidence: III	Original BMI: 45.8 kg/m²					
Mahawar et al. [14]	N = 16,055	Method: Various	14 studies including 2 RCT's investigating weight loss vs pouch and/or stoma size	EWL% Δ: N/A	Large pouch offers no benefit in weight loss, may increase marginal ulcer risk. Quality of data does not allow optimal size of pouch to be determined.	Width of pouch may be more determinant for weight loss than volume. Surgical and pouch measurement techniques differ widely.
Year: 2019	Mean age: 45.27	Pouch size: Various		BMI Δ: N/A		
Design: Systematic review	Female (%): 75.87%					
Follow up: N/A	Original BMI: 44.99 kg/m²			Complications N/A		
Level of evidence: III						

Study	Method / Pouch size	Study details	Description	Outcomes	Findings	Comments
Ren et al. [18] Year: 2014 Design: Single-site RCT Follow up: 12 months Level of evidence: II	Method: Intraoperative measurements Large pouch size: 25-35 cc Small pouch size: 10-20 cc	N = 69 Mean age: 44.5 Female (%): 43% Original BMI: 33.7 kg/m²	Randomized controlled trial to evaluate if pouch size had any effect on T2DM in RYGB patients.	EWL% △: 9.8% BMI △: −0.9 kg/m² Complications: N/A	Small (△0.9 kg/m²) but statistically significant (p = 0.04) greater weight loss in smaller pouch group at 12 months.	Low N (69) and preoperative BMI (33.7 kg/m²) with minimal difference between groups (△0.9 kg/m²).
Roberts et al. [21] Year: 2007 Design: Retrospective comparative Follow up: 12 months Level of evidence: III	Method: UGI Large pouch size: 60-120 cm² Small pouch size: 30-59 cm²	N = 320 Mean age: 41.2 Female (%): 81.6% Original BMI: 51 kg/m²	Patients categorized based on pouch size and followed for 1 year post-RYGB to compare weight loss.	EWL% △: 15.8% BMI △: N/A Complications: N/A	Negative correlation (r = −0.302 p < 0.02) between pouch size and EWL% at 12 months.	Precop BMI and pouch size positive correlation r = 0.19 P < 0.01
Tran et al. [23] Year: 2016 Design: Systematic review Follow up: N/A Level of evidence: III	Method: Various Pouch size: Various	N = 87 Mean age: 45 Female(%): 75% Original: BMI:51.7 kg/m²	Systematic review of various revisional operations for weight recidivism following RYGB, including 5 studies measuring pouch resizing.	EWL% △: N/A BMI △: −2.9 kg/m² Complications 17%	3/5 studies only followed 12 months post revision. 1 study followed 36 months, showed higher BMI post-revision (BMI△ + 3 kg/m² at 36 months post-revision).	Pouch revision studies underpowered (n = 5–25).

(continued)

Table 31.2 (continued)

Author/design	Subjects	Pouch size	Revision/method	Weight △/ complications	Findings	Comments
Uitenbogaart et al. [24] Year: 2019	N = 202 Mean age: 43.2 Female (%): 83%	Method: UGI Large pouch size: Width or length >×2 size of adjacent vertebrae	Group of weight loss failure (<50% EWL) following RYGB were compared to controls with successful weight loss.	Weight △ not compared.	Pouch dilation: Present in 23% of weight loss failure group.	Interobserver reliability with kappa of 0.25 (p = 0.01) on assessment of pouch size on UGI contrast study questions that UGI is a poor assessment of pouch size.
Design: Retrospective case-control Follow up: 44.7 months Level of evidence: III	Original BMI: 42.4 kg/m²	Small pouch size: Width or length <×2 size of adjacent vertebrae	Pouch size was evaluated with UGI.	Complications: N/A	Present in 11% of control group. (p = 0.024)	

Iannelli et al. [12] demonstrated that weight loss was greater (BMI $\triangle$ −7.6 kg/m^2 vs BMI $\triangle$ −3.1 kg/m^2) if the revised pouch was categorized as large immediately following index-RYGB versus slowly enlarging over time following index-RYGB. One single-site randomized controlled trial [18] with short (12 month) follow-up and low number of subjects (69) with a low preoperative BMI (average BMI 33.27 kg/m^2) demonstrated a small (BMI $\triangle$ −0.9 kg/m^2) but increased weight loss following slightly smaller (10-20 cc vs 25-35 cc) pouch volumes following RYGB. Although this was a randomized controlled trial the applicability of the patient population studied and their results may not transfer well to the level of obesity treated in the general American and European population. Two systematic reviews including most of the studies referenced in this manuscript evaluated the evidence of pouch size on weight loss and concluded that although the data suggests that smaller pouch size leads to greater weight loss, at least in the short term (12 months or less) that the quality of the data published does not currently support recommendations for an optimal pouch size.

Overall there is little consensus in methodology on how to determine pouch size and no uniformity in categorizing what determines a large versus a small pouch among the studies. Furthermore, Uittenbogaart et al. [24] demonstrated that there is poor inter-observer reliability (kappa = 0.25 (p = 0.01)) when assessing the pouch size with the most commonly used method, the upper gastrointestinal contrast study.

31.4 Recommendations

If the gastric pouch is to be fashioned or revised for optimal weight loss, either a very small (10-20 cc) or large but elongated (10 cm length) gastric pouch should be created, preferably at index-operation. (Evidence quality low; weak recommendation).

For patients experiencing poor weight loss following RYGB (<50% EWL) or weight regain (>30% EWL from nadir), laparoscopic gastric pouch size revision could offer short-term (<24 month) weight loss but at an elevated perioperative morbidity. (Evidence quality low; weak recommendation).

For patients experiencing poor weight loss following RYGB (<50% EWL) or weight regain (>30% EWL from nadir), a thorough multi-modality investigation should be pursued to determine both behavioral, psychosocial, and anatomical (pouch size, gastrojejunal stoma, and roux-limb length) and the appropriate interventions should be tailored to the individual patient's needs. (Evidence quality low; weak recommendation).

Laparoscopic pouch size revision carries significant morbidity and offers modest short-term and minimal long-term weight recidivism benefit for the patient. (Evidence quality low; weak recommendation).

31.5 Personal View on Data

The data reviewed in this manuscript demonstrates a lack of unity in both measuring and defining what entails a large pouch. The most commonly used modality for measuring pouch size, an upper gastro-intestinal contrast study, is dynamic over time in relation to pouch emptying time and has data to suggest poor inter-observer reliability. Historically, a smaller pouch has been considered to lead to greater weight loss and as such has been studied as a component of revisional bariatric surgery. However, one recent randomized controlled trial demonstrated that a larger pouch size was associated with greater weight loss [6]. The quality of the data evaluating the effect of pouch size on weight loss is additionally rather poor; only two randomized controlled trials are included in this manuscript, but they demonstrate conflicting evidence of pouch size on weight loss outcomes and the study finding reduction in pouch size beneficial for weight loss lacks practical applicability to the level of obesity currently treated in our population. Most of the remaining studies evaluated in this manuscript demonstrate a shorter follow-up and are mostly retrospective in design.

The included studies depicting pouch size revision all employed laparoscopic techniques and demonstrated a significant and fairly harmful morbidity rate [5, 7, 12]. This would suggest that revisional laparoscopic surgery for pouch size is prohibitive on two levels, the risk of harm for the patient, and the lack of effective long-term weight recidivism treatment.

Weight recidivism following RYGB is multi-faceted, which some of the data in this manuscript describes. Factors such as original BMI, duration from index RYGB, an enlarged pouch immediately following RYGB versus slowly enlarging over time, gastrojejunal stoma size, and psychological factors strongly influence weight loss outcomes following RYGB.

Gastrojejunal stoma size has been demonstrated as a strong independent risk factor for weight regain following RYGB [25–30] and was not controlled for in a majority of the studies included in this manuscript. In fact, two studies demonstrating an association between revision of pouch size and increased weight loss for weight recidivism also concurrently refashioned the GJ-stoma size, questioning the effect of pouch size revision on weight recidivism [5, 7].

31.6 Summarized Recommendations

Optimal pouch size for RYGB should either not exceed 10-20 cc in volume or be constructed in a narrow and elongated (10 cm length) fashion.

Poor weight loss (<50% EWL) or weight regain (>30% EWL from nadir) following RYGB should not be treated by laparoscopic pouch size revision due to increased morbidity and lack of successful long term (>24 month) outcomes.

Weight recidivism is more likely successfully treated by a multi-modal approach including behavioral, psychological, dietary, exercise and endoscopic measures to address gastrojejunal stoma size.

References

1. Benotti PN, Forse RA. The role of gastric surgery in the multidisciplinary management of severe obesity. Am J Surg. 1995;169(3):361–7.
2. Colquitt JL, Pickett K, Loveman E, Frampton GK. Surgery for weight loss in adults. Cochrane Database Syst Rev. 2014;8:CD003641.
3. Karmali S, Brar B, Shi X, Sharma AM, de Gara C, Birch DW. Weight recidivism post-bariatric surgery: a systematic review. Obes Surg. 2013;23(11):1922–33.
4. King WC, Belle SH, Hinerman AS, Mitchell JE, Steffen KJ, Courcoulas AP. Patient behaviors and characteristics related to weight regain after roux-en-Y gastric bypass: a multicenter prospective cohort study. Ann Surg. 2019;4
5. Al-Bader I, Khoursheed M, Al Sharaf K, Mouzannar DA, Ashraf A, Fingerhut A. Revisional laparoscopic gastric pouch resizing for inadequate weight loss after roux-en-Y gastric bypass. Obes Surg. 2015;25(7):1103–8.
6. Boerboom A, Cooiman M, Aarts E, Aufenacker T, Hazebroek E, Berends F. An extended pouch in a roux-en-Y gastric bypass reduces weight regain: 3-year results of a randomized controlled trial. Obes Surg. 2020;30(1):3–10.
7. Borbély Y, Winkler C, Kröll D, Nett P. Pouch reshaping for significant weight regain after roux-en-Y gastric bypass. Obes Surg. 2017;27(2):439–44.
8. Campos GM, Rabl C, Mulligan K, Posselt A, Rogers SJ, Westphalen AC, et al. Factors associated with weight loss after gastric bypass. Arch Surg. 2008;143(9):8.
9. Edholm D, Ottosson J, Sundbom M. Importance of pouch size in laparoscopic roux-en-Y gastric bypass: a cohort study of 14,168 patients. Surg Endosc. 2016;30(5):2011–5.
10. Hamdi A, Julien C, Brown P, Woods I, Hamdi A, Ortega G, et al. Midterm outcomes of Revisional surgery for gastric pouch and Gastrojejunal anastomotic enlargement in patients with weight regain after gastric bypass for morbid obesity. Obes Surg. 2014;24(8):1386–90.
11. Heneghan HM, Yimcharoen P, Brethauer SA, Kroh M, Chand B. Influence of pouch and stoma size on weight loss after gastric bypass. Surg Obes Relat Dis. 2012;8(4):408–15.
12. Iannelli A, Schneck A-S, Hébuterne X, Gugenheim J. Gastric pouch resizing for roux-en-Y gastric bypass failure in patients with a dilated pouch. Surg Obes Relat Dis. 2013;9(2):260–7.
13. Madan AK, Tichansky DS, Phillips JC. Does Pouch Size Matter? Obes Surg. 2007;17(3):317–20.
14. Mahawar K, Sharples AJ, Graham Y. A systematic review of the effect of gastric pouch and/or gastrojejunostomy (stoma) size on weight loss outcomes with Roux-en-Y gastric bypass. Surg Endosc [Internet]. 2019 Nov 19 [cited 2020 Feb 9].
15. Nishie A, Brown B, Barloon T, Kueh D, Samuel I. Obes Surg. 2007;17(9):1183–8.
16. O'Connor EA, Carlin AM. Lack of correlation between variation in small-volume gastric pouch size and weight loss after laparoscopic roux-en-Y gastric bypass. Surg Obes Relat Dis. 2008;4(3):399–403.
17. Parikh M, Heacock L, Gagner M. Laparoscopic "Gastrojejunal sleeve reduction" as a revision procedure for weight loss failure after roux-en-Y gastric bypass. Obes Surg. 2011;21(5):650–4.
18. Ren Y, Yang W, Yang J, Wang C. Effect of roux-en-Y gastric bypass with different pouch size in Chinese T2DM patients with BMI 30–35 kg/m2. Obes Surg. 2015;25(3):457–63.
19. Riccioppo D, Santo MA, Rocha M, Buchpiguel CA, Diniz MA, Pajecki D, et al. Small-volume, fast-emptying gastric pouch leads to better long-term weight loss and food tolerance after roux-en-Y gastric bypass. Obes Surg. 2018;28(3):693–701.
20. Robert M, Pechoux A, Marion D, Laville M, Gouillat C, Disse E. Relevance of roux-en-Y gastric bypass volumetry using 3-dimensional gastric computed tomography with gas to predict weight loss at 1 year. Surg Obes Relat Dis. 2015;11(1):26–31.
21. Roberts K, Duffy A, Kaufman J, Burrell M, Dziura J, Bell R. Size matters: gastric pouch size correlates with weight loss after laparoscopic roux-en-Y gastric bypass. Surg Endosc. 2007;21(8):1397–402.

22. Topart P, Becouarn G, Ritz P. Pouch size after gastric bypass does not correlate with weight loss outcome. Obes Surg. 2011;21(9):1350–4.
23. Tran DD, Nwokeabia ID, Purnell S, Zafar SN, Ortega G, Hughes K, et al. Revision of roux-en-Y gastric bypass for weight regain: a systematic review of techniques and outcomes. Obes Surg. 2016;26(7):1627–34.
24. Uittenbogaart M, Leclercq WKG, Smeele P, van der Linden AN, Luijten AAPM, van Dielen FMH. Reliability and usefulness of upper gastro intestinal contrast studies to assess pouch size in patients with weight loss failure after roux-en-Y gastric bypass. Acta Chir Belg. 2019;27:1–5.
25. Abu Dayyeh BK, Lautz DB, Thompson CC. Gastrojejunal stoma diameter predicts weight regain after roux-en-Y gastric bypass. Clin Gastroenterol Hepatol. 2011;9(3):228–33.
26. Hedberg HM, Trenk A, Kuchta K, Linn JG, Carbray J, Ujiki MB. Endoscopic gastrojejunostomy revision is more effective than medical management alone to address weight regain after RYGB. Surg Endosc. 2018;32(3):1564–71.
27. Sharma V, Sharma A. A capsule or a tablet. Clin Gastroenterol Hepatol. 2011;9(9):804.
28. Shukla AP, He D, Saunders KH, Andrew C, Aronne LJ. Current concepts in management of weight regain following bariatric surgery. Expert Rev Endocrinol Metab. 2018;13(2):67–76.
29. Thompson CC, Chand B, Chen YK, DeMarco DC, Miller L, Schweitzer M, et al. Endoscopic suturing for Transoral outlet reduction increases weight loss after roux-en-Y gastric bypass surgery. Gastroenterology. 2013;145(1):129–137.e3.
30. Thompson CC, Jacobsen GR, Schroder GL, Horgan S. Stoma size critical to 12-month outcomes in endoscopic suturing for gastric bypass repair. Surg Obes Relat Dis. 2012;8(3):282–7.

Does Stoma Size Matter After Gastric Bypass?

32

Michael Keating and Philip Omotosho

32.1 Introduction

Though the question "does stoma size matter after gastric bypass?" would seem a relatively straightforward one, the technical approach to creating the gastrojejunal anastomosis introduces significant complexity. This is because technique varies widely. Nevertheless, the technique employed in creating the anastomosis primarily determines stoma size and therefore features prominently in the discussion. Stoma size carries potential implications for both weight loss outcomes and complication rates. The effect of gastrojejunostomy size on both weight loss and complication rates has been extensively evaluated in the literature, though with somewhat contradictory and inconclusive results. Through a review of the current literature, this chapter addresses the role anastomotic size might play in the weight loss outcomes and anastomotic complication rates following Roux-en-Y gastric bypass.

32.2 Search Strategy

A literature search of publications from 2000 to 2019 was conducted in PubMed to identify data concerning the effect of gastrojejunostomy size on weight loss and complications (especially stenosis) in patients who underwent Roux-en-Y gastric bypass. Search terms used included ("gastrojejunostomy" OR gastrojejunal

M. Keating
Department of Surgery, Rush University, Chicago, IL, USA
e-mail: Michael_R_Keating@rush.edu

P. Omotosho (✉)
Minimally Invasive and Bariatric Surgery, Department of Surgery, Rush University, Chicago, IL, USA
e-mail: Philip_Omotosho@rush.edu

© Springer Nature Switzerland AG 2021
J. Alverdy, Y. Vigneswaran (eds.), *Difficult Decisions in Bariatric Surgery*,
Difficult Decisions in Surgery: An Evidence-Based Approach,
https://doi.org/10.1007/978-3-030-55329-6_32

anastomosis OR gastroenterostomy OR gastrojejunal) AND ("bariatric surgery" OR "gastric bypass" OR "Roux-en-Y") AND ("size" OR "stricture" OR "stenosis" OR "complication" OR "weight loss"). Fourteen retrospective reviews, two randomized controlled trials, two meta-analyses, one systematic review. The data was classified using the GRADE system.

Additional articles were also discovered from the references of relevant articles found using the above search criteria.

32.3   Results

32.3.1 Effect of Stoma Size on Weight Loss

The effect of gastrojejunostomy stoma size on weight loss after laparoscopic Roux-en-Y gastric bypass has been a matter of significant interest in the literature since the procedure was first adopted. This is commonly evaluated by comparing postoperative weight loss (using a number of methodologies, including: % excess weight loss (EWL), total weight loss, % excess BMI lost, etc.) between various anastomotic techniques, rather than a direct comparison of stoma sizes. Stoma size is generally deduced from the anastomotic technique utilized, with many papers citing internal diameters for different circular staplers and thus different stoma aperture areas (Table 32.1). The stoma size in the linear stapled technique is particularly difficult to assess for several reasons. First, the amount of tissue included in the stapler is often not reliably reflected by the size of the stapler load (for example, a 45 mm GIA cartridge is commonly used, but some surgeons apply only 15 mm of the cartridge length, whereas others might use the entire length). Second, the size of the common gastroenterotomy that must be closed with suture is variable to a degree. Finally, the technique of closure of the gastroenterotomy (single versus double layer, etc.) may also impact the stoma size.

Unfortunately, only a few studies have evaluated this question in a prospective manner, and the studies generally have relatively small numbers of patients included. In 2000 Stahl et al. performed a retrospective review which compared weight loss between patients who had a 21 mm circular stapled gastrojejunostomy (CSA) (n = 31) versus 25 mm circular stapled gastrojejunostomy (n = 19) in open gastric bypass [1]. They found no significant difference in weight loss or subjective complaints (nausea, vomiting, dysphagia) between the two groups (average %EWL

Table 32.1 Summary of stoma sizes as relating to gastrojejunostomy technique

Technique	Internal diameter	X-Sectional area
21-mm circular	12 mm [6]	113 mm² [6]
	11 mm [4]	70 mm² [19]
25-mm circular	16 mm [6]	201 mm² [6]
	13 mm [4]	99.5 mm² [19]
45-mm linear	17.5–19 mm [8]	

61%, 65%, and 64% at 12, 15, and 18 months for 21 mm group, vs. 61%, 67%, and 69% in 25 mm group). Several other studies that evaluated weight loss between patients with 21 mm CSA compared to a 25 mm CSA also found no significant difference in weight loss [2–6].

A 2003 study by Shope et al. retrospectively compared results for circular stapled anastomosis to linear stapled anastomosis (LSA) in laparoscopic gastric bypass [7]. A total of 61 patients were included in the study, with 32 anastomoses created with 25 mm EEA stapler, and 29 anastomoses created with a 60 mm GIA stapler fired with 4 cm of the cartridge. Weight loss was found to be similar between the two groups (at 6–8 months, %EWL 46.7% for EEA group vs. 51.4% for GIA group). A retrospective review by Owens and Sczepaniak comparing 21 mm CSA (n = 124) vs. 45 mm LSA (n = 100) found weight loss to be less with the LSA technique at 18 months (%EWL 86% in CSA group vs. 77% in LSA group); this difference was statistically significant [8]. They estimated the size of the linear anastomosis to be larger than the 25 mm CSA anastomosis, and postulated that the smaller stoma lead to greater weight loss in the CSA group. Schneider et al. performed a retrospective analysis of prospectively collected data, and found no difference in average excess BMI lost (EBMIL) at 1 and 2 years between the CSA and LSA techniques [9]. Two meta-analyses comparing outcomes between CSA and LSA in laparoscopic gastric bypass did not detect any difference in weight loss between the two groups [10, 11]. Two more recent studies by Lee et al. and Lois et al. compared hand-sewn anastomosis (HSA) to CSA as well as LSA, with no significant differences found in excess weight loss [12, 13].

A unique study by Ramos et al. in 2017 compared weight loss between patients who underwent bypass with LSA with different lengths of firing of GIA stapler (either 15 mm fire, or full 45 mm fire) [14]. Data was collected prospectively, with 64 patients in each arm. Both groups had significant weight loss, but weight loss was significantly higher in the 15 mm fire group at 24 months (37% BMI reduction vs. 33.3% in the 45 mm group). There was a single case of stenosis, which was in the 15 mm group.

A 2019 systematic review by Mahawar et al. also examined the effect of gastric pouch and stoma size on weight loss in RYGB [15]. Included were ten studies that evaluated the effect of the size of the GJ at time of surgery on weight loss. Six studies showed no significant effect of stoma size on weight loss. Four studies found larger stoma size to be associated with worse weight loss. Overall the quality and heterogeneity of data was deemed too poor to perform a meta-analysis, however.

Most of the literature reviewed focused on the effect of stoma size on initial weight loss. However there is some evidence to suggest that enlarged GJ diameter is likely associated with weight recidivism as well. A retrospective review from 2011 by Abu Dayyeh et al. analyzed a large consecutive series of patients who underwent endoscopy after RYGBP with recording of the GJ stoma diameter and serial weight measurements [16]. The study included 165 patients, 59% of whom had significant weight regain, defined as ≥20% of maximum weight lost after gastric bypass. Enlarged GJ stoma diameter was associated with weight regain on univariate and multivariate analysis. There was no correlation between pouch size and

GJ stoma diameter. This information was used to create a scoring system (variables included GJ diameter, race, % maximal body weight lost after RYGB) to predict weight regain. Heneghan et al. also reviewed patients who underwent upper endoscopy for GI symptoms or weight regain after gastric bypass; patients were grouped into those with successful weight loss (Group A, 175 pts) or weight regain (Group B, 205 pts) [17]. Pouch and stoma measurements were collected during endoscopy; the stoma was considered enlarged if it was >2 cm in diameter; the pouch was considered enlarged if >6 cm long or >5 cm wide. Pouch and stoma size were found to be normal in 63% of patients in Group A compared to only 29% in Group B. The most common abnormality was found to be an enlarged stoma, and stoma diameter was independently related to weight regain after gastric bypass in multivariate analysis. One challenge in interpreting these data is that in the absence of baseline stomal measurements, it is difficult to ascertain the degree to which (or even if) stomal dilation has occurred. More investigation is warranted to further elucidate this relationship between stoma enlargement and weight regain, and there likely are additional factors (e.g., genetic, behavioral, environmental) at play.

32.3.2 Effect of Stoma Size on Rates of Stenosis/Stricture

Another important consideration is the impact of anastomotic technique (and consequently) stoma size on anastomotic stricture. As discussed by Takata et al, the etiology of stricture formation is thought to be multifactorial, with local tissue ischemia, tension on the anastomosis, subclinical leak, submucosal hematoma, acid/peptic ulceration, early experience with RYGBP, and method of gastrojejunostomy creation all potentially contributing [18] (Table 32.2).

An early examination of whether anastomotic technique/size affected stricture rates came from Nguyen et al. in 2003 [2]. This study retrospectively compared the incidence of GJ stricture after laparoscopic gastric bypass with 21 mm vs. 25 mm EEA stapled gastrojejunostomy. Of 185 total patients, 29 developed stricture. The stricture rate amongst those with 21 mm CSA was 26.8%, compared to 8.8% in the 25 mm CSA group. Gould et al. found similar results when comparing rates of stenosis between 21 and 25 mm EEA stapled gastrojejunostomies, with a stenosis rate of 15.9% in 21 mm group vs. 6.2% in the 25 mm group [3]. Another study by Suggs et al. (stenosis rate of 9.4% with 21 mm EEA vs. 2.9% with 25 mm EEA) had very similar findings [4]. Perhaps most resoundingly, in a randomized, prospective blinded study from 2007, Fisher et al. also found a significantly lower stricture rate in patients who had a 25 mm EEA GJ compared to a 21 mm EEA GJ (7% vs. 17% respectively) [19].

Sczepaniak and Owens retrospectively compared GJ stricture rate between 21 mm CSA with 45 mm LSA (using half the staple load) [20]. They estimated the size of the linear anastomosis to be slightly larger than the CSA, and found the LSA technique to have significantly fewer strictures (0/100 patients) compared to CSA (16/124 patients). Similarly, a retrospective review from Schneider et al. found the LSA technique to have a lower stricture rate (0%) compared to CSA (7%) [9]. Two

Table 32.2 Summary of effect of stoma size on weight loss and stenosis

Author (year)	N	Techniques compared	Effect of stoma size on weight loss	Effect of stoma size on stenosis	Study type	Grade of Evidence
Stahl et al. (2000) [1]	50	21 mm CSA (n = 31) vs. 25 mm CSA (n = 19)	No significant impact		Retrospective review	Low
Shope et al. (2003) [7]	61	25 mm CSA (n = 32) vs. LSA	No significant impact		Retrospective review	Low
Nguyen et al. (2003) [2]	185	21 mm CSA (n = 71) vs. 25 mm CSA (n = 114)	No significant impact	Increased rate of stenosis with 21 mm (26.8%) vs. 25 mm (8.8%)	Retrospective review	Low
Gould et al. (2006) [3]	226	21 mm CSA (n = 145) vs. 25 mm CSA (n = 81)	No significant impact	Increased rate of stenosis with 21 mm (15.9%) vs. 25 mm (6.2%)	Retrospective review	Low
Fisher et al. (2007) [19]	200	21 mm CSA (n = 100) vs. 25 mm CSA (n = 100)		Increased rate of stenosis with 21 mm (17%) vs. 25 mm (7%)	Randomized prospective blinded study	Moderate
Suggs et al. (2007) [4]	438	21 mm CSA (n = 64) vs. 25 mm CSA (n = 374)	No significant impact	Increased rate of stenosis with 21 mm (9.4%) vs. 25 mm (2.9%)	Retrospective review	Low
Cottam et al. (2009) [5]	200	21 mm CSA (n = 100) vs. 25 mm CSA (n = 100)	No significant impact		Randomized prospective blinded study	Moderate
Owens and Sczepaniak (2009) [8]	224	21 mm CSA (n = 124) vs. 45 mm LSA (n = 100)	Less weight loss with LSA		Retrospective review	Low
Sczepaniak and Owens (2009) [20]	224	21 mm CSA (n = 124) vs. 45 mm LSA (n = 100)		Decreased rate of stenosis with 45 mm LSA (0%) vs. 21 mm CSA (12.9%)	Retrospective review	Low
Smith et al. (2011) [6]	261	21 mm CSA (n = 145) vs. 25 mm CSA (n = 116)	No significant impact		Retrospective analysis of prospectively collected data	Low

(continued)

Table 32.2 (continued)

Author (year)	N	Techniques compared	Effect of stoma size on weight loss	Effect of stoma size on stenosis	Study type	Grade of Evidence
Abu Dayyeh (2011) [16]	165	Stoma size in pts with significant weight regain	Larger stoma size associated with significant weight regain		Retrospective review	Low
Giordano et al. (2011) [10]	1321	LSA vs. CSA	No significant impact	Decreased stenosis with LSA compared to CSA	Meta-analysis	High
Penna et al. (2012) [11]	9374	LSA (n = 2946) vs. CSA (n = 6428)	No significant impact	Increased rate of stricture with CSA	Meta-analysis	High
Heneghan et al. (2012) [17]	380	Successful weight loss (n = 175) vs. weight regain (n = 205)	Larger stoma diameter independently related to weight regain		Retrospective review	Low
Lee et al. (2014) [12]	468	HSA (n = 174) vs. CSA (n = 110) vs. LSA (n = 142)	No significant impact	No significant impact	Prospective database study	Low
Lois et al. (2015) [13]	190	CSA (n = 55) vs. HSA (n = 135)	No significant impact	Increased rate of stenosis with CSA (16.4%) vs. HSA (3%)	Retrospective review	Low
Schneider et al. (2016) [9]	228	25 mm CSA (n = 57) vs. LSA (n = 171)	No significant impact	Decreased rate of stenosis with LSA (0%) vs. 25 mm CSA (7%)	Retrospective analysis of prospectively collected data	Low
Ramos et al. (2017) [14]	128	15 mm LSA (n = 64) vs. 45 mm LSA (n = 64)	Increased weight loss with 15 mm stapler fire compared to 45 mm stapler fire	Stenosis similar between 15 mm fire (1.56%) vs. 45 mm fire (0%)	Prospective database study	Low
Mahawar et al. (2019) [15]			Larger stomas associated with worse weight loss		Systematic review	Moderate
Edholm (2019) [21]		CSA vs. LSA		No significant impact	Systematic review and Meta-analysis	High

meta-analyses by Giordano et al. and Penna et al. comparing LSA and CSA also found significantly decreased risk of GJ stricture using linear rather than circular stapled anastomoses [10, 11]. However, as discussed in Penna et al, there were several limitations to the studies involved in these meta-analyses. First, none of the included studies described the inner-diameter of the linear-stapled GJ, so it is difficult to correlate size of GJ to decreased stricture rate. Secondly, studies using linear stapler describe highly variable depths of stapler insertion which may confound the influence of anastomotic diameter on post-operative stricture. Lastly, studies comparing linear to circular staplers were somewhat inconsistent in their use of 21 mm vs. 25 mm EEA staplers, with some not mentioning circular staple size at all.

Interestingly, a more recent systematic review and meta-analysis by Edholm [21] comparing complications rates between CSA and LSA did not find a significant difference in stricture or leak rate between the two techniques. Stricture rates were reported in 11 of the 13 included studies, and 3 of these 11 studies used 21 mm CSA rather than 25 mm CSA. While the relative risk of stricture in LSA was 74% that of CSA, there was overlap of the 95% confidence interval, therefore no significant difference was found. It should be noted, however, that the two largest cohorts included in this meta-analysis did not have data on stricture rates.

A prospective database study comparing stricture rates for hand-sewn anastomosis (HSA), CSA, and LSA by Lee et al. found no significant difference in stricture rates between the three different anastomotic techniques [12]. However, a retrospective review by Lois et al. comparing anastomotic complications between CSA and HSA found a significantly higher rate of stenosis in CSA (16.4%) compared to HSA (3%) [13]. Clearly, similar challenges exist with ascertaining the true size of a fully hand-sewn anastomosis in these analyses. Ramos et al. compared linear stapled anastomosis with 15 mm vs. 45 mm stapler fires; there were no incidences of stenosis with the 45 mm stapler fire (0/64) compared to 1/64 in the 15 mm stapler fire group [14].

32.4 Conclusions

The size of the gastrojejunostomy in a laparoscopic gastric bypass is largely dictated by the anastomotic technique utilized by the surgeon. Therefore, the technical approach remains an important surrogate for stomal size. Circular stapled anastomosis is favored by many surgeons for its relative ease of use. This may also give a more consistent stomal size compared to hand-sewn or linear stapled anastomoses. Linear stapled anastomoses may provide more flexibility, but perhaps less consistency in the size of the stoma. Though there is conflicting evidence, most of the available data suggest that the anastomotic technique (and therefore stoma size) does not appear to have a significant impact on overall weight loss. There is a possible association between larger stoma size and increased weight regain, though more investigation is required to better elucidate this relationship. The evidence seems to indicate that the 21 mm stapler has a significantly higher rate of stenosis relative to the 25 mm stapler. As such, the 21 mm EEA stapler appears to have fallen out of favor for creating the GJ in gastric bypass. There is also moderate evidence that the linear stapled technique leads to less stenosis than circular stapled anastomoses. As shown by Ramos et al, the length of staple firing in linear stapled anastomoses does seem to impact weight loss, with greater weight loss with shorter stapler firings, and no significant impact on stenosis, though more data is needed [14].

32.4.1 A Personal Approach to the Data

The stoma size in a Roux-en-Y gastric bypass is directly related to the technique employed in creating the gastrojejunostomy. Thus stoma size is most commonly documented in the literature in this manner, and evaluation of stoma size is by inference and estimation. Irrespective of technical approach (SC, LS, fully hand-sewn) most surgeons aim for a final internal stoma diameter of 16–20 mm. Available evidence is supportive of this inclination, as weight loss outcomes are not significantly improved by creating a smaller stoma, but they might be negatively impacted by a wider stoma. Lastly, stoma diameters smaller than 16 mm have been associated with a higher rate of anastomotic stricture requiring intervention.

32.4.2 Recommendations

1. If a circular stapler approach is preferred, the 25 mm device is recommended over the 21 mm, as the latter does not appear to confer an outcome benefit while being more commonly associated with anastomotic complications, namely stricture (Evidence quality high; strong recommendation).
2. If a linear stapled anastomosis is preferred, we would recommend against deploying the full length of a 45 mm staple cartridge, as this has been associated with diminished weight loss. A 25 mm portion of such a cartridge is commonly utilized amongst surgeons who employ this technique (Evidence quality low; weak recommendation).

References

1. Stahl RD, Sherer RA, Seevers CE, Johnston D. Comparison of 21 vs. 25 mm gastrojejunostomy in the gastric bypass procedure—early results. Obes Surg. 2000;10(6):540–2. https://doi.org/10.1381/096089200321593751.
2. Nguyen NT, Stevens CM, Wolfe BM. Incidence and outcome of anastomotic stricture after laparoscopic gastric bypass. J Gastrointest Surg Off J Soc Surg Aliment Tract. 2003;7(8):997–1003. Discussion 1003. https://doi.org/10.1016/j.gassur.2003.09.016
3. Gould JC, Garren M, Boll V, Starling J. The impact of circular stapler diameter on the incidence of gastrojejunostomy stenosis and weight loss following laparoscopic Roux-en-Y gastric bypass. Surg Endosc. 2006;20(7):1017–20. https://doi.org/10.1007/s00464-005-0207-5.

4. Suggs WJ, Kouli W, Lupovici M, Chau WY, Brolin RE. Complications at gastrojejunostomy after laparoscopic Roux-en-Y gastric bypass: comparison between 21- and 25-mm circular staplers. Surg Obes Relat Dis Off J Am Soc Bariatr Surg. 2007;3(5):508–14. https://doi.org/10.1016/j.soard.2007.05.003.

5. Cottam DR, Fisher B, Sridhar V, Atkinson J, Dallal R. The effect of stoma size on weight loss after laparoscopic gastric bypass surgery: results of a blinded randomized controlled trial. Obes Surg. 2009;19(1):13–7. https://doi.org/10.1007/s11695-008-9753-y.

6. Smith C, Garren M, Gould J. Impact of gastrojejunostomy diameter on long-term weight loss following laparoscopic gastric bypass: a follow-up study. Surg Endosc. 2011;25(7):2164–7. https://doi.org/10.1007/s00464-010-1516-x.

7. Shope TR, Cooney RN, McLeod J, Miller CA, Haluck RS. Early results after laparoscopic gastric bypass: EEA vs GIA stapled gastrojejunal anastomosis. Obes Surg. 2003;13(3):355–9. https://doi.org/10.1381/096089203765887651.

8. Owens ML, Sczepaniak JP. Size really does matter-role of gastrojejunostomy in postoperative weight loss. Surg Obes Relat Dis Off J Am Soc Bariatr Surg. 2009;5(3):357–61. https://doi.org/10.1016/j.soard.2008.08.020.

9. Schneider R, Gass J-M, Kern B, et al. Linear compared to circular stapler anastomosis in laparoscopic Roux-en-Y gastric bypass leads to comparable weight loss with fewer complications: a matched pair study. Langenbecks Arch Surg. 2016;401(3):307–13. https://doi.org/10.1007/s00423-016-1397-0.

10. Giordano S, Salminen P, Biancari F, Victorzon M. Linear stapler technique may be safer than circular in gastrojejunal anastomosis for laparoscopic Roux-en-Y gastric bypass: a meta-analysis of comparative studies. Obes Surg. 2011;21(12):1958–64. https://doi.org/10.1007/s11695-011-0520-0.

11. Penna M, Markar SR, Venkat-Raman V, Karthikesalingam A, Hashemi M. Linear-stapled versus circular-stapled laparoscopic gastrojejunal anastomosis in morbid obesity: meta-analysis. Surg Laparosc Endosc Percutan Tech. 2012;22(2):95–101. https://doi.org/10.1097/SLE.0b013e3182470f38.

12. Lee S, Davies AR, Bahal S, et al. Comparison of gastrojejunal anastomosis techniques in laparoscopic Roux-en-Y gastric bypass: gastrojejunal stricture rate and effect on subsequent weight loss. Obes Surg. 2014;24(9):1425–9. https://doi.org/10.1007/s11695-014-1219-9.

13. Lois AW, Frelich MJ, Goldblatt MI, Wallace JR, Gould JC. Gastrojejunostomy technique and anastomotic complications in laparoscopic gastric bypass. Surg Obes Relat Dis Off J Am Soc Bariatr Surg. 2015;11(4):808–13. https://doi.org/10.1016/j.soard.2014.11.029.

14. Ramos AC, Marchesini JC, de Souza Bastos EL, et al. The role of gastrojejunostomy size on gastric bypass weight loss. Obes Surg. 2017;27(9):2317–23. https://doi.org/10.1007/s11695-017-2686-6.

15. Mahawar K, Sharples AJ, Graham Y. A systematic review of the effect of gastric pouch and/or gastrojejunostomy (stoma) size on weight loss outcomes with Roux-en-Y gastric bypass. Surg Endosc. 2019; https://doi.org/10.1007/s00464-019-07277-w.

16. Abu Dayyeh BK, Lautz DB, Thompson CC. Gastrojejunal stoma diameter predicts weight regain after Roux-en-Y gastric bypass. Clin Gastroenterol Hepatol Off Clin Pract J Am Gastroenterol Assoc. 2011;9(3):228–33. https://doi.org/10.1016/j.cgh.2010.11.004.

17. Heneghan HM, Yimcharoen P, Brethauer SA, Kroh M, Chand B. Influence of pouch and stoma size on weight loss after gastric bypass. Surg Obes Relat Dis Off J Am Soc Bariatr Surg. 2012;8(4):408–15. https://doi.org/10.1016/j.soard.2011.09.010.

18. Takata MC, Ciovica R, Cello JP, Posselt AM, Rogers SJ, Campos GM. Predictors, treatment, and outcomes of gastrojejunostomy stricture after gastric bypass for morbid obesity. Obes Surg. 2007;17(7):878–84. https://doi.org/10.1007/s11695-007-9163-6.

19. Fisher BL, Atkinson JD, Cottam D. Incidence of gastroenterostomy stenosis in laparoscopic Roux-en-Y gastric bypass using 21- or 25-mm circular stapler: a randomized prospective blinded study. Surg Obes Relat Dis Off J Am Soc Bariatr Surg. 2007;3(2):176–9. https://doi.org/10.1016/j.soard.2006.11.014.

20. Sczepaniak JP, Owens ML. Results of gastrojejunal anastomotic technique designed to reduce stricture. Surg Obes Relat Dis Off J Am Soc Bariatr Surg. 2009;5(1):77–80. https://doi.org/10.1016/j.soard.2008.10.005.
21. Edholm D. Systematic review and meta-analysis of circular- and linear-stapled gastrojejunostomy in laparoscopic Roux-en-Y gastric bypass. Obes Surg. 2019;29(6):1946–53. https://doi.org/10.1007/s11695-019-03803-w.

Part VIII

The Pediatric Population

Indications, Choice of Operations and Outcomes of Metabolic and Bariatric Surgery in Children

33

Katherine S. Blevins and Janey S. A. Pratt

33.1 Introduction

Metabolic and Bariatric Surgery (MBS) has been shown to be an effective and durable treatment for severe obesity is adults. The use of this treatment in children has lagged due primarily to lack of understanding of childhood obesity and implicit bias against surgical therapy. However, there now exists significant high-quality evidence confirming the safety and efficacy of Metabolic and Bariatric surgery for the treatment of severe obesity in children. The most recent American Academy of Pediatrics Statement on the use of Metabolic and Bariatric surgery [1] suggests that surgery is indicated for a BMI of 120% of the 95th percentile with a co-morbidity or a BMI of 140% of the 95th percentile, reguardless of age. These cut offs reflect the CDC growth charts and definitions of obesity that correspond to the adult definitions of a BMI of 35 and 40 respectively. There remain difficult decisions in pediatric bariatric surgery namely due to the challenges of defining which operations to use and how much of the success or failure of an operation is a result of physiology or psychology. There is almost no data on whether inadequate weight loss or co-morbidity resolution is due to socio-environmental factors (i.e. food insecurity, childhood trauma, lack of compliance, parenting issues, etc.) versus inadequate physiologic change induced by MBS [2].

K. S. Blevins · J. S. A. Pratt (✉)
Division of Pediatric Surgery, Stanford University School of Medicine, Stanford, CA, USA

Lucile Packard Children's Hospital, Palo Alto, CA, USA
e-mail: jsapratt@stanford.edu

© Springer Nature Switzerland AG 2021
J. Alverdy, Y. Vigneswaran (eds.), *Difficult Decisions in Bariatric Surgery*,
Difficult Decisions in Surgery: An Evidence-Based Approach,
https://doi.org/10.1007/978-3-030-55329-6_33

Table 33.1 PICO search terms

P (Patients)	I (Intervention)	C (Comparator)	O (Outcomes)
Pediatric and adolescent patients (Age < 18) with obesity	Bariatric and metabolic surgery (RYGB, VSG)	Medical management	Weight loss and resolution of comorbidities

33.2 Search Strategy

A literature search of English language publications from 2000 to 2019 was used to identify published data on bariatric and metabolic surgery on pediatric or adolescent patients. We performed a focused search in the PubMed database of literature published between 2000 and 2019. Search terms included "pediatrics", "obesity", and "bariatric surgery". See Table 33.1. Randomized controlled trials, prospective and retrospective cohort studies were identified to examine primary data. Reviews and meta-analyses were examined, but results from primary data were selected in the data review [3]. Recent guidelines for Pediatric Metabolic and Bariatric Surgery [1, 4] were also reviewed and incorporated into recommendations.

33.3 Results

For the purpose of this article—and in alignment with recent guideline statements—the term "pediatric" refers to a person under 18 years of age. The term "adolescent" is defined differently in various settings, for the purpose of this review the term "adolescent" refers to a person aged 10–19 years.

Obesity is defined as a BMI $\geq$ 120% of the 95th percentile or an absolute BMI $\geq$ 35 kg/m^2, whichever is lower based on age and sex [5]. The definition of severe obesity includes class I, II, and III obesity as defined by the American Heart Association criteria: obesity class I ($\geq$95th percentile to <120% of the 95th percentile); obesity class II ($\geq$120% to 140% of the 95th percentile) or a BMI $\geq$ 35 to 39 kg/m^2, whichever is lower; and obesity class III ($\geq$140% of the 95th percentile) or BMI $\geq$ 40 kg/m^2, whichever was lower [6].

The prevalence of obesity is increasing, with nearly 10% of adolescents in 2014 having class II obesity [6]. This, in conjunction with the high probability of obesity in adulthood [7], identifies an opportunity for early intervention for patients to prevent a lifetime of poor health and quality of life [8]. Several large clinical trials have been identified as the foundation for current guideline statements from the ASMBS and the AAP.

Teen-LABS (NCT00465829): Designed as an ancillary study to the Longitudinal Assessment of Bariatric Surgery Study [9], consecutive adolescents aged $\leq$19 years undergoing bariatric surgery at each of 5 Teen-LABS centers between February 28, 2007 and December 30, 2011 were offered enrollment. Two hundred forty-two patients were enrolled in the study. These patients had a mean age of 17.1 (1.56 SD) years at surgery, had a median BMI of 50.5, and a median waist circumference of 145.9 cm at baseline. The cohort was primarily non-Hispanic (93%), white (72%), and female (76%) with 66.5% undergoing Roux-en-Y gastric bypass (RYGB), 5.8% undergoing adjustable gastric band (AGB), and 27.7% undergoing vertical sleeve gastrectomy (VSG). Within 30 days of surgery, 19 patients (7.9%) experienced 20 major complications and 36 (14.9%) experienced 47 minor complications. There were no deaths. Procedure-specific rates of patients with major complications were as follows: RYGB = 9.3% (95% CI, 5.3–14.9); VSG = 4.5% (95% CI, 0.9–12.5); and AGB = 7.1% (95% CI, 0.2–33.9). Comparable rates for minor events were as follows: RYGB = 16.8% (95% CI, 11.4–23.5); VSG = 11.9% (95% CI, 5.3–22.2); and AGB = 7.1% (95% CI, 0.2–33.9).

Three year follow-up data [10] revealed the mean weight had decreased by 27% in the total cohort; 28% by those who underwent RYGB, and 26% by those who underwent sleeve gastrectomy. Remission of Type 2 Diabetes Mellitus (T2DM) had occurred in 95%, abnormal kidney function in 86%, prediabetes in 76%, an elevated blood pressure in 74%, and dyslipidemia in 66%. 5-year data for RYGB patients (161 patients) was reported compared to a cohort of adult patients with a 26% weight loss in the adolescent patients, with adolescents more likely than adults to have remission of type 2 diabetes (86% vs. 53%) and hypertension (68% vs. 41%) [11].

AMOS (NCT00289705): The Adolescent Morbid Obesity Surgery (AMOS) study is a prospective, controlled, nonrandomized interventional study comparing 81 adolescents with severe obesity undergoing RYGB with a matched control group of adolescents undergoing conventional medical treatment of obesity, as well as a matched cohort of adults undergoing metabolic and bariatric surgery in Sweden. The adolescent patients had a mean 29% weight loss after 5 years, similar to the matched adult group. A majority of control patients (69%) gained weight [12, 13]. In adolescent patients, resolution of comorbidities occurred as follows: Type 2 diabetes (100%, 3/3), disturbed glucose homeostasis (86%, 18/21), dyslipidemia (83%, 43/52), elevated blood pressure (92%, 11/12), inflammation with CRP ≥ 2 mg/L (74%, 45/61), and elevated liver enzymes (100%, 19/19).

FABS-5+ (NCT00776776): The Follow-up of Adolescent Bariatric Surgery at 5 Plus years (FABS-5+) is a prospective follow-up analysis of a cohort of adolescents who underwent RYGB for severe obesity between 2001 and 2007. Seventy four patients underwent surgery, with 5+ year follow-up in 58 patients. At a mean follow-up of 8 years, the average weight loss of 29.2%. Resolution of comorbidities were as follows, with long term data compared to baseline: elevated blood pressure (27/57 [47%] vs. 9/55 [16%]; p = 0.001), dyslipidemia (48/56 [86%] vs. 21/55 [38%]; p < 0.0001), and type 2 diabetes (9/56 [16%] vs. 1/55 [2%]; p = 0.03) [14].

The results of these trials show that MBS is appropriate management for children with severe obesity and results in 29% total body weight loss on average. See Table 33.2.

Table 33.2 Summary of key trials

Study	Patients	Outcome classification	Primary Outcome	Length of Follow-up	Quality of evidence
[24] Comparison of Surgical and Medical Therapy for Type 2 Diabetes in Severely Obese Adolescents 2018	Teen-LABS and TODAY study patients (secondary review of data)	Glycemic control, BMI, prevalence of elevated blood pressure, dyslipidemia, abnormal kidney function, clinical adverse events	Mean weight loss of 27%	5 years	High quality
[14] Long-term outcomes of bariatric surgery in adolescents with severe obesity (FABS-5+): a prospective follow-up analysis 2017	74 patients aged 13–21 years who underwent RYGB, prospective follow-up analysis 5+ years (FABS 5+)	BMI, comorbidities, micronutrient status, safety	Mean weight loss of 29.2%	Mean follow-up 8 years; All 5+ years	High quality
[12] Laparoscopic Roux-en-Y gastric bypass in adolescents with severe obesity (AMOS): a prospective, 5-year, Swedish nationwide study 2017	81 adolescents undergoing RYGB with matched control group of adolescents undergoing medical treatment of obesity, as well as adults undergoing MBS in Sweden	Change in BMI, anthropometry, biochemistry, quality of life evaluation and clinical outcomes	Mean weight loss of 29%	5 years	High quality

33.4   Recommendations Based on the Data

Based on review of the data and best practices, the indications for pediatric metabolic and bariatric surgery are outlined in recent guidelines including the ASMBS pediatric metabolic and bariatric surgery guidelines [4] and the Pediatric Metabolic and Bariatric Surgery Best Practices statement [1]. Indications are as follows:

- Class II obesity with clinically significant disease, including obstructive sleep apnea (OSA), T2DM, Idiopathic Intercranial Hypertension (IIH), Non-Alcoholic Steato-Hepatitis (NASH), Blount disease, Slipped Capital Femoral Epiphysis (SCFE), Gastro Esophogeal Reflux Disease (GERD), and hypertension (high quality)
- Class III obesity (high quality)

Contraindications to surgery are as follows:

- A medically correctable cause of obesity (low quality)
- An ongoing substance abuse problem (within the preceding 1 year) (no data)
- A medical, psychiatric, psychosocial, or cognitive condition that prevents adherence to postoperative dietary and medication regiments (no data)
- Current or planned pregnancy within 12–18 months of the procedure (low quality)

An interdisciplinary team is essential to build a successful Pediatric Metabolic and Bariatric Surgery program [15]. This team at minimum consists of a high-volume bariatric and/or pediatric surgeon, pediatrician, pediatric psychologist, program coordinator, and dietician (moderate quality). Other support services like pediatric Anesthesia, Endocrine, GI, Pulmonary, Radiology, Child life, Physical Therapy, Social Services, and Psychiatry are helpful. The Metabolic and Bariatric Surgery Accreditation and Quality Improvement Program (MBSAQIP) accredits pediatric MBS programs, and their guidelines should be followed even if accreditation is not sought [16–19] (moderate quality).

Obesity is a life-long disease, therefore a transition plan to an adult program is necessary [20–22] (high quality). Any child with obesity and a significant comorbidity should be considered for MBS to prevent end organ damage from the disease: T2DM [23, 24](high quality), OSA [25–27] (high quality), GERD [28] (moderate quality), Blount's (low quality), Slipped capital femoral epiphysis (SCFE) [29] (low quality), Idiopathic intracranial hypertension (IIH) [30, 31] (moderate quality), Non-alcoholic fatty liver disease [32–34] (high quality), Hypertension [35] (high quality). Surgery early in the onset of these diseases can prevent progression and end organ damage and may prevent the need for other surgeries (moderate quality).

Choice of operation should be guided by current guidelines around MBS in the pediatric and adolescent populations [4]:

- Vertical Sleeve Gastrectomy (VSG): this has become the most used and most recommended operation in adolescents for several reasons: near equivalent weight loss to the Roux en y Gastric Bypass (RYGB) in adolescents, fewer reoperations, better iron absorption, and near equivalent effect on comorbidities as RYGB in adolescents. However, given the more extensive long-term data available for RYGB, we can recommend the use of either RYGB or VSG in adolescents. Long term outcomes of GERD after VSG are still not well understood (high quality).
- The use of emerging technologies in adolescents should be considered when standard procedures are unavailable or anatomically inappropriate, but when done in adolescents they must be used in the setting of an age appropriate multidisciplinary team that treats obesity and under an IRB approved trial. Companies should be encouraged to fund trials of new devices in children with obesity at least as soon as a device is FDA approved in adults (low quality).

In summary, the choice of a VSG in children has a lower risk profile, similar weight loss and comorbidity resolution as RYGB and allows for future operations as needed if obesity is unresponsive or returns over time. For patients with severe GERD and severe obesity the RYGB may be a more effective operation, but the most important recommendation based on surgical risk and complications is to avoid Fundoplication's in these patients [4].

33.5   A Personal View of the Data

Pediatric obesity is a chronic disease that starts in childhood and continues into adulthood in at least 85% of patients [36, 37]. Only about one third of adult patients with obesity had obesity in childhood. Childhood onset obesity is clearly different from adult onset obesity—it can start at birth, around 8 years old, or later in adolescence. The future treatment of this disease will likely be a multifaceted approach involving the use of MBS, pharmacotherapy, and socio-environmental interventions. The holy grail is to identify which patients will respond to MBS alone, and which need adjunct interventions. Further study is needed to identify the level and order of supportive therapies such as lifestyle changes (exercise and food choices and eating patterns) and pharmacotherapies that can be used to improve outcomes.

Currently data is reported as a percentage of total body weight loss and comorbidity resolution, however in practice what we see is that each operation has patients who respond well to surgery, and those for whom surgery has almost no effect on weight loss or comorbidity resolution. We see patients with inadequate weight loss as defined in adults to be <30–50% excess BMI loss or in children we propose <15–20% total BMI loss. Studies have showed that in adults inadequate weight loss occurs after VSG in 21–36% and after RYGB in 5–15% [38, 39].

In practice, with children we have started with the lowest risk procedure—the VSG in any patient who meets weight criteria, can make lifestyle changes and wants surgery. When one in four patients doesn't lose weight, we initiate medications—Metformin, Topamax and Phentermine have all been used in children and adolescents. Many feel that GLP-1 uptake inhibitors may soon be approved for use in children; this medication may be particularly effective after VSG given the variable increase in GLP-1. The timing and effectiveness of medication usage in children is still unknown. The VSG can be converted to RYGB or Biliopancreatic Diversion with duodenal switch (BPD-DS) at a later date if obesity is refractory to medications as well. This step wise approach reduces the risk exposure of children to vitamin deficiencies, alcohol addiction, kidney stones and internal hernias all seen after RYGB or BPD-DS.

The interdisciplinary team is key to success of these patients. Full workup of children is time consuming, and many who present to the clinic will require pulmonary, gastrointestinal, endocrine and psychological evaluation prior to MBS. It is helpful to have simple, age appropriate goals that children can learn and follow. One helpful mantra that our clinic developed is the 60-60-60 rule. Eat 60 g of protein, drink 60 oz. of water and exercise 60 min every day.

Timing of surgery in children is also important, as many children may not feel ready when they first present to clinic. If their BMI is already above 140% of the 95th percentile, it is imperative to perform surgery as soon as possible to prevent lifelong obesity. Most children will only lose 20–30% of their total body weight and if they are starting above 300 lb, they will likely always have obesity. It is important to have a longitudinal program with regular visits with a dietician and an MD or APP who can reinforce the importance of exercise, lifestyle changes and environmental modification. Relegating families to "diet and exercise" without regular reinforcement will fail every time.

There is no reason to exclude children who have developmental delay, autism or psychiatric illness that is treated and stable. These children are often more compliant than neurotypical individuals and tend to lose significant weight [40, 41]. They also are less able to be compliant with interventions like CPAP and insulin and other treatment options for comorbidities. In our practice, a pre-operative trial of a liquid diet for 3 days is completed to determine if caregiver and child are able to comply to post-operative changes in diet prior to pursuing surgery. We also obtain an ethics consult on patients who are not able to ascent to surgery.

Some of the most important future areas of investigation include if MBS is more appropriate treatment than alternative surgeries for OSA, SCFE, and Blount's. T2DM is most likely best approached by early MBS in children with concurrent severe obesity than metformin and insulin, as has been proven in adults [24], but this is not yet considered standard of care in endocrinology clinics. Further, the role of support interventions (lifestyle and pharmacotherapy) and the socio-ecologic environment before and after MBS has on patient outcomes remain elusive. More studies using mixed research methods including Patient Reported Outcomes Measures may allow us to identify the best approach to adjunct therapy to optimize outcomes following MBS for the treatment of severe pediatric obesity.

Abstracted Recommendations

- Indications: Children with a BMI of 120% of the 95th percentile and a comorbidity or a BMI of 140% of the 95th percentile should be referred to an interdisciplinary pediatric obesity clinic to be considered for MBS.
- Indications: Syndromic Obesity, Developmental Delay, ASD and treated psychiatric disorders are not contraindications to MBS.
- Choice of MBS: The VSG is most frequently used procedure due to its low risk profile and comparable outcomes to the RYGB in Adolescents.
- Outcomes: For T2DM MBS is superior to medical management in adults and most likely also in children.
- Outcomes: For severe reflux in children with concurrent severe obesity, the RYGB is superior to the Nissen Fundoplication, but some patients will respond to VSG.
- Outcomes: Remission occurs for Type 2 Diabetes Mellitus (T2DM) in 95%, abnormal kidney function in 86%, prediabetes in 76%, an elevated blood pressure in 74%, and dyslipidemia in 66% after MBS.

References

1. Armstrong SC, Bolling CF, Michalsky MP, Reichard KW, Section on Obesity, Section on Surgery. Pediatric metabolic and bariatric surgery: evidence, barriers, and best practices. Pediatrics. 2019;144(6).
2. Messiah SE, Sacher PM, Yudkin J, Qureshi FG, Hoelscher DM, Barlow SE. Partnering support interventions with bariatric surgery to maximize health outcomes in adolescents with severe obesity. Obes Silver Spring Md. 2019;27(11):1784–95.
3. Paulus GF, de Vaan LEG, Verdam FJ, Bouvy ND, Ambergen TAW, van Heurn LWE. Bariatric surgery in morbidly obese adolescents: a systematic review and meta-analysis. Obes Surg. 2015;25(5):860–78.
4. Pratt JSA, Browne A, Browne NT, et al. ASMBS pediatric metabolic and bariatric surgery guidelines, 2018. Surg Obes Relat Dis Off J Am Soc Bariatr Surg. 2018;14(7):882–901.
5. Kelly AS, Barlow SE, Rao G, et al. Severe obesity in children and adolescents: identification, associated health risks, and treatment approaches: a scientific statement from the American Heart Association. Circulation. 2013;128(15):1689–712.
6. Skinner AC, Skelton JA. Prevalence and trends in obesity and severe obesity among children in the United States, 1999-2012. JAMA Pediatr. 2014;168(6):561–6.
7. Freedman DS, Mei Z, Srinivasan SR, Berenson GS, Dietz WH. Cardiovascular risk factors and excess adiposity among overweight children and adolescents: the Bogalusa Heart Study. J Pediatr. 2007;150(1):12–7.e2.
8. Twig G, Yaniv G, Levine H, et al. Body-mass index in 2.3 million adolescents and cardiovascular death in adulthood. N Engl J Med. 2016;374(25):2430–40.
9. Inge TH, Zeller MH, Jenkins TM, et al. Perioperative outcomes of adolescents undergoing bariatric surgery: the Teen-Longitudinal Assessment of Bariatric Surgery (Teen-LABS) study. JAMA Pediatr. 2014;168(1):47–53.
10. Inge TH, Courcoulas AP, Jenkins TM, et al. Weight loss and health status 3 years after bariatric surgery in adolescents. N Engl J Med. 2016;374(2):113–23.
11. Inge TH, Courcoulas AP, Jenkins TM, et al. Five-year outcomes of gastric bypass in adolescents as compared with adults. N Engl J Med. 2019;380(22):2136–45.

12. Olbers T, Beamish AJ, Gronowitz E, et al. Laparoscopic Roux-en-Y gastric bypass in adolescents with severe obesity (AMOS): a prospective, 5-year, Swedish nationwide study. Lancet Diabetes Endocrinol. 2017;5(3):174–83.
13. Göthberg G, Gronowitz E, Flodmark C-E, et al. Laparoscopic Roux-en-Y gastric bypass in adolescents with morbid obesity—surgical aspects and clinical outcome. Semin Pediatr Surg. 2014;23(1):11–6.
14. Inge TH, Jenkins TM, Xanthakos SA, et al. Long-term outcomes of bariatric surgery in adolescents with severe obesity (FABS-5+): a prospective follow-up analysis. Lancet Diabetes Endocrinol. 2017;5(3):165–73.
15. Inge TH, Garcia V, Daniels S, et al. A multidisciplinary approach to the adolescent bariatric surgical patient. J Pediatr Surg. 2004;39(3):442–7. Discussion 446–7
16. Nguyen NT, Nguyen B, Nguyen VQ, Ziogas A, Hohmann S, Stamos MJ. Outcomes of bariatric surgery performed at accredited vs nonaccredited centers. J Am Coll Surg. 2012;215(4):467–74.
17. Gebhart A, Young M, Phelan M, Nguyen NT. Impact of accreditation in bariatric surgery. Surg Obes Relat Dis Off J Am Soc Bariatr Surg. 2014;10(5):767–73.
18. Michalsky M, Reichard K, Inge T, Pratt J, Lenders C. American Society for Metabolic and Bariatric Surgery. ASMBS pediatric committee best practice guidelines. Surg Obes Relat Dis Off J Am Soc Bariatr Surg. 2012;8(1):1–7.
19. Altieri MS, Pryor A, Bates A, Docimo S, Talamini M, Spaniolas K. Bariatric procedures in adolescents are safe in accredited centers. Surg Obes Relat Dis Off J Am Soc Bariatr Surg. 2018;14(9):1368–72.
20. Kumar S, Kelly AS. Review of childhood obesity: from epidemiology, etiology, and comorbidities to clinical assessment and treatment. Mayo Clin Proc. 2017;92(2):251–65.
21. Whitaker RC, Wright JA, Pepe MS, Seidel KD, Dietz WH. Predicting obesity in young adulthood from childhood and parental obesity. N Engl J Med. 1997;337(13):869–73.
22. Juonala M, Magnussen CG, Berenson GS, et al. Childhood adiposity, adult adiposity, and cardiovascular risk factors. N Engl J Med. 2011;365(20):1876–85.
23. Inge TH, Miyano G, Bean J, et al. Reversal of type 2 diabetes mellitus and improvements in cardiovascular risk factors after surgical weight loss in adolescents. Pediatrics. 2009;123(1):214–22.
24. Inge TH, Laffel LM, Jenkins TM, et al. Comparison of surgical and medical therapy for type 2 diabetes in severely obese adolescents. JAMA Pediatr. 2018;172(5):452–60.
25. Kalra M, Inge T, Garcia V, et al. Obstructive sleep apnea in extremely overweight adolescents undergoing bariatric surgery. Obes Res. 2005;13(7):1175–9.
26. Ashrafian H, Toma T, Rowland SP, et al. Bariatric surgery or non-surgical weight loss for obstructive sleep apnoea? a systematic review and comparison of meta-analyses. Obes Surg. 2015;25(7):1239–50.
27. Amin R, Simakajornboon N, Szczesniak R, Inge T. Early improvement in obstructive sleep apnea and increase in orexin levels after bariatric surgery in adolescents and young adults. Surg Obes Relat Dis Off J Am Soc Bariatr Surg. 2017;13(1):95–100.
28. Dewberry LC, Khoury JC, Ehrlich S, et al. Change in gastrointestinal symptoms over the first 5 years after bariatric surgery in a multicenter cohort of adolescents. J Pediatr Surg. 2019;54(6):1220–5.
29. Griggs CL, Perez NP, Chan MC, Pratt JS. Slipped capital femoral epiphysis and Blount disease as indicators for early metabolic surgical intervention. Surg Obes Relat Dis. 2019;15(10):1836–41.
30. Andrews LE, Liu GT, Ko MW. Idiopathic intracranial hypertension and obesity. Horm Res Paediatr. 2014;81(4):217–25.
31. Chandra V, Dutta S, Albanese CT, Shepard E, Farrales-Nguyen S, Morton J. Clinical resolution of severely symptomatic pseudotumor cerebri after gastric bypass in an adolescent. Surg Obes Relat Dis Off J Am Soc Bariatr Surg. 2007;3(2):198–200.
32. Manco M, Mosca A, De Peppo F, et al. The benefit of sleeve gastrectomy in obese adolescents on nonalcoholic steatohepatitis and hepatic fibrosis. J Pediatr. 2017;180:31–7.e2.

33. Xanthakos SA, Jenkins TM, Kleiner DE, et al. High prevalence of nonalcoholic fatty liver disease in adolescents undergoing bariatric surgery. Gastroenterology. 2015;149(3):623–34.e8.
34. Lassailly G, Caiazzo R, Buob D, et al. Bariatric surgery reduces features of nonalcoholic steatohepatitis in morbidly obese patients. Gastroenterology. 2015;149(2):379–88; quiz e15–6.
35. Michalsky MP, Inge TH, Jenkins TM, et al. Cardiovascular risk factors after adolescent bariatric surgery. Pediatrics. 2018;141(2).
36. Ogden CL, Carroll MD, Fryar CD, Flegal KM. Prevalence of obesity among adults and youth: United States, 2011-2014. NCHS Data Brief. 2015;219:1–8.
37. Ogden CL, Carroll MD, Curtin LR, Lamb MM, Flegal KM. Prevalence of high body mass index in US children and adolescents, 2007-2008. JAMA. 2010;303(3):242–9.
38. Snyder B, Nguyen A, Scarbourough T, Yu S, Wilson E. Comparison of those who succeed in losing significant excessive weight after bariatric surgery and those who fail. Surg Endosc. 2009;23(10):2302–6.
39. Arman GA, Himpens J, Dhaenens J, Ballet T, Vilallonga R, Leman G. Long-term (11+years) outcomes in weight, patient satisfaction, comorbidities, and gastroesophageal reflux treatment after laparoscopic sleeve gastrectomy. Surg Obes Relat Dis Off J Am Soc Bariatr Surg. 2016;12(10):1778–86.
40. Goddard GR, Kotagal M, Jenkins TM, Kollar LM, Inge TH, Helmrath MA. Weight loss after sleeve gastrectomy in developmentally delayed adolescents and young adults. Surg Obes Relat Dis Off J Am Soc Bariatr Surg. 2019;15(10):1662–7.
41. Matheson BE, Colborn D, Bohon C. Bariatric surgery in children and adolescents with cognitive impairment and/or developmental delay: current knowledge and clinical recommendations. Obes Surg. 2019;29(12):4114–26.

Pediatric Bariatric Surgery and Sexual Developmental Milestones

34

Kimberley Eden Steele

34.1 Background

On October 28, 2019, the American Academy of Pediatrics (AAP) released a policy statement entitled: *Pediatric Metabolic and Bariatric Surgery: Evidence, Barriers, and Best Practices,* in response to the urgency of the escalating obesity epidemic among pediatric patients [1].

In the United States alone, 4.5 million children and adolescents are affected by obesity and the resulting associated comorbidities [2, 3]. While traditional methods of weight loss including diet, exercise, family counseling, behavioral therapy, and sometimes pharmacotherapy have always been the first line treatment options, these non-invasive approaches are rarely successful [4]. Unfortunately, children with obesity have a high probability of carrying this health burden into adulthood [5, 6]. Longitudinal studies of adult bariatric surgical patients, and a growing literature on pediatric bariatric surgery, have demonstrated that these procedures lead to significant and durable weight loss [7, 8]. Further, recent studies comparing traditional weight loss options to bariatric surgery in adolescents have demonstrated that earlier intervention leads to resolution or remission of comorbid conditions, thereby preventing end organ damage and the further complications [9].

While bariatric surgery is certainly invasive and therefore not without risks, there is an increased acknowledgment that its proven efficacy may justify its use to address the growing pediatric obesity epidemic. In an effort to reduce biases and allay fears towards bariatric surgery [10], the AAP released guidelines to assist

K. E. Steele (✉)
The Johns Hopkins Center for Bariatric Surgery, Department of Surgery, The Johns Hopkins University School of Medicine, Baltimore, MD, USA

© Springer Nature Switzerland AG 2021
J. Alverdy, Y. Vigneswaran (eds.), *Difficult Decisions in Bariatric Surgery*,
Difficult Decisions in Surgery: An Evidence-Based Approach,
https://doi.org/10.1007/978-3-030-55329-6_34

pediatricians in the selection of appropriate patients, assist adolescents and their families in the decision making process, identify accredited programs that offer these procedures, and advocate for coverage by insurance companies and expanded access [1, 4].

Bariatric surgery achieves its effect in part by reducing caloric intake. However, maintenance of a normal energy balance between intake in the form of a balanced and nutritious diet, and expenditure through regular exercise and thermoregulation, is essential as children develop and mature [11]. Energy imbalance leading to extremes of body weight disturb the hypothalamic-pituitary-gonadal axis and can affect sexual development. For children and adolescents, this may take the form of a premature pubertal state in females or an altered pubertal state in males [12].

The objective of this review is to summarize the existing knowledge on the relationship between bariatric surgery and sexual developmental milestones.

Does bariatric surgery affect sexual development milestones in adolescents with obesity?

PICO: Do adolescents with obesity undergoing bariatric surgery compared to those who do not undergo bariatric surgery have alterations in sexual developmental milestones? (Table 34.1).

P: Do adolescents with obesity
I: Undergoing bariatric surgery
C: Compared to adolescents with obesity not undergoing bariatric surgery
O: Have alterations in sexual developmental milestones

Table 34.1 PICO

PICO elements	Keywords	Search terms	Search strategy
Population	Adolescents with obesity (BMI ≥35) undergoing bariatric surgery	Human Adolescent Obesity	Obesity Human (filter) Adolescent (filter)
Intervention	Bariatric surgery	Bariatric surgery	Bariatric Surgery Or Surgery
Comparison	Adolescents with obesity not undergoing bariatric surgery	Diet Exercise Pharmacotherapy Behavioral therapy	Diet Or Exercise Or Pharmacotherapy or Behavioral Therapy
Outcome	Effects sexual developmental milestones	Sexual developmental milestones	Sexual developmental milestones Or Puberty Or Reproductive axis

*It is merely to bring attention to the fact that in this review adolescent refers to ages 13 to 18 years of age as per the American Academy of Pediatric's (AAP) definition.

34.2 Search Strategy

We searched MEDLINE (via PUBMED), EMBASE and SCOPUS for papers containing synonyms for both the terms "bariatric surgery" and "sexual developmental milestones" Synonyms were compiled using both a controlled vocabulary and free text (Table 34.1). Published literature through January 27, 2020 were included. We also searched for systematic reviews and meta-analyses using the clinical queries tool in Pubmed. The specific search strings included:

34.2.1 Concept

- ("paediatrics"[All Fields] OR "pediatrics"[MeSH Terms] OR "pediatrics"[All Fields]) AND ("bariatrics"[MeSH Terms] OR "bariatrics"[All Fields]) AND ("puberty"[MeSH Terms] OR "puberty"[All Fields])

Hand-searching was performed by compiling a list of the top pediatric and bariatric surgery journals based on the 2019 impact factor in two major areas: surgery and pediatrics. From this list we chose the six most pertinent journals: Academic Pediatrics, JAMA Pediatrics, The Journal of Pediatrics, and Pediatrics, Surgery of Obesity And Related Diseases, Obesity Surgery. Each of these journals was searched back six months for articles that were not identified in our database search. Duplicates were removed and titles and abstracts reviewed. Articles were excluded if they were case reports, editorials, animal studies, or published in a language other than English. The full text of articles selected by the above process were retrieved.

34.3 Criteria for Considering Studies for This Review

Our research question is to determine whether bariatric surgery affects sexual developmental milestones in adolescents with obesity.

In the United States, randomization to bariatric surgery would be inappropriate and not ethical, and therefore we considered only observational studies. We included prospective or retrospective cohort studies and case-control studies. We did not include any cross-sectional studies, as these studies do not provide temporality.

34.4 Types of Participants

Study participants who met the following criteria for exposure and outcome were included:

1. Patients up until the age of 18 years old who underwent elective bariatric surgery using open or laparoscopic technique.

We did not exclude based on race, ethnicity, gender, geographical location, health care setting, or type of bariatric surgery (laparoscopic adjustable gastric band, vertical sleeve gastrectomy, Roux-en Y gastric bypass, duodenal switch).

34.5   Type of Intervention

We included any participant who underwent elective bariatric surgery of any technique (open, laparoscopic or robotic). We included the most common procedures: laparoscopic adjustable gastric band, vertical sleeve gastrectomy, Roux-en Y gastric bypass and duodenal switch.

34.6   Type of Outcome Measures

34.6.1 Primary Outcome

The primary outcome is the attainment of sexual developmental milestones based on any of the following: clinical diagnosis, self-report, chart review, administrative database coding, radiographic diagnosis, and ICD-10 code.

34.7   Results

Relevant search strings were searched in MEDLINE, EMBASE, AND SCOPUS. An initial search yielded 2237 candidate records. No additional records were identified from hand searching. All duplicates were dropped, and records were transferred to EndNote X9 and reviewed. Only one manuscript was identified that included a pediatric population undergoing bariatric surgery and investigating sexual developmental milestones.

Table 34.2 summarizes the findings.

34.8   Obesity and the Reproductive Axis

The detrimental effects of obesity on the human body are well established in both the adult and pediatric populations. While not commonly discussed, alterations in sexual developmental milestones in the pediatric population and in the reproductive axis in adolescents and adults, are plausible consequences of the altered physiology of the obese state. Evidence suggests that excess body weight (adipose tissue) in childhood effects both growth development and puberty [12].

Table 34.2 Summary results of search

Author/Year Published/ Study	Study Type	Setting	Population	Outcome	Quality of evidence
Chin et al. 2018 Long-term follow-up of gonadal dysfunction in morbidly obese adolescent boys after bariatric surgery	Longitudinal Cohort Study Before and After Bariatric Surgery (laparoscopic adjustable gastric banding)	Academic Center for Bariatric Surgery	Total n = 54 16/54 prepubertal boys with diagnosis of gonadal dysfunction (low total testosterone <350 ng/dL at Tanner 5 Stage, followed to 2 years post-op	1. BMI, weight, waist circumference and % excess weight decreased at 2 years. Post-op 2. Mean total testosterone improved from baseline = 268– 368 ng/dL post-op 3. Negative correlation between BMI and testosterone after 2 years (r = −0.81, p = 0.003)	The only study identified during literature search investigating the effects bariatric surgery has on sexual development milestones There was no comparison group Future rigorous studies are needed to investigate the effect bariatric surgery may have on sexual developmental milestones in the pediatric/ adolescent population

Puberty marks the transition from childhood into adolescence and adulthood. Physiologic, biologic, and psychologic changes lead to development of secondary sexual characteristics (breast tissue, facial and pubic hair, voice changes, menarche), gonadal development and the ability to reproduce [13, 14].

The timing of puberty has a significant impact on the health of the individual [15].

Adipose tissue is a very important endocrine organ with many vital functions including energy storage and metabolism. The adipocyte plays a crucial role in the storage, release and regulation of energy (glucose and fatty acids) and the metabolism of sex hormones [16].

Obesity is thought to alter the hormone milieu including secretion and sensitivity of sex hormones, leptin and insulin [16]. In childhood, excess body weight (excess adipose tissue) may influence normal pubertal development and therefore alter sexual developmental milestones and ultimately the health of the individual. In girls, the timing of puberty and hormone levels provides direct evidence of the association between obesity and the onset of early puberty and increased risk of hyperandrogenism. In boys, the evidence is less clear, but there is evidence that obesity does indeed alter sexual developmental milestones, with some reports demonstrating that excess adiposity is associated with early puberty while others report a delay in puberty [17].

While sex hormones have been implicated in pubertal development, insulin [18], leptin [19] and gut hormones [20] such as ghrelin, the orexigenic "hunger hormone," and the anorexigenic PYY, are among the contributors to this process.

Treatment options to address alterations in sexual developmental milestones and puberty focus on weight loss and maintenance of a healthy weight for age. These include lifestyle modifications such as nutritional counselling for the individual and family, routine monitoring of body weight, consistent exercise, pharmacologic adjunct therapy and bariatric surgery [21].

34.9   Pediatric Bariatric Surgery and Effects on Sexual Developmental Milestones

Pediatric bariatric surgery is an increasingly proven weight-loss intervention for children and adolescents under 18 years of age who have failed traditional methods of weight loss. Nearly one in ten children and adolescents, in the United States are classified within the definition of Class II obesity with a body mass index (BMI) ≥ 35 kg/m^2 or $\geq 120\%$ of the 95th percentile values. This translates into nearly 4.5 million children and adolescents in the United States that are physically, psychologically and medically burdened by enormous fat reserves and physiologic toll this takes on their developing bodies. Today, there is strong evidence demonstrating the effectiveness of pediatric bariatric surgery. In 2017, the Endocrine Society published up to date clinical guidelines in the assessment, treatment and prevention of pediatric obesity. In their opinion, bariatric surgery could be considered in patients with the following criteria: "who attained Tanner 4 or 5 pubertal development and final or near-final adult height, the patient has a BMI of >40 kg/m^2 or has a BMI of >35 kg/m^2 and significant, extreme comorbidities" [22].

Alqahtani et al set out to challenge the concerns of pediatricians by demonstrating that bariatric surgery in prepubertal children was safe and effective. In a retrospective study using data from the investigators' program database, 116 children age ≤ 14 years (excluding syndromic cases of obesity) were identified who underwent laparoscopic vertical sleeve gastrectomy (VSG). These cases were matched on age, sex, and height with non-surgical weight management and further the cohort was compared to adolescents ages >14 who also underwent laparoscopic VSG. Investigators found significant improvement in linear growth of pediatric patients undergoing VSG when compared with matched controls of similar BMI. Interestingly, the younger children (≤ 14 years) had a lower prevalence of existing comorbidities, yet when compared to the older children who underwent VSG, they had similar resolution rates of existing comorbidities and there was no significant difference in complication rates [23].

Based on this study and an extensive systematic review conducted by the American Society of Bariatric and Metabolic Surgeons (ASMBS) entitled ASMBS Pediatric Metabolic and Bariatric Surgery Guidelines 2018, the pediatric surgery committee reported that there was no strong evidence to suggest that pediatric bariatric surgery adversely effects linear growth or puberty as measured by Tanner staging. They concluded that adolescents *should not* be denied access to bariatric surgery based on bone growth or Tanner staging [2].

In searching for published literature specifically citing any effects that bariatric surgery may have on puberty/sexual developmental milestones, only one study was identified.

In 2018, Chin et al. reported the first study in the literature to determine the effects of bariatric surgery on gonadal dysfunction. Fifty-four adolescent boys diagnosed with preoperative gonadal dysfunction were followed for 2 years following laparoscopic gastric banding. While not statistically significant, the investigators did find a trend that suggested at both 1 and 2 years following bariatric surgery, testosterone levels improved from preoperative baseline values. The improvement in testosterone levels was associated with weight loss and decreased waist circumference, hemoglobin A1C, and fasting insulin levels [24] (Table 34.2).

While there is a dearth of published literature investigating the association between bariatric surgery and sexual developmental milestones, one could extrapolate from papers describing the detrimental effects of obesity on puberty and sexual development, and the ability of weight loss to reverse or improve these negative effects, that pediatric bariatric surgery resulting in successful weight loss and resolution or improvement in comorbidities associated with obesity should improve altered sexual developmental milestones of boys and premature puberty in girls.

34.10 A Personal View of the Data

Pediatricians, bariatric surgeons, and obesity researchers alike can all agree that longitudinal outcome data are needed to assess the long-term safety and medical outcomes of children and adolescents undergoing bariatric surgery. Long term outcome data are needed to improve the care of our patients and should include anthropometric (weight loss and body mass index), medical (remission, resolution and relapse of obesity related comorbidities such as type 2 diabetes obstructive sleep apnea, chronic kidney and liver disease,) and psychosocial issues.

As evident by the dearth of paper identified by the present systematic review, it is essential that future studies include data collection on how bariatric surgery affects sexual developmental milestones and their implications for sexuality, body image, fertility, pregnancy, and quality of life.

Finally, adolescents being considered for bariatric surgery should be referred to an accredited center that offers an experienced comprehensive program including lifestyle therapy, behavioral and nutritional counselling, exercise, and extensive follow-up support. Further, the adolescent should have a cohesive plan to effectively transition them to adult bariatric care.

Obesity is a chronic disease and it requires a lifetime of responsible care.

References

1. Armstrong SC, Bolling CF, Michalsky MP, Reichard KW, Section on Obesity SOS. Pediatric metabolic and bariatric surgery: evidence, barriers, and best practices. Pediatrics. 2019;144(6):e20193223.

2. Pratt JSA, Browne A, Browne NT, Bruzoni M, Cohen M, Desai A, et al. ASMBS pediatric metabolic and bariatric surgery guidelines, 2018. Surg Obes Relat Dis. 2018;14(7):882–901.
3. Skinner AC, Ravanbakht SN, Skelton JA, Perrin EM, Armstrong SC. Prevalence of obesity and severe obesity in US children, 1999–2016. Pediatrics. 2018;141(3):e20173459.
4. Bolling CF, Armstrong SC, Reichard KW, Michalsky MP, Section On Obesity SOS. Metabolic and bariatric surgery for pediatric patients with severe obesity. Pediatrics. 2019;144(6):e20193224.
5. Freedman DS, Khan LK, Dietz WH, Srinivasan SR, Berenson GS. Relationship of childhood obesity to coronary heart disease risk factors in adulthood: the Bogalusa Heart Study. Pediatrics. 2001;108(3):712–8.
6. Di Cesare M, Sorić M, Bovet P, Miranda JJ, Bhutta Z, Stevens GA, et al. The epidemiological burden of obesity in childhood: a worldwide epidemic requiring urgent action. BMC Med. 2019;17(1):212.
7. Inge TH, Jenkins TM, Xanthakos SA, Dixon JB, Daniels SR, Zeller MH, et al. Long-term outcomes of bariatric surgery in adolescents with severe obesity (FABS-5+): a prospective follow-up analysis. Lancet Diabetes Endocrinol. 2017;5(3):165–73.
8. Inge TH, Courcoulas AP, Jenkins TM, Michalsky MP, Brandt ML, Xanthakos SA, et al. Five-year outcomes of gastric bypass in adolescents as compared with adults. N Engl J Med. 2019;380(22):2136–45.
9. Olbers T, Beamish AJ, Gronowitz E, Flodmark C-E, Dahlgren J, Bruze G, et al. Laparoscopic Roux-en-Y gastric bypass in adolescents with severe obesity (AMOS): a prospective, 5-year, Swedish nationwide study. Lancet Diabetes Endocrinol. 2017;5(3):174–83.
10. Woolford SJ, Clark SJ, Gebremariam A, Davis MM, Freed GL. To cut or not to cut: physicians' perspectives on referring adolescents for bariatric surgery. Obes Surg. 2010;20(7):937–42.
11. Das JK, Salam RA, Thornburg KL, Prentice AM, Campisi S, Lassi ZS, et al. Nutrition in adolescents: physiology, metabolism, and nutritional needs. Ann N Y Acad Sci. 2017;1393(1):21–33.
12. Chung S. Growth and puberty in obese children and implications of body composition. J Obes Metab Syndr. 2017;26(4):243–50.
13. Vijayakumar N, Op de Macks Z, Shirtcliff EA, Pfeifer JH. Puberty and the human brain: Insights into adolescent development. Neurosci Biobehav Rev. 2018;92:417–436.
14. Abreu AP, Kaiser UB. Pubertal development and regulation. Lancet Diabetes Endocrinol. 2016;4(3):254–64.
15. Golub MS, Collman GW, Foster PMD, Kimmel CA, Rajpert-De Meyts E, Reiter EO, et al. Public health implications of altered puberty timing. Pediatrics. 2008;121(Suppl 3):S218–S30.
16. Trayhurn P, Beattie JH. Physiological role of adipose tissue: white adipose tissue as an endocrine and secretory organ. Proc Nutr Soc. 2001;60(3):329–39.
17. Marcovecchio ML, Chiarelli F. Obesity and growth during childhood and puberty. World Rev Nutr Diet. 2013;106:135–41.
18. Moriarty-Kelsey M, Harwood JEF, Travers SH, Zeitler PS, Nadeau KJ. Testosterone, obesity and insulin resistance in young males: evidence for an association between gonadal dysfunction and insulin resistance during puberty. J Pediatr Endocrinol Metab. 2010;23(12):1281–7.
19. Shalitin S, Kiess W. Putative effects of obesity on linear growth and puberty. Horm Res Paediatr. 2017;88(1):101–10.
20. Horner K, Lee S. Appetite-related peptides in childhood and adolescence: role of ghrelin, PYY, and GLP-1. Appl Physiol Nutr Metab. 2015;40(11):1089–99.
21. Michalakis K, Mintziori G, Kaprara A, Tarlatzis BC, Goulis DG. The complex interaction between obesity, metabolic syndrome and reproductive axis: a narrative review. Metabolism. 2013;62(4):457–78.
22. Styne DM, Arslanian SA, Connor EL, Farooqi IS, Murad MH, Silverstein JH, et al. Pediatric obesity-assessment, treatment, and prevention: an Endocrine Society clinical practice guideline. J Clin Endocrinol Metab. 2017;102(3):709–57.
23. Alqahtani A, Elahmedi M, Qahtani ARA. Laparoscopic sleeve gastrectomy in children younger than 14 years: refuting the concerns. Ann Surg. 2016;263(2):312–9.
24. Chin VL, Willliams KM, Donnelley T, Censani M, Conroy R, Lerner S, et al. Long-term follow-up of gonadal dysfunction in morbidly obese adolescent boys after bariatric surgery. J Pediatr Endocrinol Metab. 2018;31(11):1191–7.

Which Surgical Specialist Should Perform Metabolic Bariatric Surgery in Children and Adolescents?

35

Alexander Trenk and Mark B. Slidell

35.1 Introduction

As the incidence of obesity has risen in North American children and adolescents, there has been a concomitant rise in the number of pediatric patients who undergo metabolic bariatric surgery (MBS). Over the past 3 decades there has been a three-fold increase in the incidence of childhood obesity [1]. For adolescents age 12 to 19 years, the prevalence of obesity and extreme obesity is estimated at 20.5% and 7.8% respectively, and for children as young as 6 to 11 years of age it is estimated to be 17.5% and 5.6% [2]. While metabolic and bariatric surgery (MBS) has a proven record of success in the treatment of adults with morbid obesity, it is only over the past decade or so that we have seen a similar rise in literature supporting MBS for the pediatric population. Adolescents undergoing MBS exhibit similar improvements in obesity-related conditions, such as diabetes type II, hypertension and obstructive sleep apnea [3–7]. For the most part, the result of MBS mirror the successes seen in adult populations, and a growing body of evidence similarly supports a multidisciplinary approach to MBS in pediatric patients. The American Society for Metabolic and Bariatric Surgery (ASMBS) Pediatric Committee continues to put out pediatric-specific recommendations for MBS programs with respect to how a program is staffed. With respect to the surgeon performing the procedures, it recommends a "moderate volume metabolic and bariatric surgeon, either adult or pediatric, and a transition plan into an adult program [8]." The question we will consider in this review is whether the training background of that surgical specialist affects outcomes, and whether it makes a difference if that is a pediatric general surgeon or an adult surgeon with minimally invasive surgical (MIS) training?

A. Trenk · M. B. Slidell (✉)
The University of Chicago, Chicago, Illinois, USA
e-mail: mslidell@surgery.bsd.uchicago.edu

© Springer Nature Switzerland AG 2021

401

J. Alverdy, Y. Vigneswaran (eds.), *Difficult Decisions in Bariatric Surgery*,
Difficult Decisions in Surgery: An Evidence-Based Approach,
https://doi.org/10.1007/978-3-030-55329-6_35

35.2   Search Strategy

A search of English language publications from 2005 to 2020 was performed to identify articles to answer the question of "which specialist should perform bariatric surgery in adolescents?" Databases searched were PubMed, and Cochrane Evidence Based Medicine. Terms used in our search included (Bariatric Surgery OR Metabolic Surgery OR Bariatric Surgical Procedures OR Weight loss surgery) AND (Child or Adolescent or Pediatric) AND, "Outcomes", "specialty", "hospital", "volumes", "specialty". The World Health Organization definition of an adolescent is a person who falls between the ages of 10 and 19 years of age [9], however we will also consider any evidence regarding children ages 6 to 10 in our evaluation of the literature.

P (Patients)	I (Intervention)	C (Comparator)	O (Outcomes)
Children and adolescents suffering from morbid obesity	Bariatric surgery	Adult general surgeons, adult MIS and bariatric surgeons, and pediatric surgeons with bariatric training.	Mortality, surgical complications, weight loss, long-term improvement in comorbidities, QOL, costs

35.3   Results

Our PICO literature search did not uncover any studies evaluating differences in MBS outcomes for children operated on by adult versus pediatric surgeons. There are studies comparing the outcomes for children versus adults undergoing the same procedure, but none addressing our question of who ought to be performing the operations. In the absence of any such literature, it is not possible to give evidence-based recommendations that are specific to MBS. Nonetheless, this is an important question to consider and we hope it is taken up as a research question so that we may soon have an evidence-based approach specific to MBS.

In the absence of dedicated MBS data on this subject, we can begin by reviewing expert consensus recommendations from bariatric societies. While surgery volumes are relatively low for adolescent bariatric procedures, the number of children undergoing MBS is rising, and awareness of surgical obesity treatment and its long-term benefits is necessary to ensure bariatric programs optimize physiologic and social outcomes. As espoused by Wilson et al., 'Bariatric surgery programs with a primary focus on adults may be well equipped to provide safe and effective perioperative care for adolescents but may be less equipped to handle these patients unique metabolic and challenging psychological needs' [10]. In adult MBS centers, surgeons may find it difficult to manage the long-term care of adolescent patients without close collaboration with pediatric specialists (dieticians, psychologists, pediatricians, etc.). The American Society for Metabolic and Bariatric Surgery (ASMBS) Pediatric Committee has weighed in on this and recently updated their guidelines for MBS in adolescents to provide some guidance on the best approach to these patients [8].

The ASMBS guidelines recommend that both freestanding pediatric programs and adult programs with adolescent teams undergo the process of clinical accreditation through the Metabolic and Bariatric Surgery Accreditation and Quality Improvement Program (MBSAQIP) [8]. The process of accreditation has been shown to improve quality and safety for programs caring for obese adolescents [11, 12]. In order to become an accredited bariatric program for children, there are specific requirements for a number of pediatric specialists to provide that care. The guidelines state there must be, a pediatric or adolescent-trained medical physician as the "pediatric medical advisor," and also a psychologist, psychiatrist, or otherwise adolescent-trained licensed counselor who can provide care as a "behavioral specialist" for pediatric patients. There must also be a plan in place for orderly transition into an adult program as they age out of the pediatric center. The ASMBS guidelines do not specify whether the surgeon needs to be a pediatric surgeon or an adult MIS surgeon with experience operating on adolescents. The guidelines simply state that the surgeon "may be either an adult or pediatric surgeon with a moderate volume of experience in MBS." [8]. This implies that the relevant surgical skills and training of an adult bariatric surgeon will readily transfer to operations on adolescent patients, and that a pediatric surgeon with advanced MIS training is fully capable of performing MBS. At the root of this, is a belief that adolescent anatomy and physiology closely approximates that of young adults, and that the surgical skills of these two specialties are for the most part equivalent. This seems reasonable on its face, but there is a paucity of MBS research on this question, and we must look to other areas of overlap in care provided by different surgical specialties in order to answer these questions.

If there proves to be a difference in outcomes, then the next question will be whether the different sub-specialty surgical training paths are what determines outcomes for adolescents undergoing MBS. Are the MIS skills themselves what matter the most, or is it the experience with bariatric patients, the various surgical approaches and their associated complications that ensures good outcomes?

In an effort to determine which surgical specialists might be best prepared to care for adolescent MBS patients, we reviewed literature from other areas of surgery where there is significant overlap between adult and pediatric surgeons providing the same medical and surgical care to adolescents. An excellent example of this is in the trauma and acute care surgery literature which has attempted to address this specific question about potentially overlapping areas of expertise in the care of acutely ill or traumatically injured adolescents.

There are a number of studies showing that injured children treated at pediatric trauma centers (PTCs) have a lower mortality risk when compared to children treated in and adult trauma center (ATC) or a mixed trauma center (MTC) which cares for adult and pediatric patients. The younger the child, the greater the benefits of being cared for in a PTC [13–17]. One problem with these trauma studies is that the primary outcome of interest in all of them is patient mortality. Even in severely injured children, overall mortality is very low and it is a limited outcome measure. There is very little data comparing other outcome measures between adult and pediatric surgeons caring for children, so we must look at this data for guidance, while recognizing its limitations.

One of the earliest high-quality studies comparing mortality rates based upon the surgical training of the treating trauma team, showed an 8% reduction in the likelihood of mortality among pediatric trauma patients (<18 years of age) treated at PTCs instead of ATCs in Florida [13]. Another study that followed found that adult trauma surgeons had better outcomes when the trauma center went through a formal process to obtain certification to care for injured children. Improved overall survival from injuries was seen when pediatric trauma patients were treated at ATCs who had undergone a pediatric-specific verification process similar to what the ABMBS suggests for MBS. The benefits of lowered mortality rates were greatest in the youngest children [15].

If we look specifically at injured adolescents, we see that these findings persist even in patients aged 15 to 19 years [18, 19, 20]. The mortality rates, and the adjusted odds ratio of mortality were lowest at PTCs (0.4%) vs. ATCs (3.2%) or MTCs (3.5%); (p < .001), and PTCs (reference) ATCs (OR, 4.19; 95% CI, 1.30–13.51); MTCs (odds ratio, 6.68; 95% CI, 2.03–21.99) respectively [16].

All of this trauma and acute care literature can really be summed up as two key points that we can consider applying to MBS. The first is that traumatically injured children cared for in designated pediatric trauma centers had improved outcomes compared to children treated in adult trauma centers. The younger the child, the stronger this effect appears to be. The reasons for this are unclear, but it is believed to be the benefit of the pediatric systems of care as a whole, rather than something attributable to a single surgeon's expertise. The second point is that ATCs obtain some form of certification or qualifications to treat children outperform those who do not seek additional qualifications. This suggests that the process of obtaining and maintaining these additional credentials may convey a protective effect to those injured children. The implication of this observation for other specialties such as MBS, is that adult MIS surgeons in any specialty may also manage to provide better care for children if they seek additional qualifications or designations as a certified pediatric MBS center. While this is different than directly comparing outcomes for adult and pediatric surgeons performing MBS for obese children, we do not have any MBS publications that have examined this question. Without bariatric-specific data on this subject, we are forced to look elsewhere to answer these questions.

Another way to look at this question is to ask whether a pediatric surgeon performing a low volume of MBS cases each year, can have similar outcomes to an adult MBS surgeon who has a busy bariatric practice. The answer to this question lies somewhere at an intersection of the debate around the bariatric volume/outcomes relationship, and a separate debate about the transferability of surgical skills from one procedure to a different one.

It has been shown that a high-volume surgeon is not the only factor in the volume/outcome relationship. A number of studies suggest it is more than simply the quality of the operation that predicts successful weight loss and long-term health outcomes following MBS. Rather it is the combined efforts of a multidisciplinary team including primary care physicians, mental health specialists, dieticians and health coordinators that all contribute to the success of each patient [21–23]. Adolescent bariatric programs that undergo ASMBS certification will have this multidisciplinary team around them that will help ensure good outcomes even if the surgical volumes are not as high as the busiest adult MBS centers.

The question of transferability of surgical skills matters more to the pediatric surgeon who is performing MBS. There are simply fewer children and adolescents requiring MBS than there are adults. There are very few high volume adolescent MBS practices where the primary surgeon is a pediatric surgeon. This means most pediatric surgeons performing MBS cases are not what would be considered a high volume surgeon in an adult MBS center. The question is whether the advanced MIS skills from the other cases they do will result in transferable skills for an MBS procedure, or whether most pediatric surgeons should simply leave adolescent MBS cases to the adult surgeons taking care of obese adolescents within a formal MBS center.

Unlike our first question, there is a growing body of evidence suggesting that skills and experience acquired from other complex MIS procedures may be transferrable to a different complex index operation. For example, the advanced MIS skills developed by pediatric surgeons who perform MIS procedures in neonates, appear to be transferrable between the various index operations on newborns. Surgeons who perform laparoscopic duodenal atresia (DA) repairs are typically also completing thoracoscopic esophageal atresia with tracheoesophageal fistula (EA/TEF) repairs. Neither of these cases can actually be "high volume" cases for most individual surgeons since they are inherently rare cases with most surgeons performing no more than 2–4 of each index procedures each year. Pediatric surgeons would argue that their advanced MIS skills are readily transferrable from case to case, and that this would also apply to MBS procedures. This may not always be the case in MBS procedures. There is a recent study that aimed to determine whether a "surrogate volume effect" could be detected in adult surgeons who perform common laparoscopic general surgery procedures as well as MBS cases. Their interpretation of the data was that skills acquired performing non-bariatric laparoscopic procedures did not affect all-cause morbidity in bariatric surgery [24]. We do not have evidence specifically addressing the question of whether a pediatric surgeon's advanced MIS skills will also translate to good outcomes in adolescent MBS cases.

35.4   Recommendations Based on the Data

In the end it is very difficult to answer the question of which surgical specialist is best suited to perform MBS for adolescents and children. There is a paucity of MBS data to answer whether the training background of the surgical specialist affects outcomes at all, and at this point it is unclear whether it makes a difference if that is a pediatric general surgeon or an adult surgeon with minimally invasive surgical (MIS) training. We cannot meaningfully discriminate between the impact of the surgeon's specialty training as compared with the structural benefits of the entire pediatric-specific infrastructure supporting an MBS patient. Our opinion is that future research into this question would support the argument that it is the surrounding infrastructure that has the greatest impact on overall outcomes.

Our primary recommendation is to support the guidance provided by the American Society for Metabolic and Bariatric Surgery (ASMBS) Pediatric Committee, which recommends that this care should be provided by a "moderate volume metabolic and bariatric surgeon, either adult or pediatric, [with] a transition plan into an adult program [8]." This recommendation is in line with a growing body of evidence supporting a multidisciplinary approach to MBS in pediatric patients.

At this point, there is insufficient evidence to conclude that a freestanding pediatric program is superior to an adult program with a specific adolescent team, nor is the opposite true. We believe that as the field of adolescent bariatric surgery grows and evolves, the adolescent centers would benefit from alignment with higher volume adult programs and/or higher volume pediatric surgery hospitals/centers that have the capacity for close collaboration. This can ensure adequate perioperative support for a successful program.

35.5   A Personal View of the Data

There has been very gradual growth in centers providing MBS to adolescents, and this hinders our ability to accumulate sufficient data directly comparing outcomes for adolescents treated by pediatric surgeons versus adult surgeons with expertise in caring for adolescents. One of the barriers to starting a MBS program for children and adolescents is that it requires significant investment of clinical resources and time to get a center up and off the ground and this can be a significant challenge given the lower potential case volumes of a pediatric MBS center compared to those for adults. That said, outcomes for adolescents undergoing MBS closely mirror those of adult patients in moderate volume centers. We feel that there is tremendous opportunity to develop adolescent MBS programs in children's hospitals by closely collaborating with existing adult MBS programs. This will enable the adolescent program to build off of the experience and success of the adult program and provides practitioners with resources and institutional knowledge to help with particularly challenging patients. This recommendation is in-line with the overall recommendations of the ASMBS pediatric subcommittee and we believe a collaborative approach such as this will lower the bar for developing more adolescent MBS centers and ultimately improve access to care for these children.

In the absence of any clinical studies comparing outcomes between different surgical specialists performing these operations, it is not possible to give evidence-based recommendations at this time. For now, a collaborative approach as outlined above will be the best way to provide high quality care for these children, but we believe this is an important research question to taken up soon, so that we may soon have an evidence-based recommendations specific to MBS.

35.5.1 Recommendations in Order of Preference

1. Comprehensive adolescent MBS program integrated within a pediatric hospital with a dedicated, moderate volume metabolic and bariatric surgeon. The surgeon (pediatric surgeon with extra MBS training or an adult MBS surgeon) will participate in the ASMBS certification process.
2. Adult surgeon in an adult MBS center with pediatric medical sub-specialty support. The adult MBS surgeon will participate in the ASMBS certification process.

References

1. Skinner AC, Skelton JA. Prevalence and trends in obesity and severe obesity among children in the United States, 1999–2012. JAMA Pediatr. 2014;168(6):561–6.
2. Ogden CL, Carroll MD, Lawman HG, et al. Trends in obesity prevalence among children and adolescents in the United States, 1988-1994 through 2013-2014. JAMA. 2016;315(21):2292–9.
3. Inge TH, Courcoulas AP, Jenkins TM, et al. Weight loss and health status 3 years after bariatric surgery in adolescents. N Engl J Med. 2016;374(2):113–23.
4. Olbers T, Beamish AJ, Gronowitz E, et al. Laparoscopic roux-en-Y gastric bypass in adolescents with severe obesity (AMOS): a prospective, 5-year, Swedish nationwide study. Lancet Diabetes Endocrinol. 2017;5(3):174–83.
5. Inge TH, Laffel LM, Jenkins TM, et al. Comparison of surgical and medical therapy for type 2 diabetes in severely obese adolescents. JAMA Pediatr. 2018;172(5):452–60.
6. Amin R, Simakojornboon N, Szczesniak R, Inge T. Early improvement in obstructive sleep apnea and increase in orexin levels after bariatric surgery in adolescents and young adults. Surg Obes Relat Dis. 2017;13(1):95–100.
7. Manco M, Mosca A, De Peppo F, et al. The benefit of sleeve gastrectomy in obese adolescents on nonalcoholic steatohepatitis and hepatic fibrosis. J Pediatr. 2017;180:31–7.e32.
8. Pratt JSA, et al. ASMBS pediatric metabolic and bariatric surgery guidelines, 2018. Surg Obes Relat Dis. 2018 Jul;14(7):882–901.
9. Adolescent health [homepage on the Internet] Geneva: World Health Organization, cc2018. [updated 2018]. Available from: http://www.who.int/topics/adolescent_health/en/.
10. Tsai WS, Inge TH, Burd RS. Bariatric surgery in adolescents. Recent National Trends in use and in hospital outcome. Arch Pediatr Adolesc Med. 2007;161:217–21.
11. Nguyen NT, Nguyen B, Nguyen VQ, Ziogas A, Hohmann S, Stamos MJ. Outcomes of bariatric surgery performed at accredited vs nonaccredited centers. J Am Coll Surg. 2012;215(4):467–74.
12. Gebhart A, Young M, Phelan M, Nguyen NT. Impact of accreditation in bariatric surgery. Surg Obes Relat Dis. 2014;10(5):767–73.
13. Pracht EE, Tepas JJ, Langland-Orban B, Simpson L, Pieper P, Flint LM. Do pediatric patients with trauma in Florida have reduced mortality rates when treated in designated trauma centers? J Pediatr Surg. 2008 Jan;4(1):212–21.
14. Petrosyan M, Guner YS, Emami CN, Ford HR. Disparities in the delivery of pediatric trauma care. J Trauma. 2009 Aug;67(2 Suppl):S114–9.
15. Oyetunji TA, Haider AH, Downing SR, Bolorunduro OB, Efron DT, Haut ER, Chang DC, et al. Treatment outcomes of injured children at adult level 1 trauma centers: are there benefits from added specialized care? Am J Surg. 2011 Apr;201(4):445–9.
16. Webman RB, Carter EA, Mittal S, Wang J, Sathya C, Nathens AB, Nance ML, Madigan D, Burd RS. Association between trauma center type and mortality among injured adolescent patients. JAMA Pediatr. 2016 Aug 1;170(8):780–6.
17. McCarthy A, Curtis K, Holland AJ. Pediatric trauma systems and their impact on the health outcomes of severely injured children: an integrative review. Injury. 2016 Mar;47(3):574–85.

18. Walther AE, Falcone RA, Pritts TA, Hanseman DJ, Robinson BRH. Pediatric and adult trauma centers differ in evaluation, treatment and outcomes for severely injured adolescents. J Pediatr Surg. 2016;51:1346–50.

19. Matsushima K, Schaefer EW, Won EJ, Nichols PA, Frankel HL. Injured adolescents, not just large children: difference in care and outcome between adult and pediatric trauma centers. Am Surg. 2013;79:267–73.

20. Matsushima K, Kulaylat AN, Won EJ, et al. Variation in the management of adolescent patients with blunt abdominal solid organ injury between adult versus pediatric trauma centers: an analysis of a statewide trauma database. J Surg Res. 2013;183:808–13.

21. Michalsky M, Reichard K, Inge T, Pratt J, Lenders C. ASMBS pediatric committee best practice guidelines. Surg Obes Relat Dis. 2012 Jan-Feb;8(1):1–7.

22. Pratt JSA, Lenders CM, Dionne EA, Hoppin AG, Hsu GLK, Inge TH, Lawlor DF, Marino MF, Meyers AF, Rosenblum JL, Sanchez VM. Best practice updates for pediatric/adolescent weight loss surgery. Obesity. 2009;17(5):901–10.

23. Jamal MK, DeMaria EJ, Johnson JM, et al. Impact of major comorbidities on mortality and complications after gastric bypass. Surg Obes Relat Dis. 2005;1:511–6.

24. Hunt KD, Doumouras AG, Lee Y, Gmora S, Anvari M, Hong D. The effect of surrogate procedure volume on bariatric surgery outcomes: do common laparoscopic general surgery procedures matter? Surg Endosc. 2020 Mar;34(3):1278–84. https://doi.org/10.1007/s00464-019-06897-6.

Part IX

The Future

Deep Brain Stimulation as a Treatment for Obesity

36

Micaela Esquivel, Casey Halpern, and Dan Azagury

36.1 Introduction

Bariatric surgery is widely recognized as the only effective long-term treatment for severe obesity. Some studies have shown significant weight loss in over 90% of patients treated [1]. That being said, bariatric surgery has its limitations, and long-term weight regain and metabolic syndrome recurrence has been shown to occur in 10–40% of patients in some studies [2–4], with laparoscopic sleeve gastrectomy accounting for the higher end of that range. The recidivism rates after Laparoscopic Roux-en-Y Gastric Bypass (LRYGB) are lower than after sleeve gastrectomy and their causes are multifactorial. Studies have shown that bariatric surgery not only impacts anatomical restriction to food consumption, but also has neuroendocrinological effects that impacts weight loss [5].

Would future treatments be able to take advantage of the increasing understanding of the neuroanatomic and neuropsychiatric basis for obesity? Could neuromodulation have a role in treatment of obesity?

36.2 What Is Deep Brain Stimulation?

Deep brain stimulation (DBS) administers reversible electrical stimulation to specific portions of the brain, making those areas of the brain inactive without ablating them (or destroying them). This high-frequency electrical stimulation mimics the

M. Esquivel · D. Azagury (✉)
Department of Surgery, Stanford University School of Medicine, Stanford, CA, USA
e-mail: mesquive@stanford.edu; dazagury@stanford.edu

C. Halpern
Department of Neurosurgery, Stanford University School of Medicine, Stanford, CA, USA
e-mail: chalpern@stanford.edu

© Springer Nature Switzerland AG 2021
J. Alverdy, Y. Vigneswaran (eds.), *Difficult Decisions in Bariatric Surgery*,
Difficult Decisions in Surgery: An Evidence-Based Approach,
https://doi.org/10.1007/978-3-030-55329-6_36

effects of previously used ablative procedures, with the benefit of not only being able to turn off the stimulation (reverse the effect), but also being able to titrate the effect.

DBS surgery is a neurosurgical operation that is performed on awake patients to ensure neurologic and mental function is maintained throughout the procedure. It is completed stereotactically with the use of an MRI or CT attached to a stereotactic head frame. Two electrodes are inserted into specific areas of the brain, one on each side of the brain, and are placed through two quarter sized burr holes. The leads are then attached to extension wires that attach to a neurostimulator device that is placed in the subcutaneous tissue of the chest or abdomen. During and after electrode placement, neurologic and mental function is assessed. The device is then programmed and turned on at the post-operative visit.

DBS has been shown to be not only effective, but also safe, for the treatment of Parkinson's Disease, Chronic Obsessive-Compulsive Disorder, and Dystonia, among a variety of other neurologic disorders [6–8]. Additionally, several more recent DBS clinical trials have targeted the hypothalamus specifically for the treatment of Alzheimer's disease, depression, cluster headaches [9, 10]. Though studies have shown the role of the hypothalamus in satiety and feeding since the 1960's [11], more recent studies confirm the same relationship [12]. With this information, it can be inferred that deep brain stimulation may be effective in treating obesity.

36.3   How can Deep Brain Stimulation Be Used for Obesity?

We will discuss two focal areas of the brain that are associated with the neural circuitry of obesity: the Lateral Hypothalamus (LH) and the Nucleus Accumbens (NAc) (see Fig. 36.1). These two areas could be the targets for neuromodulation in the treatment of obesity.

36.3.1 Lateral Hypothalamus: The Feeding Center of the Brain

The LH is the hunger and satiety center of the brain. The LH produces two neuropeptides: orexin and melanin-concentrating hormone (MCH), both of which are anabolic and elicit feeding [13]. In experimental models, MCH over expression is associated with obesity and insulin resistance, while MCH-knockout mice are associated with hypophagia and are slim [14]. A lesion to this area of the brain in rats has also caused leanness and weight loss [15–17], and it is felt that chronic DBS would mimic the same effect as these lesions (removal/ablation of that area).

Due to the convincing evidence, DBS of the LH was piloted in three humans, all of which were obese after failed response to bariatric surgery. The study showed an increase in resting metabolism at the 3-year follow-up and weight loss in two of individuals [18]. These findings also speak to the size and specific location of DBS, as the size of DBS target can be as small as 2 mm to reach an effect, while the LH

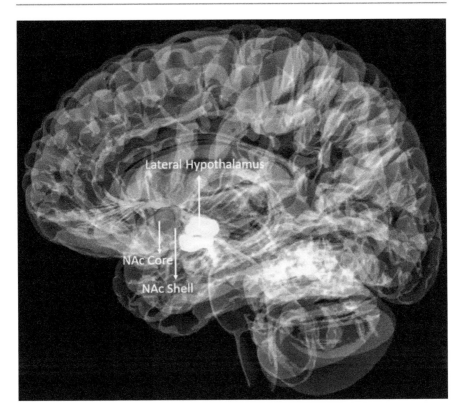

Fig. 36.1 Schematic representation of the feeding and reward circuitry pathways intersecting the Lateral Hypothalamus and Nucleus Accumbens (NAc). The streamlines intersecting the NAc and Lateral Hypothalamus were rendered using deterministic tractography in the Human Connectome Project diffusion MRI template. The analysis was conducted using DSI Studio (http://dsi-studio. labsolver.org)

measures 6 mm in its largest dimension. Additionally, the position of the probe was demonstrated to be suboptimal on post-operative imaging in the patient with no response (Fig. 36.2).

36.3.2 Nucleus Accumbens: The Reward Center of the Brain

We like to think of the NAc as the dopamine superhighway of the brain, where all the dopaminergic wiring converges. Reward anticipation, cravings, consumption driven reward, withdrawal and addiction-like behavior all meet at the NAc [19, 20]. Some of these behaviors, such as food addiction, are due to dysfunctional reward wiring in the brain [21, 22]. When rodents have access to high calorie and highly appetizing food, their dopamine levels increase, which has been shown to trigger binge-eating behavior [23]. Mice accustomed to a high fat diet will intentionally

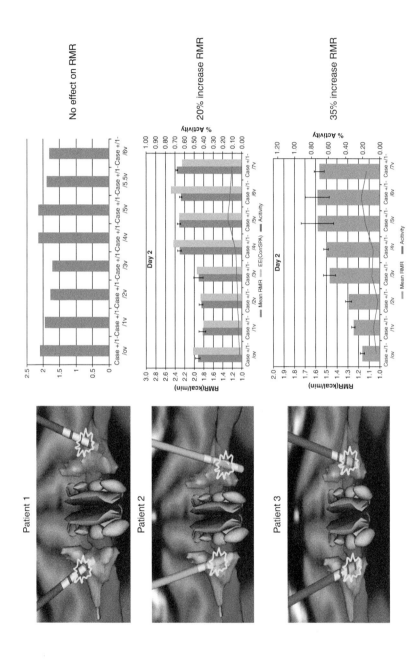

Fig. 36.2 Probe placement and effect on resting metabolic rate (RMR) in the three patients of the original trial by Whiting et al. Adapted with permission from D. Whiting, MD

withstand harsh environments to obtain this diet, and show evidence of withdrawal when removed from the diet [24].

Similar findings have been shown in humans with the use of functional MRI's of the brain [25, 26]. These findings are particularly interesting in bariatric patients, where post roux-en-Y gastric bypass patients 1 month after surgery had a decrease response of the NAc to high calorie food images [27]. Two additional studies also showed alterations in the dopamine response after bariatric surgery [28, 29]. In regards to the NAc and DBS specifically, obese mice (diet induced) with chronic DBS to the NAc showed decrease caloric intake and sustained weight loss [30].

Based off of the information above, both the LH and NAc are two potential targets. The LH to primarily control the feeding and satiety response, and the NAc to target the reward pathway.

36.4 Ethical Considerations

The use of DBS to manipulate the reward wiring of the brain in obese patients may result in nonadaptive behavior if neural modulation is imperfectly executed, as has been seen in DBS use in addiction [31]. Though it is generally felt that informed consent can be obtained on obese patients prior to treatment [32], is autonomy threatened due to this behavior-changing treatment? This is an interesting question when linking obesity and addiction, that altered reward pathways actually disrupts these patients' baseline autonomy and daily decision-making. And as described by Caplan, what are the ethics in "denying autonomy in order to create it: the paradox of forcing treatment upon addicts" [33] In addition, there have been reports of threatened autonomy during DBS treatment, with some studies showing increased impulsivity and even suicidality [34].

As argued by Halpern et al., that though there is concern for DBS in controlling one's actions in the context of treatment, they argue that *through* treatment patients may finally gain the self control in regards to food consumption [35].

36.5 Conclusions

The use of DBS for treatment of obesity is compelling. And as shown from the bariatric literature, not all patients have sustained weight loss or improved metabolic responses to surgery. Although DBS may not be suitable for all patients, there are likely subsets of patients who would greatly benefit from such therapy. The scope of obesity impacting our population is large and is having an increasing global impact. Further trials of the use of DBS at the LH and NAc targets to treat obesity are needed. The more tools we have to fight this disease, the greater benefits we can offer our patients.

Acknowledgments Daniel A. N. Barbosa, a Postdoctoral Research Scholar in the M.D. Halpern-Malenka Lab in the Department of Neurosurgery at Stanford University School of Medicine, for generating the schematic in Fig. 36.1.
    Donald M. Whiting M.D., M.S.,FACS. Chief Medical Officer, Allegheny Health Network. Pittsburgh, for Fig. 36.2.

References

1. Magro DO, Geloneze B, Delfini R, Pareja BC, Callejas F, Pareja JC. Long-term weight regain after gastric bypass: a 5-year prospective study. Obes Surg. 2008;18:648–51. https://doi.org/10.1007/s11695-007-9265-1.
2. Christou NV, Look D, Maclean LD. Weight gain after short- and long-limb gastric bypass in patients followed for longer than 10 years. Ann Surg. 2006;244:734–40. https://doi.org/10.1097/01.sla.0000217592.04061.d5.
3. Gracia-Solanas JA, Elia M, Aguilella V, Ramirez JM, Martinez J, Bielsa MA, Martinez M. Metabolic syndrome after bariatric surgery. Results depending on the technique performed. Obes Surg. 2011;21:179–85. https://doi.org/10.1007/s11695-010-0309-6.
4. King WC, Hinerman AS, Belle SH, Wahed AS, Courcoulas AP. Comparison of the performance of common measures of weight regain after bariatric surgery for association with clinical outcomes. JAMA. 2018;320(15):1560–9. https://doi.org/10.1001/jama.2018.14433.
5. Orlando FA, Goncalves CG, George ZM, Halverson JD, Cunningham PR, Meguid MM. Neurohormonal pathways regulating food intake and changes after roux-en-Y gastric bypass. Surg Obes Relat Dis. 2005;1:486–95. https://doi.org/10.1016/j.soard.2005.05.009.
6. Halpern C, Hurtig H, Jaggi J, Grossman M, Won M, Baltuch G. Deep brain stimulation in neurologic disorders. Parkinsonism Relat Disord. 2007;13:1–16. https://doi.org/10.1016/j.parkreldis.2006.03.001.
7. Tagliati M, Krack P, Volkmann J, Aziz T, Krauss JK, Kupsch A, Vidailhet AM. Long-term management of DBS in dystonia: response to stimulation, adverse events, battery changes, and special considerations. Mov Disord. 2011;26:54–62. https://doi.org/10.1002/mds.23535.
8. Toft M, Lilleeng B, Ramm-Pettersen J, Skogseid IM, Gundersen V, Gerdts R, Pedersen L, Skjelland M, Roste GK, Dietrichs E. Long-term efficacy and mortality in Parkinson's disease patients treated with subthalamic stimulation. Mov Disord. 2011;26:1931–4. https://doi.org/10.1002/mds.23817.
9. Mayberg HS, Lozano AM, Voon V, McNeely HE, Seminowicz D, Hamani C, Schwalb JM, Kennedy SH. Deep brain stimulation for treatment-resistant depression. Neuron. 2005;45:651–60.
10. Schoenen J, Di Clemente L, Vandenheede M, Fumal A, De Pasqua V, Mouchamps M, Remacle JM, de Noordhout AM. Hypothalamic stimulation in chronic cluster headache: a pilot study of efficacy and mode of action. Brain. 2005;128:940–7. https://doi.org/10.1093/brain/awh411.
11. Wyrwicka W, Dobrzecka C. Relationship between feeding and satiation centers of the hypothalamus. Science. 1960;132:805–6. https://doi.org/10.1126/science.132.3430.805.
12. van de Sande-Lee S, Pereira FR, Cintra DE, Fernandes PT, Cardoso AR, Garlipp CR, Chaim EA, Pareja JC, Geloneze B, Li LM, Cendes F, Velloso LA. Partial reversibility of hypothalamic dysfunction and changes in brain activity after body mass reduction in obese subjects. Diabetes. 2011;60:1699–704. https://doi.org/10.2337/db10-1614.
13. Griffond B, Risold PY. MCH and feeding behavior-interaction with peptidic network. Peptides. 2009;30:2045–51. https://doi.org/10.1016/j.peptides.2009.07.008.
14. Ludwig DS, Tritos NA, Mastaitis JW, Kulkarni R, Kokkotou E, Elmquist J, Lowell B, Flier JS, Maratos-Flier E. Melanin-concentrating hormone overexpression in transgenic mice leads to obesity and insulin resistance. J Clin Invest. 2001;107:379–86. https://doi.org/10.1172/JCI10660.
15. Harrell LE, Decastro JM, Balagura S. A critical evaluation of body weight loss following lateral hypothalamic lesions. Physiol Behav. 1975;15:133–6.
16. Keesey RE, Powley TL. Self-stimulation and body weight in rats with lateral hypothalamic lesions. Am J Phys. 1973;224:970–8.
17. Sani S, Jobe K, Smith A, Kordower JH, Bakay RA. Deep brain stimulation for treatment of obesity in rats. J Neurosurg. 2007;107:809–13.
18. Whiting DM, Tomycz ND, Bailes J, de Jonge L, Lecoultre V, Wilent B, Alcindor D, Prostko ER, Cheng BC, Angle C, Cantella D, Whiting BB, Mizes JS, Finnis KW, Ravussin E, Oh

MY. Lateral hypothalamic area deep brain stimulation for refractory obesity: a pilot study with preliminary data on safety, body weight, and energy metabolism. J Neurosurg. 2013;119:56–63. https://doi.org/10.3171/2013.2.JNS12903.

19. Kenny PJ. Reward mechanisms in obesity: new insights and future directions. Neuron. 2011;69:664–79. https://doi.org/10.1016/j.neuron.2011.02.016.

20. Volkow ND, Wang GJ, Telang F, Fowler JS, Logan J, Childress AR, Jayne M, Ma Y, Wong C. Cocaine cues and dopamine in dorsal striatum: mechanism of craving in cocaine addiction. J Neurosci. 2006;26:6583–8. https://doi.org/10.1523/JNEUROSCI.1544-06.2006.

21. Johnson PM, Kenny PJ. Dopamine D2 receptors in addiction-like reward dysfunction and compulsive eating in obese rats. Nat Neurosci. 2010;13:635–41. https://doi.org/10.1038/nn.2519.

22. Gearhardt AN, Yokum S, Orr PT, Stice E, Corbin WR, Brownell KD. Neural correlates of food addiction. Arch Gen Psychiatry. 2011;68:808–16. https://doi.org/10.1001/archgenpsychiatry.2011.32.

23. Volkow ND, Li TK. Drug addiction: the neurobiology of behaviour gone awry. Nat Rev Neurosci. 2004;5:963–70. https://doi.org/10.1038/nrn1539.

24. Maldonado-Irizarry CS, Swanson CJ, Kelley AE. Glutamate receptors in the nucleus accumbens shell control feeding behavior via the lateral hypothalamus. J Neurosci. 1995;15:6779–88.

25. Stoeckel LE, Weller RE, Cook EW 3rd, Twieg DB, Knowlton RC, Cox JE. Widespread reward-system activation in obese women in response to pictures of high-calorie foods. NeuroImage. 2008;41:636–47. https://doi.org/10.1016/j.neuroimage.2008.02.031.

26. O'Doherty JP, Deichmann R, Critchley HD, Dolan RJ. Neural responses during anticipation of a primary taste reward. Neuron. 2002;33:815–26. https://doi.org/10.1016/S0896-6273(02)00603-7.

27. Ochner CN, Kwok Y, Conceicao E, Pantazatos SP, Puma LM, Carnell S, Teixeira J, Hirsch J, Geliebter A. Selective reduction in neural responses to high calorie foods following gastric bypass surgery. Ann Surg. 2011;253:502–7. https://doi.org/10.1097/SLA.0b013e318203a289.

28. Dunn JP, Cowan RL, Volkow ND, Feurer ID, Li R, Williams DB, Kessler RM, Abumrad NN. Decreased dopamine type 2 receptor availability after bariatric surgery: preliminary findings. Brain Res. 2010;1350:123–30. https://doi.org/10.1016/j.brainres.2010.03.064.

29. Steele KE, Prokopowicz GP, Schweitzer MA, Magunsuon TH, Lidor AO, Kuwabawa H, Kumar A, Brasic J, Wong DF. Alterations of central dopamine receptors before and after gastric bypass surgery. Obes Surg. 2010;20:369–74. https://doi.org/10.1007/s11695-009-0015-4.

30. Halpern CH, Tekriwal A, Santollo J, Keating JG, Wolf JA, Daniels D, Bale TL. Amelioration of binge eating by nucleus accumbens shell deep brain stimulation in mice involves D2 receptor modulation. J Neurosci. 2013;33:7122–9. https://doi.org/10.1523/JNEUROSCI.3237-12.2013.

31. Carter A, Hall W. Proposals to trial deep brain stimulation to treat addiction are premature. Addiction. 2011;106:235–7. https://doi.org/10.1111/j.1360-0443.2010.03245.x.

32. Unterrainer M, Oduncu FS. The ethics of deep brain stimulation (DBS). Med Health Care Philos. 2015 Jan;18

33. Caplan A. Denying autonomy in order to create it: the paradox of forcing treatment upon addicts. Addiction. 2008;103:1919–21. https://doi.org/10.1111/j.1360-0443.2008.02369.x.

34. Voon V, Krack P, Lang AE, Lozano AM, Dujardin K, Schupbach M, D'Ambrosia J, Thobois S, Tamma F, Herzog J, Speelman JD, Samanta J, Kubu C, Rossignol H, Poon YY, Saint-Cyr JA, Ardouin C, Moro E. A multicentre study on suicide outcomes following subthalamic stimulation for Parkinson's disease. Brain. 2008;131:2720–8. https://doi.org/10.1093/brain/awn214.

35. Ho AL, Sussman ES, Zhang M, et al. Deep brain stimulation for obesity. Cureus. 2015, March 25;7(3):e259. https://doi.org/10.7759/cureus.259.

How Manipulating the Microbiome Can Affect the Outcome Following Bariatric Surgery

37

Romina Pena and José M. Balibrea

37.1 Introduction

Obesity and its correlated comorbidities represent a global health problem that requires a complex multidisciplinary treatment strategy. Although lifestyle modifications including nutrition improvement and exercise can help achieve clinically substantial weight loss, their efficacy on comorbidity resolution is questionable. To this day, bariatric surgery remains the best treatment for obesity. The improvement on glucose intolerance, lipid profiles and blood pressure, among other health benefits have led to adopt the more appropriate concept of *metabolic surgery*. Nevertheless, the mechanisms that lay behind the success of these procedures are still poorly understood, as the latter entail much more than anatomical modifications to induce calorie restriction.

There is extensive ongoing research focusing on the outcomes of bariatric surgery. The bile acid metabolism, intestinal barrier and gut microbiome suffer important alterations after surgery that according to evidence, play a role in its results. It is known that Roux-en-Y gastric bypass (RYGB), among other procedures, causes a shift in the gut microbiota *composition*, increasing its diversity and gene richness, but more importantly, enhances its *function* [1]. Studies show differences in microbial metabolites than can affect host metabolism, improving hormone secretion and insulin sensitivity through gut-modulated signaling involving the microbiome-gut-brain-axis [2].

R. Pena
Gastrointestinal Surgery Department, Hospital Clínic de Barcelona, University of Barcelona, Barcelona, Spain

J. M. Balibrea (✉)
Bariatric and Upper Gastrointestinal Surgery, Gastrointestinal Surgery Department, Hospital Clínic de Barcelona, University of Barcelona, Barcelona, Spain

© Springer Nature Switzerland AG 2021
J. Alverdy, Y. Vigneswaran (eds.), *Difficult Decisions in Bariatric Surgery*,
Difficult Decisions in Surgery: An Evidence-Based Approach,
https://doi.org/10.1007/978-3-030-55329-6_37

Obesity-related microbiome is heavily influenced by diet. Low-fiber and fat-enriched diets (prevalent in Western countries) cause a severe dysbiosis that relates to detrimental effects, such as the absorption of bacterial lipopolysaccharides resulting in a chronic inflammatory state triggered by low-grade endotoxemia [3]. Recent studies show that bariatric surgery only *partially* rescues the gut microbiome, so other interventions such as specialized diets, probiotics or fecal microbiota transplant should be considered to further restore gut ecology in obese patients and possibly improve bariatric surgery outcomes.

37.2 Search Strategy

We performed a literature search of English language publications from 2007 to 2020 on PubMed. Terms used in the search were "bariatric surgery, bariatric surgery outcomes" AND "gut microbiome, gut microbiota, microbiome modulation". Various types of studies were included in our analysis (randomized controlled trials, cohort studies systematic reviews, and guidelines).

37.3 How Bariatric Surgery Changes the Gut Microbiome

The gastrointestinal tract has a great microbial diversity, with a specific ecosystem housed in each region, specialized in gene expression and function to control every stage of the digestive process. As expected, the anatomical reconfiguration after bariatric surgery changes the down-stream gut microbiome with beneficial or detrimental consequences for the host. The majority of the information on the relationship between gut microbiota and health and disease is derived from stool analysis, as it is believed to be representative of all gut population. Nevertheless, the gut microbiota from stomach to distal ileum, main object of bariatric surgery, remains largely unexplored as endoscopic diagnostic procedures are required. More sophisticated and less invasive techniques are under rapid development to further define the foregut microbiome [4].

37.3.1 Changes in Microbial Richness

Low microbial gene richness is found in overweight to severely obese patients with increasing prevalence in each group. It is associated with low-grade inflammation, adverse adipose tissue repartition, type-2 diabetes and blood hypertension. Gene richness increases after bariatric surgery, associating with an improvement in bioclinical parameters as previous studies have shown [5].

37.3.2 Changes in Composition

In addition to diminished gene richness, gut microbiome in obese patients presents phylogenetic   differences   to   lean   subjects,   mainly   a   decreased Bacteroidetes:Firmicutes ratio. According to a recent meta-analysis by Guo et al.

[6] this ratio is higher after bariatric surgery. Evidence showed an increase in *Bacteroidetes, Fusobacteria,* Verrucomicrobia *(Akkermansia)* and Proteobacteria *(Escherichia),* and a decrease in the phylum *Firmicutes (Clostridiaceae).* Studies in animals have suggested the role of intestinal microbiota in weight loss, as the transfer of post-RYGB microbiota to germ-free mice induces weight loss when compared with sham surgery microbiota. However, evidence on the exact mechanisms involved in gut microbiome-mediated weight loss and metabolic improvements is still limited [7].

37.3.3 Changes in Function

Functional changes mirror the taxonomical changes in the gut microbiome. After bariatric surgery the smaller stomach and duodenal bypass cause malabsorption of vitamins, minerals and drugs. Bacteria show an increased potential for oxygen tolerance and to assimilate essential compounds and energy substrates to compensate the reduce food intake after RYGB [8].

There is extensive literature describing the association between functional changes in gut microbiome and clinical parameters, but mechanistic explanation is still immature. Targeted metabolomics to measure circulating biomarkers have shed light on microbial pathways that contribute to post bariatric surgery outcomes. One example is the activation of the Farnesoid X Receptor (FXR) by enteral bile acid, stimulating the production of the fibroblast growth factor 19 (FGF19), delivered to the liver via the portal system to modulated bile acid, glucose and lipid metabolism. Gut microbiota is responsible for bile acid transformation and regulation of the synthesis by FXR suppression. Some studies show an increase in circulating bile acids, higher levels of FXR and FGF19 after RYGB and sleeve gastrectomy (SG) [9].

37.4   How we Can Alter the Microbiome before and after Surgery

It is logical to think that the gut microbiome heavily interacts with and influences the host metabolism, as the intestinal metagenome contains more than three million genes, with a 100:1 ratio to the entire human genome. The architecture of the gut microbiome is determined by a myriad of factors, some of them modifiable, including environmental elements, drugs, diseases, exercise, and nutrition [10]. The gut microbiota then seems to be an accessible target for modulation, meaning *pre-habilitation* prior to surgery or *rehabilitation* after the procedure to improve outcomes.

37.4.1 Diet

As published data shows, diet is the key factor in short-term and long-term composition and function of the intestinal bacteria. Western diets are classically fat-enriched and low in fiber. Traditional diets are characterized by high fiber, low sugar and fat, offering a much healthier environment for bacteria to prosper, favoring diversity. Fiber offers indigestible carbohydrates to bacteria, that process them into beneficial metabolites, such as short-chain fatty acids. Health benefits associated with a high-fiber diet include enhanced intestinal barrier integrity, decreased inflammation and improved lipid metabolism and insulin sensitivity [11].

A previously published study offers an example of how a dietary intervention correlates to better metabolic outcomes through gut microbiome alteration. A calorie restrictive diet found an increase in fecal *Akkermansia muciniphila* and microbial gene richness and was associated with an improvement in glucose homeostasis, lipid profile and body composition [12]. Another study demonstrated how a 6-week energy-restricted high-protein diet improved gene richness and corelated to metabolic improvements [13]. Nevertheless, research has shown that modulations of the microbiome can prevail in time, and long-term dietary patterns translate to specific enterotypes. Dietary intervention leads to rapid and significant changes but insufficient in magnitude, as showed by Wu et al. [14]. Further investigation in nutritional genomics is needed to design a personalized dietary strategy that would be capable of switching the obese phenotype in high-risk individuals into a long-term healthier microbiome profile [15].

37.4.2 Probiotics

Probiotics are live microorganisms that when administered in a certain amount, offer health benefits to the host. There are studies that suggest that probiotics might have a role in modifying the gut microbiome in obese patients. Most common probiotic bacteria that have shown anti-obesity effects including weight loss, lower BMI and body fat, are Bifidobacterium and *Lactobacillus* [11].

The research on probiotics regarding bariatric surgery is scarce and mostly directed to their use in the postoperative period. In 2008, Woodard et al. [16] found a significant reduction in bacterial overgrowth after RYGB with the daily administration of *Lactobacillus*. They also reported the unexpected result of statistically significant greater percent excess weight loss at 6 weeks and 3 months in the probiotic group. Other studies have reported the reduction of gastrointestinal symptoms and better quality of life after RYGB [17].

Probiotics have also been tested as a treatment for nonalcoholic fat liver disease (NAFLD) and type-2 diabetes showing some protective effect [18]. Nevertheless, a randomized controlled trial by Sherf-Dagan et al. [19] found no improvement in hepatic, inflammatory or clinical outcomes at 6 and 12-months after a 6-month treatment with probiotics in patients who underwent SG. Microbial diversity was increased during treatment in both groups and decreased again at 12-month follow-up. Evidence suggests that probiotics have a direct beneficial effect on the gut microbiome, but more research is needed to validate their use in the context of bariatric surgery.

37.4.3 Prebiotics and Symbiotics

Prebiotics are non-digestible compounds that are metabolized by the gut microbiota and can modulate its composition and function. Most commonly used prebiotics are inulin, fructo-oligosaccharides, and galacto-oligosaccharides. Symbiotics are the combination of probiotics and prebiotics. Prebiotics promote the growth of beneficial bacteria over hostile commensals, help preserve intestinal barrier integrity and improve glucose and lipid metabolism. Fernandes et al. [20] conducted a randomized controlled triple-blind trial that reported that supplementation with prebiotics for 14 days increased weight loss, whereas both prebiotics and symbiotics were unable to improve inflammation markers after RYGB.

37.4.4 Other Strategies

An interesting study interrogated the role of *H. pylori* eradication in the response to bariatric surgery. Prevalence of *H. pylori* varies from 15 to up to 85%, although its role in the pathophysiology of the disease is still controversial. Previous data stated that *H. pylori* infection did not influence bariatric surgery outcomes, but eradication with antibiotic treatment correlated with subsequent short-term metabolic improvement, including lower BMI, a better lipid profile and lower blood glucose levels, mainly in non-diabetic patients [21]. In the future, targeted antibiotic administration after personalized microbiome profiling might be feasible, switching the broad-kill strategy to a highly selective decontamination of the gut microbiome in search of better postoperative outcomes.

There is recent evidence on novel treatments that modify gut microbiome and could influence the evolution of weight loss and metabolic markers in obese patients. A promising strategy for healthy microbiome restoration in obese patients might be the fecal microbiota transplant (FMT). The effectiveness of this strategy in the treatment of *C. difficile* infections offered hope as a therapeutic intervention for other gastrointestinal diseases. FMT through a duodenal tube from healthy donors with a normal BMI to obese patients diagnosed with type-2 diabetes increased insulin sensitivity, fecal microbiota diversity and butyrate-producing bacteria, according to Vrieze et al. [22]. FMT should be investigated as an adjuvant strategy in bariatric surgery patients.

Given the fact that the majority of the human microbiome resides in the intestine, the role of a newly redesigned bowel prep 2.0 outside of colorectal surgery has been contemplated in recent literature. Alverdy et al. [23] proposed a comprehensive workflow for the prevention of surgical site infection and anastomotic leakage, including a microbiome-preserving bowel preparation, preoperative high fiber diet, microbial screening for high-risk pathogens, targeted antibiotics and dietary rehabilitation. Considering obese patients have a markedly dysbiotic microbiome, designing a similar protocol for bariatric surgery seems appropriate.

37.5   Role of the Microbiome in Bariatric Surgery Complications

37.5.1 Short-Term Complications

Big data analysis reveal that anastomotic leak, wound infection, pulmonary and urinary tract infections and deep venous thromboembolism are some of the most common, yet fortunately infrequent complications of bariatric procedures, that translate to prolonged hospital stay and increased costs [24]. Advances in perioperative care including minimally invasive techniques and the implementation of an enhanced recovery after surgery (ERAS) protocol have brought down these complications at an all-time low in all surgical fields, including bariatrics [25]. Avoiding opioids, abstaining from drains and catheters, mindful antibiotic administration, early oral feeding and mobilization have proven effective measures for this achievement.

Nevertheless, microbiome science has acutely reminded us that the efforts on lowering postoperative complications lack mechanistic analysis, as a great deal of these events might be best studied and treated at a molecular level. Alverdy et al. [26] have been successful advocates for this statement, encouraging disruptive thinking on the pathophysiology of common complications after gastrointestinal surgery, including surgical site infections (SSIs) and anastomotic leaks (AL), both of which represent a burden in bariatric surgery.

Through *quorum sensing*, bacteria can detect surgical injury and change phenotype into a *pathobiome*, adapting to a more hostile environment provided by broad spectrum antibiotics, physiologic stress, change in diet during hospitalization and the anatomical rearrangement of bariatric surgery. Depending on the host basal microbiome and magnitude of the surgical injury, certain pathogens might bloom in the postoperative period and be responsible for adverse outcomes, especially if the refaunation is inadequate [27].

There is no strong evidence that confirms that SSIs are due to a breach in aseptic technique with contamination of the field during or after surgery, as demonstrated by the lack of culture positivity. Additional causal factors are being considered, including local wound trauma that might act as a chemoattractant for both immune cells and bacteria [28]. Minimally invasive approaches and certain wound protectors that evenly distribute pressure and avoid local ischemia could prevent SSIs in this context [29]. Even though skin bacteria are the usual offenders on SSIs in clean surgeries such as bariatric procedures, intestinal microbiota might also play a role. This concept was beautifully proven by Krezalek et al. [30] who demonstrated the *Trojan Horse hypothesis*, by which gut-derived Methicillin-resistant *Staphylococcus aureus* silently travel inside immune cells to successfully cause wound infection in mice who underwent colorectal surgery.

In regard to AL, they are one of the most devastating complication of bariatric procedures. The classical notion of a faulty technique has dominated the literature, focusing on the mechanical aspects as culprit. Nevertheless, there is mounting evidence on the role of gut microbiome in the pathogenesis of AL. It is known that specific bacteria can express a collagenolytic phenotype and impair anastomotic healing to the point of dehiscence, as Shogan et al. [31] stated regarding the collagen degradation and MMP9 activation by *E. faecalis*. Targeted strategies are under investigation to mitigate the deleterious potential of collagenolytic bacteria without damaging the microbiome structure. A more recent study by Hyoju et al. [32] showed how oral polyphosphate suppresses collagenase production by *P. aeruginosa* and *S. marcescens*, successfully preventing AL in mice undergoing colorectal surgery.

Most importantly, Gaines et al. [33] recently demonstrated that Western diet promotes intestinal colonization by collagenolytic microbes and promotes tumor formation and that administration of Pi-PEG reduced tumor formation maintaining microbial diversity. Little is known of the role of gut bacteria in leaks on RYGB or SG. If we can extrapolate the knowledge obtained from the colorectal field to bariatrics, it is logical to think that modulation of both the upper and lower gastrointestinal microbiome, possibly through diet and supplementation of specific compounds, could prevent postoperative complications.

37.5.2 Long-Term Complications/Unsatisfactory Results

Obese patient present different responses to bariatric surgery. One of the possible explanations for this phenomenon lies in the gut microbiome. As an example, Seridi et al. [34] findings showed that IL-6 did not respond to RYGB, possible reflecting complex inflammatory patterns of obese and diabetic patients and uncontrolled environmental variables. A study by Aron-Wisnesky et al. [35] investigated several cohorts of severely obese patients after different bariatric procedures. Despite major weight loss and metabolic improvement, gene richness was not fully rescued, as it was still considered low at 1 year after surgery and did not improve a 5-years follow-up. Both SG and RYGB severely alter a dysbiotic microbiome, but the association of compositional and functional changes with patient outcomes in the long-term is under interrogation.

37.6   Role of Microbial Monitoring in Post-Bariatric Surgery Follow-Up

Identifying metabolomic signatures and circulating biomarkers could represent a new and more sophisticated way to track response to treatment, as specific microbial metabolites correlate with post-bariatric surgery outcomes. SCFA, branched chained amino acids (BCAAs), circulating bile acids and trimethylamine-N-oxide (TMAO) are some examples, but current results are contradictory [36]. Further research is needed to refine the interpretation of these tests and accurately correlate them to patient outcomes.

37.7   Conclusions and Recommendations

Bariatric surgery and gut microbiome have a complex relationship. Anatomical modifications inevitably alter the regional microbial architecture and bacterial metabolites have an effect on host metabolism. Microbial gene richness and diversity increase after bariatric surgery, corelating with improvement in clinical and metabolic features, including BMI, fat tissue distribution and insulin sensitivity.

Diet has proven fundamental in determining the fitness of the gut microbiome. Western diets are linked to severe dysbiosis, prevalent in obese patients. A high-fiber low-fat diet induces a healthier phenotype that associates with favorable outcomes and is thus recommended. The use of probiotics, prebiotics or symbiotics, similar to dietary interventions, seems to have beneficial effects through modulation of the gut microbiota. More studies are required to fully validate their administration in this context. Time of application or treatment duration is also a matter of discussion. The non-obese phenotype has been proven transferable through FMT in animals and humans with promising results, but larger studies are required to endorse this new indication of the procedure.

Finally, the application of the ERAS protocol and minimizing trauma to the wound through minimally invasive surgery are recommended as standard practice to prevent postoperative complications such as SSIs and AL, but the role of the gut microbiome in this context has been extrapolated from colorectal surgery and is still to be determined.

A Personal Approach to the Data

Bariatric surgery undoubtedly generates changes in the gut microbiome that partially explain metabolic outcomes. Microbiome manipulation through diet, supplements or direct microbial exchange seems promising but evidence is not strong enough to support the systematic use of these strategies. The vast majority of bariatric procedures are being performed with depurated, minimally invasive techniques and under the greatest postoperative care, so putting gut microbiome on the spotlight and redirecting resources to precision medicine might be the key to further improve post bariatric surgery outcomes. Identification of high-risk microbial profiles preoperatively may allow for a personalized approach including non-invasive targeted therapies to rescue gut ecology and aid the resensitazion of the gut-brain axis. The evolution of metagenomics and metabolomics is rendering an immense amount of information that is challenging to comprehend, but big data analysis and artificial intelligence may be useful tools in this matter. Making this technology cost-effective and readily available seems light-years ahead, but as Dr. Mandela said, "it's always seems impossible until it's done".

37.8   Recommendations

- Obese patients should follow a high-fiber low-fat diet before and after bariatric surgery (Evidence quality high; strong recommendation).
- Probiotics, prebiotics and symbiotics may be useful in further improving the gut microbiome as adjuvant treatment to bariatric surgery (Evidence quality moderate; weak recommendation).

- Novel strategies such as fecal microbiota may be validated in the treatment of obese-induced dysbiosis and help improve post bariatric surgery outcomes (Evidence quality moderate; weak recommendation).

Disclosures
The authors have nothing to disclose.

References

1. Graessler J, Qin Y, Zhong H, Zhang J, Licinio J, Wong M-L, et al. Metagenomic sequencing of the human gut microbiome before and after bariatric surgery in obese patients with type 2 diabetes: correlation with inflammatory and metabolic parameters. Pharmacogenomics J [Internet]. 2013;13(6):514–22. Available from: http://www.nature.com/articles/tpj201243
2. Torres-Fuentes C, Schellekens H, Dinan TG, Cryan JF. The microbiota–gut–brain axis in obesity. Lancet Gastroenterol Hepatol [Internet]. 2017;2(10):747–56. Available from: https://linkinghub.elsevier.com/retrieve/pii/S2468125317301474
3. Cani PD, Amar J, Iglesias MA, Poggi M, Knauf C, Bastelica D, et al. Metabolic Endotoxemia initiates obesity and insulin resistance. Diabetes [Internet]. 2007;56(7):1761–72. Available from: http://diabetes.diabetesjournals.org/cgi/doi/10.2337/db05-1367
4. Martinez-Guryn K, Leone V, Chang EB. Regional diversity of the gastrointestinal microbiome. Cell Host Microbe [Internet]. 2019;26(3):314–24. Available from: https://linkinghub.elsevier.com/retrieve/pii/S1931312819304202
5. Kong L-C, Tap J, Aron-Wisnewsky J, Pelloux V, Basdevant A, Bouillot J-L, et al. Gut microbiota after gastric bypass in human obesity: increased richness and associations of bacterial genera with adipose tissue genes. Am J Clin Nutr [Internet]. 2013;98(1):16–24. Available from: https://academic.oup.com/ajcn/article/98/1/16/4578316
6. Liou AP, Paziuk M, Luevano J-M, Machineni S, Turnbaugh PJ, Kaplan LM. Conserved shifts in the gut microbiota due to gastric bypass reduce host weight and adiposity. Sci Transl Med [Internet]. 2013;5(178):178ra41. Available from: https://www.ncbi.nlm.nih.gov/pmc/articles/PMC3624763/pdf/nihms412728.pdf
7. Guo Y, Huang Z-P, Liu C-Q, Qi L, Sheng Y, Zou D-J. Modulation of the gut microbiome: a systematic review of the effect of bariatric surgery. Eur J Endocrinol [Internet]. 2018;178(1):43–56. Available from: https://eje.bioscientifica.com/view/journals/eje/178/1/EJE-17-0403.xml
8. Palleja A, Kashani A, Allin KH, Nielsen T, Zhang C, Li Y, et al. Roux-en-Y gastric bypass surgery of morbidly obese patients induces swift and persistent changes of the individual gut microbiota. Genome Med [Internet]. 2016;8(1):67. Available from: http://genomemedicine.biomedcentral.com/articles/10.1186/s13073-016-0312-1
9. Jansen PLM, van Werven J, Aarts E, Berends F, Janssen I, Stoker J, et al. Alterations of hormonally active fibroblast growth factors after Roux-en-Y gastric bypass surgery. Dig Dis [Internet]. 2011;29(1):48–51. Available from: https://www.karger.com/Article/FullText/324128
10. Li J, Riaz Rajoka MS, Shao D, Jiang C, Jin M, Huang Q, et al. Strategies to increase the efficacy of using gut microbiota for the modulation of obesity. Obes Rev [Internet]. 2017;18(11):1260–71. Available from: http://doi.wiley.com/10.1111/obr.12590
11. Guyton K, Alverdy JC. The gut microbiota and gastrointestinal surgery. Nat Rev Gastroenterol Hepatol [Internet]. 2017;14(1):43–54. https://doi.org/10.1038/nrgastro.2016.139.
12. Dao MC, Everard A, Aron-Wisnewsky J, Sokolovska N, Prifti E, Verger EO, et al. Akkermansia muciniphila and improved metabolic health during a dietary intervention in obesity: relationship with gut microbiome richness and ecology. Gut [Internet]. 2016;65(3):426–36. Available from: http://gut.bmj.com/lookup/doi/10.1136/gutjnl-2014-308778

13. Cotillard A, Kennedy SP, Kong LC, Prifti E, Pons N, Le Chatelier E, et al. Dietary intervention impact on gut microbial gene richness. Nature [Internet]. 2013;500(7464):585–8. Available from: http://www.nature.com/articles/nature12480
14. Wu GD, Chen J, Hoffmann C, Bittinger K, Chen Y-Y, Keilbaugh SA, et al. Linking long-term dietary patterns with gut microbial Enterotypes. Science (80-) [Internet]. 2011;334(6052):105–8. Available from: http://www.sciencemag.org/cgi/doi/10.1126/science.1208344
15. Nicoletti C, Cortes-Oliveira C, Pinhel M, Nonino C. Bariatric surgery and precision nutrition. Nutrients [Internet]. 2017;9(9):974. Available from: http://www.mdpi.com/2072-6643/9/9/974
16. Woodard GA, Encarnacion B, Downey JR, Peraza J, Chong K, Hernandez-Boussard T, et al. Probiotics improve outcomes after Roux-en-Y gastric bypass surgery: a prospective randomized trial. J Gastrointest Surg [Internet]. 2009;13(7):1198–204. Available from: http://link.springer.com/10.1007/s11605-009-0891-x
17. Wagner NRF, Zaparolli MR, Cruz MR, Schieferdecker MEM, Campos ACL. Postoperative changes in intestinal microbiota and use of probiotics in Roux-en-Y gastric bypass and sleeve vertical Gastrectomy: an integrative review. ABCD Arq Bras Cir Dig (São Paulo) [Internet]. 2018;31(4):e1400. Available from: http://www.scielo.br/scielo.php?script=sci_arttext&pid=S0102-67202018000400500&lng=en&tlng=en
18. Sáez-Lara M, Robles-Sanchez C, Ruiz-Ojeda F, Plaza-Diaz J, Gil A. Effects of probiotics and Synbiotics on obesity, insulin resistance syndrome, type 2 diabetes and non-alcoholic fatty liver disease: a review of human clinical trials. Int J Mol Sci [Internet]. 2016;17(6):928. Available from: http://www.mdpi.com/1422-0067/17/6/928
19. Sherf-Dagan S, Zelber-Sagi S, Zilberman-Schapira G, Webb M, Buch A, Keidar A, et al. Probiotics administration following sleeve gastrectomy surgery: a randomized double-blind trial. Int J Obes [Internet]. 2018;42(2):147–55. https://doi.org/10.1038/ijo.2017.210.
20. Fernandes R, Beserra BTS, Mocellin MC, Kuntz MGF, da Rosa JS, de Miranda RCD, et al. Effects of prebiotic and Synbiotic supplementation on inflammatory markers and anthropometric indices after Roux-en-Y gastric bypass. J Clin Gastroenterol [Internet]. 2016;50(3):208–17. Available from: http://content.wkhealth.com/linkback/openurl?sid=WKPTLP:landingpage&an=00004836-201603000-00009
21. Goday A, Castañer O, Benaiges D, Pou AB, Ramón JM, del Iglesias M, et al. Can helicobacter pylori eradication treatment modify the metabolic response to bariatric surgery? Obes Surg [Internet]. 2018;28(8):2386–95. Available from: http://link.springer.com/10.1007/s11695-018-3170-7
22. Vrieze A, Van Nood E, Holleman F, Salojärvi J, Kootte RS, Bartelsman JFWM, et al. Transfer of intestinal microbiota from lean donors increases insulin sensitivity in individuals with metabolic syndrome. Gastroenterology [Internet]. 2012;143(4):913–916.e7. https://doi.org/10.1053/j.gastro.2012.06.031.
23. Alverdy JC, Hyman N. Bowel preparation under siege. Br J Surg [Internet]. 2020;107(3):167–70. Available from: http://doi.wiley.com/10.1002/bjs.11454
24. Balla A, Batista Rodríguez G, Corradetti S, Balagué C, Fernández-Ananín S, Targarona EM. Outcomes after bariatric surgery according to large databases: a systematic review. Langenbeck's Arch Surg [Internet]. 2017;402(6):885–99. Available from: http://link.springer.com/10.1007/s00423-017-1613-6
25. Małczak P, Wysocki M, Twardowska H, Dudek A, Tabiś J, Major P, et al. Impact of adherence to the ERAS® protocol on short-term outcomes after bariatric surgery. Obes Surg. 2020;
26. Alverdy JC. Microbiome medicine: this changes everything. J Am Coll Surg [Internet]. 2018;226(5):719–29. https://doi.org/10.1016/j.jamcollsurg.2018.02.004.
27. Alverdy JC, Hyoju SK, Weigerinck M, Gilbert JA. The gut microbiome and the mechanism of surgical infection. Br J Surg. 2017;104(2):e14–23.
28. Alverdy JC. El ambiente de la herida, la virulencia microbiana y la infección postoperatoria: lecciones prácticas para el cirujano. 2018;6.

29. Weber CE, Abbas M, Bonner G, Mustafa RR, Motamedi SMK, Khaitan L. Is it the technique or wound protection that is key to reducing wound infections in Roux-en-Y gastric bypass procedures? Surg Endosc. 2019;0123456789

30. Krezalek MA, Hyoju S, Zaborin A, Okafor E, Chandrasekar L, Bindokas V, et al. Can methicillin-resistant Staphylococcus aureus silently travel from the gut to the wound and cause postoperative infection? Modeling the "Trojan horse hypothesis". Ann Surg [Internet]. 2018;267(4):749–58. Available from: http://insights.ovid.com/crossref?an=00000658-201804000-00023

31. Shogan BD, Belogortseva N, Luong PM, Zaborin A, Lax S, Bethel C, et al. Collagen degradation and MMP9 activation by Enterococcus faecalis contribute to intestinal anastomotic leak. Sci Transl Med [Internet]. 2015;7(286):286ra68. Available from: https://linkinghub.elsevier.com/retrieve/pii/S0010782415007088

32. Hyoju SK, Klabbers RE, Aaron M, Krezalek MA, Zaborin A, Wiegerinck M, et al. Oral polyphosphate suppresses bacterial collagenase production and prevents anastomotic leak due to Serratia marcescens and Pseudomonas aeruginosa. Ann Surg. 2018;267(6):1112–8.

33. Gaines S, van Praagh JB, Williamson AJ, Jacobson RA, Hyoju S, Zaborin A, et al. Western diet promotes intestinal colonization by Collagenolytic microbes and promotes tumor formation following colorectal surgery. Gastroenterology [Internet]. 2019; https://doi.org/10.1053/j.gastro.2019.10.020.

34. Seridi L, Leo GC, Dohm GL, Pories WJ, Lenhard J. Time course metabolome of Roux-en-Y gastric bypass confirms correlation between leptin, body weight and the microbiome. PLoS One [Internet]. 2018;13(5):e0198156. https://doi.org/10.1371/journal.pone.0198156.

35. Aron-Wisnewsky J, Prifti E, Belda E, Ichou F, Kayser BD, Dao MC, et al. Major microbiota dysbiosis in severe obesity: fate after bariatric surgery. Gut [Internet]. 2019;68(1):70–82. Available from: http://gut.bmj.com/lookup/doi/10.1136/gutjnl-2018-316103

36. Jain AK, le Roux CW, Puri P, Tavakkoli A, Gletsu-Miller N, Laferrère B, et al. Proceedings of the 2017 ASPEN research workshop-gastric bypass: role of the gut. J Parenter Enter Nutr [Internet]. 2018;42(2):279–95. https://doi.org/10.1002/jpen.1121.

Index

© Springer Nature Switzerland AG 2021

J. Alverdy, Y. Vigneswaran (eds.), *Difficult Decisions in Bariatric Surgery*,
Difficult Decisions in Surgery: An Evidence-Based Approach,
https://doi.org/10.1007/978-3-030-55329-6